Facing Your Fifties

FACING YOUR FIFTIES
EVERY MAN'S REFERENCE GUIDE TO MID-LIFE HEALTH

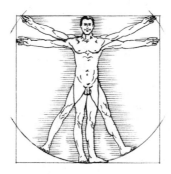

Gordon Ehlers, M.D., and Jeff Miller

M. Evans and Company, Inc.
New York

M. Evans and Company, Inc.
216 East 49th Street
New York, New York 10017

The information contained in this book is not intended to serve as a replacement for professional medical advice. Any use of the information in this book is at the reader's discretion. The author and publisher specifically disclaim any and all liability arising directly or indirectly from the use or application of any information contained in this book. A health care professional should be consulted regarding your specific situation.

Library of Congress Cataloging-in-Publication Data

Ehlers, Gordon.
    Facing your fifties : every man's reference guide to mid-life health / by Gordon Ehlers and Jeff Miller.
        p.   cm.
    ISBN 0-87131-954-3
    1. Middle aged men—Health and hygiene. I. Miller, Jeff (Jeffrey B.), 1952–   .
II. Title.
RA777.8.E35 2002
613'.04234—dc21   2002016107

Printed in the United States of America

9 8 7 6 5 4 3 2 1

ACKNOWLEDGMENTS

Gordon Ehlers, M.D.

To my parents, to whom I owe my sturdy constitution and love of learning; to my childhood doctor, the late H.B. Stapleton, M.D., who was an early inspiration; and to the faculty at the University of Nebraska College of Medicine, who have always emphasized compassionate patient care. Thanks also to my colleagues Kent Voorhees, M.D., whose many suggestions have made this a much better book, and Richard Drexelius, M.D.,whose willingness to take a chance on a veteran clinician gave me the opportunity to teach. Special thanks to my wife, Michele, without whose love and support my medical career would not have been possible.

Jeff Miller

To my mother and father, who endowed me with good health and the attitude to appreciate it; and to my wife and best friend, Susan Burdick, who fills me with love, joy, and inspiration every day. A special thanks to our agent, Nicholas Smith; the initial copy editor, Evie Newell; and the illustrator, Bill Ramsey—all of whom helped us produce the best book possible.

CONTENTS

8: What You Can Do—*A Summary of Positive Choices That Make a Difference*

WHAT AILS YOU, WHAT IT MIGHT BE, AND WHAT CHAPTER IT'S IN

PROBLEM— FROM HEAD TO TOE	MOST LIKELY CAUSE/ REASON	LESS LIKELY CAUSE/ REASON	UNUSUAL/ RARE CAUSE/ REASON	SEE CHAPTER
Headache	Sinus congestion, eye strain, stress, and tension	Sinus infection, migraine	Cluster headache, brain tumor	6
Vision Problems	Age changing the shape of the eyeball	Previously undiagnosed poor vision, diabetes	Cataracts, glaucoma	6
Hearing Loss	Wax buildup	Nerve deafness from occupational or recreational sources	Conductive deafness from infection or fused bones in the middle ear	6
Sore Neck	Muscle tension from stress	Acute injury, overuse		2

1

PROBLEM— FROM HEAD TO TOE	MOST LIKELY CAUSE/ REASON	LESS LIKELY CAUSE/ REASON	UNUSUAL/ RARE CAUSE/ REASON	SEE CHAPTER
Shoulder Pain	Degenerative conditions involving tendons and bursae	Acute injury, overuse	Arthritis, cancer	2
Chest Pain— only with bend- ing, twisting, or directly pushing on the area	Muscle or cartilage strain or tear	Fractured or broken ribs	Angina or heart attack	2, 3
Chest Pain— burning, meal related, difficul- ty swallowing	Indigestion, heartburn, acid reflux/GERD	Ulcer, gallblad- der disease	Stomach can- cer, esophageal cancer, heart attack	3, 4
Chest Pain— pressure with or without sweating, short- ness of breath	Angina and/or heart attack	Blood clot to lungs (pulmonary (embolus)	Muscle pain, indigestion	3, 4
Lower Back Pain—with pain radiating to the leg or hip	Disc problems, arthritis	Overuse, poor back mechan- ics, obesity	Cancer, infection	2
Lower Back Pain—without radiating pain	Overuse, poor back mechanics, lack of fitness	Disc problems, arthritis, obesity	Cancer, infection	2

What Ails You, What it Might Be, and What Chapter It's In

PROBLEM—FROM HEAD TO TOE	MOST LIKELY CAUSE/ REASON	LESS LIKELY CAUSE/ REASON	UNUSUAL/ RARE CAUSE/ REASON	SEE CHAPTER
Knee Pain	Acute injury, overuse	Degenerative arthritis, degenerative cartilage	Referral pain from hip or back problems	2
Sore Heel or Foot	Strained or pulled muscle, stone bruise, plantar fasciitis	High arch, obesity, arthritis	—	2
Skin Lesions —Present a Long Time, Unchanging	Benign moles, freckles	Cancer	—	2
Skin Lesions —New, Changing	Cancer (basal cell)	Cancer (squamous cell)	Cancer (melanoma, other)	7
Lack of Sexual Function— Occasional	Drug/alcohol related, lack of sleep, relationship problems	Vascular or nervous system problems	Low testosterone	5, 6
Lack of Sexual Function— Constant	Depression, vascular or nervous system problems, low testosterone	Drug/alcohol related	—	5, 6
Diarrhea— Occasional	Indigestion, bad diet, minor viral infection	Indigestion, bad diet, minor viral infection	Bacterial infection (food poisoning), malabsorption, drug/alcohol related	4, 7

PROBLEM—FROM HEAD TO TOE	MOST LIKELY CAUSE/ REASON	LESS LIKELY CAUSE/ REASON	UNUSUAL/ RARE CAUSE/ REASON	SEE CHAPTER
Diarrhea—Chronic	Stress/tension, malabsorption	Infection, parasites, drug/alcohol related	Cancer, food poisoning	4, 7
Blood in Stool—Bright Red	Hemorrhoids, ulcerlike tear of the anus (fissure)	Colon cancer, colitis	Infection	4, 7
Blood in Stool—Dark or Black	Bleeding ulcer or GERD related	Diet related (Pepto Bismol, iron, etc.)	Cancer, infection	4, 7
Blood in Urine—Visual	Bladder cancer	Kidney stone, infection (prostate, bladder)	Prostate cancer	4, 7
Blood in Urine—Microscopic	Nondisease, kidney stone, infection (prostate, bladder)	Cancer (bladder or kidney)	Prostate cancer	4, 7
Fatigue	Poor sleeping habits, lack of fitness, depression	Various disease states (e.g. diabetes, thyroid)	—	6, 7

INTRODUCTION

Do We Really Need to Know This Stuff?

Most of us men approach our health like we shop: When we need a pair of pants we go to one store, try on one pair, and if they fit, we walk out with new pants. No scouring mountains of advertising supplements, no endless comparison shopping, and no multiple trips to the changing room.

Which means, of course, that when it comes to health, most men don't want to know anything until something breaks down. Then, and only then, do we want immediate answers and are willing to take instant action.

This medical *laissez-faire* attitude served us well through our teens, twenties, and even our thirties. Late-night parties, round-the-clock studying, brutal contact sports, the occasional cold, the infrequent bout of flu, a couple of broken bones, lots of cuts, scrapes, bumps, and bruises, and the all-too-infamous hangovers never lasted long or seemed to have any permanent impact on our hectic, meteoric lives. For the vast majority of us, our bodies back then ran lean, mean, and smooth—we hardly even heard what was going on under the hood. In fact, to use another analogy, we were practically bullet-proof well into our forties.

Then came the fifties.

Now, we creak a lot. We read at arm's length. We're stiff and we ache in places we never knew existed. Muscles are vanishing nearly as fast as our hair. If we lose a couple hours of sleep, we're not worth much the next day. Even our special friend seems to be slowing down a bit—although we're definitely not prepared to acknowledge that fact just yet. And why is it we don't have the same stamina we had twenty years ago?

All in all, the fifties seem to embrace us with a vengeance, like the long-lost cousin we picked on when we were kids but who's a giant now. Some might say the fifties decade—like that cousin—is in pay-back mode.

That's an apt description. The sins of our misspent youth are definitely catching up with us. All those pizzas and beer, cigarettes and drugs (if we were into those), and the general physical punishment, or benign neglect, we put our bodies through are coming back to haunt us. And these ghosts are materializing not in the form of spooky holograms but in far scarier sights—love handles, beer guts, lack of stamina, and painful joints, tendons, and ligaments. To make matters worse, exercise for many of us is like most high school buddies—long gone and little remembered.

KNOWLEDGE TIMES ACTION EQUALS GOOD HEALTH

The good news—yep, there's definitely lots of good news—is that men in their fifties can still have a major impact on:

• Blunting the consequences of problems from the past.

• Drastically improving how we're feeling now.

• Significantly increasing the odds (not the certainty) of negotiating our senior years in good health.

• Stopping—and sometimes even reversing—what seem at times to be unstoppable forces of nature.

How can we pull off such "miracles"?

With knowledge used as a fuel for action. Former surgeon general Dr. C. Everett Koop was right when he said, "The best prescription is knowledge." We men need to know the basics of how our bodies act, react, and change with age, or we're going to end up being old before our time—or just dead before our time.

WHY THE FIFTIES ARE SO IMPORTANT

The time between fifty and sixty is a particularly critical one for males because this is when:

- Heart disease—the number one killer in America—begins to rear its ugly head.

- Joints, tendons, and ligaments start reaching the breaking point.

- Certain cancers first establish beachheads—many of them not generating symptoms or visible signs until years later, when the chances of a cure are greatly diminished.

It's no wonder the medical community has determined that fifty is the critical year to start having numerous periodic tests, exams, and screenings.

To top it all off, fifty is fast becoming the new middle age for Americans. With huge advances in science and technology, greater medical education and awareness, and an increase in the number of people wanting to actively improve their health, there will be more baby boomers reaching 100 than the world has ever seen.

The big caveat, though, is that it's up to each individual whether or not that magical 100 year mark will be reached in the midst of good health, or in the ravages of decrepitude. That's the rub, of course: Are you going to live to be 100? Which means you should take care of yourself now, or are you going to live to be only fifty-nine? Which means you don't need to bother.

Then there's an additional element that really muddies the water—the health category of "shit happens." It's conceivable, though not statistically likely, that a person can do everything right in the way of diet, exercise, and regular checkups and still be killed by an out-of-the-blue disease, accident, or illness. This is what strikes fear—and subsequent inaction—into the hearts of many stout fellows.

STACKING THE ODDS IN YOUR FAVOR

So why bother with any health efforts? Why not just let fate run its course?

Because of odds. Nearly everything in life, every decision we make, is a calculated assessment of the odds. And many times we don't even know we're working the numbers. A simple analogy: If you need something for dinner, you think nothing of getting in your car, driving to the supermarket, then driving home. But what if the street is coated with ice? The odds of an accident-free trip suddenly become very different. You might think, well, I've got something here at home I can eat instead. It all comes down to: Is the reward great enough to outweigh the risks?

The same kind of calculation applies to your health. Starting with the harshest of realities, we should face the fact that none of us is getting out of this life alive.

We're not supposed to. But it's also true that while we're living, it makes good sense to stack the odds in our favor regarding health. The rewards of good health definitely outweigh the "risks" of a little sweat, a little dietary restraint, and a little preventive effort.

For prevention, two good examples of stacking the odds in your favor are: (1) taking eighty-one milligrams of aspirin (a "baby" aspirin) daily; and (2) taking 400 IU (international units) of vitamin E daily (both mentioned later in greater detail). How likely is it that taking aspirin will cause a problem for most people? Not very. How likely is it that taking vitamin E will cause a problem for anyone? Not likely. But both help to significantly reduce the risk of a fifties male suffering a heart attack or stroke. In these two cases, the benefits far outweigh the effort and effects of taking the pills.

But even these two seemingly simple preventive measures have pitfalls. Those with a propensity for stomach ulcers should not take aspirin, while taking more than 1,000 IU of vitamin E a day can possibly cause bleeding. Additionally, some recent studies seem to indicate that an aspirin a day for a person who has not had heart trouble might increase the risk of stroke or bleeding. Other new studies on vitamin E seem to show that it is not actually as helpful as once thought in preventing coronary disease (which can cause heart attacks and strokes).

In the face of such contradictory findings, what's the average guy to do?

GOOD HEALTH CARE AND MAINTENANCE NEED A PARTNERSHIP

The taking of aspirin and vitamin E are good examples of why it's critical that proper health care be a partnership between yourself and a licensed health care professional. Besides the usual diagnoses and treatments of minor and major ailments, a doctor can help put the tremendous amount of health care information—much of it confusing, highly technical, and/or contradictory—into proper perspective. And a doctor can help with such life-changing situations as quitting smoking or developing a diet and exercise plan that will work for you.

The problem is finding—and staying with—the right partner. As many know, in the current environment of managed care and health insurance panels, people are rarely given the opportunity to form a long-term relationship with a doctor. You get the feeling (as implied in some governmental policies and insurance plans) that doctors are interchangeable, that they're like airline pilots—when you board an airplane you don't know who the pilot is, but you assume there's a minimal level of competence there.

It's true that medical education, standards, and practices are so strictly regulated that, generally speaking, all doctors do have a certain degree of competence. But what cannot be denied, or overstressed, is the tremendous health benefit that comes from having a long-term relationship with a doctor to whom you can talk openly, one who is understanding of your particular medical background and needs. With no fear of hyperbole, that relationship can definitely add tremendous quality to anyone's life and could quite literally add years as well.

This is not to say that the doctor controls your health. He or she is more the knowledgeable guidance counselor, especially when it comes to preventive measures. You are the true master of your own health—a doctor can't make you stop smoking, can't make you take that pill, can't make you eat right or exercise. In the end, it's all up to you. This is borne out by the fact that only 30 percent of your general health is attributable to genetics (family history), while a whopping 70 percent is directly related to what you do or don't do in your life.

Being the master of your own health doesn't mean, however, that you can or should do everything when it comes to your health. It's important to know when you need professional help and when you don't. *Facing Your Fifties* answers that all-important question and many others.

TIME TO PUT UP OR SHUT UP

When it comes to health issues and being sick, our female counterparts have always seen us as big babies, whiners who can't stop complaining about this ache or pain, that ailment or illness. They say men believe that every health problem— no matter how small—seems to be the harbinger of life-threatening illnesses.

Maybe there is a small grain of truth in what they say (although they'd sure feel bad if that hangnail did turn out to be a brain tumor). But, happily, our bad rap as complainers is diminishing as we take more and more personal responsibility for our bodies and what happens to them. While we are renowned for not wanting to know about our health, weren't we the ones who began the running craze? And aren't we now flocking to gyms, wellness centers, and aerobics classes? We're also reading men's health and fitness magazines, trying spa treatments, and working on our diets. We've even found ourselves watching an occasional *Oprah* TV show and enjoying it.

No doubt about it, we're changing. We're making strides that get bigger and bigger every day. And the best part is that as we change—as we learn about our health and take action to improve it—we're actually feeling better, looking better, and becoming generally happier in the process.

We're finally realizing one of life's great truths: A good life starts with a healthy life. And the beauty of it all is that we have the power to create that healthy life— it only takes a little motivation, a little self-discipline, and a little effort.

HOW TO USE THIS BOOK

Facing Your Fifties is a down-to-earth, practical, quick-reference guide for the average fifties male and/or his significant other. No unexplained medical jargon, no trivial details, and no extreme measures that few would ever follow.

Look at it as a kind of first-consult book that can quickly provide a general assessment of your problem so you'll know if you should stop worrying, start doing something specific, or get to a doctor. While not an encyclopedia (especially for those already familiar with any long-term problems), *Facing Your Fifties* does give extensive detail about specific ailments that males in this age group might experience. The entire book is dedicated to explaining and outlining the watch words that all fifties males should have imprinted in their brains:

• **Awareness**—of potential medical dangers and changes your fifties body will experience.

• **Early-warning testing**—most notably for high blood pressure, high cholesterol, prostate cancer, and colon cancer, as well as annual general checkups.

• **Preventive actions**—that include watching your diet and alcohol consumption, exercising, not smoking, and wearing sunscreen.

Facing Your Fifties, as a quick-reference guide, can be consulted when something starts going wrong ("Hey, my shoulder's hurting, I'll see what they say about shoulders"), but the book's real value comes when it's read cover-to-cover. There is a natural progression within the book's organization that starts with an assessment chapter to help you determine where you stand on the overall health scale. Then, the body is broken down into logical parts that are explained in separate chapters. These chapters contain:

• Basic background information critical to understanding the specifics of your health.

• A breakout of specific ailments men face, with an emphasis on those faced by fifties men.

• Treatment and prevention options for every ailment mentioned.

• Real-life stories about men who have faced particular medical situations.

Introduction

• Descriptions of pertinent drugs, their benefits, and side effects.

• A summary of the good news within the chapter.

Facing Your Fifties then details in three chapters the all-important issues of:

1. Sex, energy, and male menopause.

2. Mental state and changing patterns.

3. Cancer.

Ending on a positive note, *Facing Your Fifties* has an extensive chapter on what you can do to improve your health. This last chapter fully explains exercise and diet, outlining positive choices that make a difference, as well as how to stop smoking.

It should be noted that this book can only go so far in identifying and treating specific ailments. Because each person is different—and there are numerous medical factors that are affected and/or altered by the individuality of patients and ailments—it is critical that treatments mentioned in *Facing Your Fifties* be presented to your own doctor for review before trying them yourself. Additionally, the burgeoning field of alternative, or complementary, medicine (which could take up an entire book), is referred to only with items that have been scientifically proven.

For those interested in finding medical information in other places, an excellent source for drug information is *The Physician's Desk Reference,* which is available in two versions, one for physicians (found in any library) and an inexpensive consumer edition published in paperback. As for seeking advice on the Internet, care should be taken to consult only established medical sites.

1: WHERE DO YOU STAND NOW?

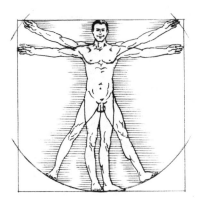

A Comprehensive Status Report

BACKGROUND BASICS

Who are you?

- A corporate executive who practically lives on the road.

- A regular guy who's trying to be health conscious but isn't getting very far.

- An avid jogger who's in better shape now than when he was thirty.

- A guy whose job keeps him on his feet all day, so he doesn't see the need for "extra" exercise.

- A former jock who hasn't worked out in twenty years.

- An ex-husband who's not very good about meal planning and taking care of himself.

• **A nutrition-conscious guy who's always munching on a granola bar.**

As long as you're a male and you're in your fifties (or nearly there), it doesn't matter. What does matter is that you picked up this book. And that you've read this far. That's the first sign that you want to know more about your health and how to maintain and/or improve it.

But where do you start?

The first step is to determine where on the general health ladder you stand right now—what rung you're on compared to the "average" or "ideal" fifties Joe. That will be a critical point of reference from which you can put the rest of this book into personal context. And we know that's important, because if you can't apply this book to your own situation, then it's not worth very much. Besides, it's always an interesting exercise to see where you stand against everyone else—even if the results might not be what you expect.

Don't worry, though, you don't have to jump through any hoops, do any push-ups, or answer any questions that involve speeding trains and velocity vectors (although one does involve math, so get out your pocket calculator). The following are *the* critical benchmarks by which doctors determine where you are when it comes to overall health. They'll tell you everything from your artery health to your body fat ratio.

So, with no further ado, pencils ready? Begin. And good luck!

WEIGHT TO HEIGHT

Level of Importance: High, because those who are overweight risk everything from heart disease to prematurely deteriorated joints.

Ideal weight ranges for men:

5'1"	123–145	5' 9"	139–175
5'2"	125–148	5'10"	141–179
5'3"	127–151	5'11"	144–183
5'4"	129–155	6' 0"	147–187
5'5"	131–159	6' 1"	158–190
5'6"	133–163	6' 2"	165–195
5'7"	135–167	6' 3"	167–200
5'8"	137–171	6' 4"	171–207

Additional Information: Your weight really should not change with age, although lack of exercise, change in eating habits, and reduction in muscle mass will all conspire to put on pounds as you put on years. Keep in mind that muscle weighs more than fat. So if you weigh the same at 55 as you did at 25, you should be proud—who wouldn't?— but you should also be aware that muscle mass generally decreases with age. All of which means that your total weight should actually decrease as you get older (unless you're pumping iron). If your weight hasn't decreased over the years, if it's stayed the same, then you're probably putting on fat. (See chapter 8 for diet and exercise details.)

BODY MASS INDEX

Level of Importance: High. It is a good general indicator of fat to body weight ratio. Too much fat can be the underlying cause of numerous health risks and serious ailments.

How to calculate BMI: Divide your weight in pounds by your height in inches squared, then multiple the result by 705. An example—a man who's 5'10" (70 inches) and weighs 175 pounds would calculate: 175 divided by 4,900 (70 × 70) = .0357142 times 705 = 25.18. That BMI means the man is slightly overweight.

Ideal BMI	24 or less
Considered Overweight	25 or more
Obese	30 or more

Additional Information: Be honest about your true height and weight—the result means nothing if those figures are inaccurate. In body mass indexing, no allowance is given for age. Calculate various weights above and below your own to see how the BMI changes, then set a goal BMI and start working toward it. (See chapter 8 for diet and exercise details.) If you have a good BMI, don't get too cocky—this index is only an indicator of fat to body weight ratio; it's not a yardstick for overall physical conditioning. For very muscular individuals, the BMI may read falsely high.

HEIGHT																
FEET		5'	5'1"	5'2"	5'3"	5'4"	5'5"	5'6"	5'7"	5'8"	5'9"	5'10"	5'11"	6'	6'1"	6'2"
INCHES		60	61	62	63	64	65	66	67	68	69	70	71	72	73	74
WEIGHT	**CM**	152	155	157	160	163	165	168	170	173	175	178	180	183	185	188
LB	**KG**															
100	45.5	19.6	18.9	18.3	17.8	17.2	16.7	16.2	15.7	15.2	14.8	14.4	14.0	13.6	13.2	12.9
110	50.0	21.5	20.8	20.2	19.5	18.9	18.3	17.8	17.3	16.8	16.3	15.8	15.4	14.9	14.5	14.2
120	54.5	23.5	22.7	22.0	21.3	20.6	20.0	19.4	18.8	18.3	17.8	17.3	16.8	16.3	15.9	15.4
130	59.1	25.4	24.6	23.8	23.1	22.4	21.7	21.0	20.4	19.8	19.2	18.7	18.2	17.7	17.2	16.7
140	63.6	27.4	26.5	25.7	24.9	24.1	23.3	22.6	22.0	21.3	20.7	20.1	19.6	19.0	18.5	18.0
150	68.2	29.4	28.4	27.5	26.6	25.8	25.0	24.3	23.5	22.9	22.2	21.6	21.0	20.4	19.8	19.3
160	72.7	31.3	30.3	29.3	28.4	27.5	26.7	25.9	25.1	24.4	23.7	23.0	22.4	21.7	21.2	20.6
170	77.3	33.5	32.2	31.2	30.2	29.2	28.3	27.5	26.7	25.9	25.2	24.4	23.8	23.1	22.5	21.9
180	81.8	35.2	34.1	33.0	32.0	31.0	30.0	29.1	28.3	27.4	26.6	25.9	25.2	24.5	23.8	23.2
190	86.4	37.2	36.0	34.8	33.7	32.7	31.7	30.7	29.8	28.9	28.1	27.3	26.6	25.8	25.1	24.4
200	90.9	39.1	37.9	36.7	35.5	34.4	33.4	32.3	31.4	30.5	29.6	28.8	28.0	27.2	26.4	25.7
210	95.5	41.1	39.8	38.5	37.3	36.1	35.0	34.0	33.0	32.0	31.1	30.2	29.4	28.5	27.8	27.0
220	100.0	43.1	41.7	40.3	39.1	37.8	36.7	35.6	34.5	33.5	32.6	31.6	30.7	29.9	2.91	28.3
230	104.5	45.0	43.5	42.2	40.8	39.6	38.4	37.2	36.1	35.0	34.0	33.1	32.1	31.3	30.4	29.6
240	109.1	47.0	45.4	44.0	42.6	41.3	40.0	38.8	37.7	36.6	35.5	34.5	33.5	32.6	31.7	30.9
250	113.6	48.9	47.3	45.8	44.4	43.0	41.7	40.4	39.2	38.1	37.0	35.9	34.9	34.0	33.1	32.2
260	118.2	50.9	49.2	47.7	46.2	44.7	43.4	42.1	40.8	39.6	38.5	37.4	36.3	35.3	34.4	33.5
270	122.7	52.8	51.1	49.5	47.9	46.4	45.0	43.7	42.4	41.1	40.0	38.8	37.7	36.7	35.7	34.7
280	127.3	54.8	53.0	51.3	49.7	48.2	46.7	45.3	43.9	42.7	41.4	40.3	39.1	38.1	37.0	36.0
290	131.8	56.8	54.9	53.2	51.5	49.9	48.4	46.9	45.5	44.2	42.9	41.7	40.5	39.4	38.3	37.3
300	136.4	58.7	56.8	55.0	53.3	51.6	50.0	48.5	47.1	45.7	44.4	43.1	41.9	40.8	39.7	38.6

BLOOD PRESSURE

Level of Importance: Highest. This is the primary indicator of how healthy your blood vessels are. In many ways, you're only as healthy as your arteries are.

Ideal	**120 over 80 (or less on both)**
Good Range	**120–129 over 80–84**

Additional Information: In theory, for those who stay fit and healthy, blood pressure should not change significantly (more than a few points) during a lifetime. However, it has been shown that numerous factors do affect blood pressure, everything from age to stress levels. It's critical to good health for those who do have high blood pressure to bring it down. This can be accomplished through the use of excellent drugs and, to a lesser degree, by exercise, proper diet, and learning how to handle stress and tension. (See chapter 3 for blood pressure and blood vessel details, chapter 6 for stress relief ideas, and chapter 8 for diet and exercise details.)

Where Do You Stand Now?

*C*HOLESTEROL *L*EVELS

Level of Importance: Highest. Research has established that those with a high level of cholesterol in their blood have a greater risk of heart disease (the number one killer of adults in the world) than those with a low cholesterol level.

Ideal range	
HDL (Good Cholesterol)	**More than 40**
LDL (Bad Cholesterol)	**0 to 100**
Total Cholesterol Count	**Less Than 200**

Additional Information: These latest figures represent new—and tougher—official government guidelines. The only way to get an accurate count of HDL and LDL is to fast for twelve hours before the test. Even the milk in a cup of coffee can affect the results. It is critical to good health that high cholesterol levels be brought down. Exercise can play an important role in this (it can actually increase your HDL), as can diet and the use of any number of excellent drugs that have been developed to lower cholesterol. (See chapter 3 for cholesterol details and chapter 8 for diet and exercise details.)

*B*LOOD *S*UGAR *(G*LUCOSE*) L*EVEL

Level of Importance: High. Any blood sugar levels out of the normal range could signify diabetes, which can lead to permanent, severe organ and/or body system damage and, ultimately, if not controlled, death.

Fasting Range 65–110

Additional Information: If a person registers a fasting blood sugar level of 110 to 125, this means he's borderline and will be monitored. If a person has two separate blood tests in which both times the fasting level is over 126, he's a diabetic. Because there are rarely any symptoms from diabetes until it has become seriously advanced, monitoring blood sugar and sugar in the urine are the only ways of detecting this potentially fatal disease. Make sure to truly fast overnight before the test. Diet and exercise can have a tremendous impact on how your body processes sugar. (See chapter 4 for diabetes details and chapter 8 for diet and exercise details.)

GETTING THE MOST OUT OF SEEING YOUR DOCTOR

We've all heard the horror story: A doctor makes a diagnosis in less than thirty seconds.

But that's like saying a singer with his first hit song is an "instant star," even though he's worked in the business for twenty years. Inside that thirty-second diagnosis are years of medical school, years of on-the-job training, and years of seeing patients.

We can all agree, though, that a visit to a doctor is usually too short—a product of many unchangeable variables. So how can you maximize the time you get with your physician? For ailments beyond the everyday colds, here are two suggestions for what you can do prior to seeing your doctor:

1. **Get the basics down.** When did the problem start? What are all the symptoms? If there's pain, exactly where is it, and what kind is it (dull, sharp, throbbing)?

2. **Do some detective work.** Every doctor is a little like Sherlock Holmes. Why not be a Doctor Watson and do some background work? Does the ailment come and go at certain times? With certain foods? Try to objectively analyze possible causes.

Suggestions while you are seeing your doctor:

- **Tell the truth**—This is no time to try to fool yourself or your doctor. Physicians know most men will lie about three topics: smoking, drinking, and sex. Be honest.

- **Mention all medications you take**—Even vitamins and herbal remedies.

- **Be concise and complete**—Respecting a doctor's limited time, you should keep the explanation brief, while including everything you think might be relevant.

The best advice? Build a long-term relationship with one doctor. The rewards are huge.

Where Do You Stand Now?

PROSTATE SPECIFIC ANTIGEN (PSA) TEST

Level of Importance: High, especially for men in our age group. This is a time when an aggressive form of prostate cancer can take its greatest toll (Frank Zappa, the rock musician who died of prostate cancer in his fifties, is a prime example). A PSA test registers a protein that is produced by the prostate. Prostate cell damage (produced by cancer or inflammation) increases the amount of protein detected in the blood.

> **Normal Range for Fifties Men: 0 to 4**

Additional Information: Testing should start at fifty (earlier in African-American males and those with a family history), and be done on a yearly basis so that any spikes in the readings (even though still in the normal range) can be caught. Increased age (especially beyond sixty) generally means higher average readings, even without cancer being present. The PSA test is controversial, because it can have both false positives (a high reading when you don't have cancer) and false negatives (a low reading when you do have cancer), but we believe the benefits of testing outweigh these relatively slight inconveniences, especially when stacked up against the aggressive, fast-moving form of prostate cancer. (See chapter 4 for prostate details.)

EXERCISE STATUS

Level of Importance: High. If your lifestyle or job does not include twenty to thirty minutes of physical activity (walking at the very least) several days a week, you are not doing what you should be doing.

Additional Information: No exercise is ever useless, but if you're not breaking even a little sweat or feeling your heart pound just a bit, it's not enough. To establish fitness, you need to sustain some form of exercise (preferably aerobic to start with) that puts at least a slight strain on you and your heart, or you're not getting full value for your exercise. (See chapter 8 for exercise details.)

2: THE MUSCULO-SKELETAL SYSTEM

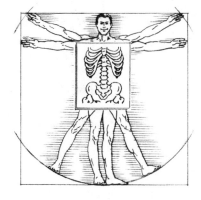

Upholding More than Its Own

Simply put, the musculoskeletal system is comprised of your bones, joints, muscles, ligaments, and tendons. As we all know, though, when it comes to those body parts, nothing is very simple—that's why these background basics are so extensive, explaining the major components in detail.

How important is your musculoskeletal system to your health and well being?

When it comes to general health maintenance, the musculoskeletal system is the key to virtually all the body's other systems and organs. It's the key to controlling cholesterol and blood pressure, the key to energy and stamina, and the key to better utilization of oxygen, which makes our hearts and lungs work more efficiently. There's even considerable evidence that, at least in rats, it's the key to increasing the number of functioning nerve cells and brain synapses (the highways for nerve impulses).

Why the Musculoskeletal System Is So Important

1. Your body's overall health comes in large part from your physical condition.

2. Your physical condition is dictated by how well you exercise.

3. How well you exercise depends on the density and durability of bones, and the strength, stretchability, and resilience of muscles, joints, tendons, and ligaments.

In this chain reaction to creating good health, you can see how the musculoskeletal system is critical and heavily influences all other reactions—thereby impacting the overall quality and duration of life.

Take, for example, a runner in his fifties who jogs a couple of miles every day. Suddenly he decides to boost his regimen to eight miles a day, without properly preparing his muscles, joints, tendons, and ligaments for the extra stress and strain. The first day he'll probably make it, because his heart and lungs are in good shape from his previous jogging. But the next day his muscles, tendons, ligaments, and joints will be so tight and painful he'll have trouble moving at all.

If he had properly conditioned and prepared his musculoskeletal system, his heart and lungs would have followed like greyhounds after the rabbit.

It's unfortunate but true that many of us see our bones, muscles, and joints as nothing more than the clichéd image of girders, beams, and cables holding up a building. While there's an obvious grain of truth to that analogy, there's a whole beach worth of reality usually missed:

• **Bones** aren't inert; they can get stronger with use.

• **Muscles, tendons, and ligaments** aren't just cables that allow your body to do things. They're living tissue that can be conditioned to survive greater stress.

• **Cartilage** can stay healthy when worked correctly.

All these components thrive on proper use, but deteriorate with overuse, misuse, or underuse.

How *should* your body feel at fifty?

The simple truth is that your muscles and joints are naturally going to feel a little tighter and achier. They will be more prone to injury, slower to heal, and generally require more maintenance than they did when you were young.

The Musculoskeletal System

How Musculoskeletal Problems Occur

• Injury

• Overuse

• Degeneration, including degenerative arthritis

All muscles, bones, joints, tendons, and ligaments are, at times, susceptible to one or a combination of these, although typically it's only the knee that suffers from all three. Some cause-and-effect relationships among the three seem evident, and in many cases, age is a determining factor—from middle age on, the likelihood of all three increases.

While injuries and overuse can be successfully treated in a variety of ways, degenerative arthritis, no matter where it attacks, has no known cure, and the cause is unknown, although possibilities include age, obesity, genetics, joint injury, overuse, and misuse.

While none of that sounds too appealing, there is good news—substantial improvement is still firmly within your grasp, and the benefits of an improved musculoskeletal system can be overwhelming. In one Tufts University study, reported in the *Journal of the American Medical Association*, a group of Boston nursing-home residents in their nineties were put on a high-intensity program of weight training. Strength gains averaged an incredible 174 percent. Two of the subjects actually stopped using canes to walk, and a third could once again get up by himself from a chair.

Obviously, keeping your musculoskeletal system in good working order is critical to good health, no matter what your age.

Bones—*The Foundation of the Team*

Bones not only make up our skeletal frame but also store mineral salts and, in their honeycombed interior, house the body's blood-forming tissue. Most of the growth and formation of the 206 bones in your body takes place by the time you're eighteen, with peak bone mass occurring around age thirty. Throughout your life, however, your bones still have the capacity to remake and strengthen themselves in a process called "remodeling."

Bones remain strong and durable and, barring injury, don't give us too much trouble. Unfortunately, two major problems that we'll have to face in the sixties, seventies, and beyond are already laying their groundwork:

1. **Osteoporosis.** This abnormal loss of bone tissue and strength is less common in men than women, but the National Osteoporosis Foundation reports that 20 percent of sufferers are men, and that one in eight men over the age of fifty will suffer some kind of fracture due to the disease during their lifetime. Hip fractures alone lay low nearly 80,000 men (mostly seniors) every year.

2. **Arthritis.** This is a condition that causes swelling, pain—many times severe— and loss of range of motion in affected joints. An umbrella term for nearly 100 different conditions, arthritis afflicts thirty-six million Americans and is the most common cause of disability in America, according to the Centers for Disease Control and Prevention. The most common form of arthritis, affecting twenty million Americans, is degenerative arthritis—also referred to as osteoarthritis and/or degenerative joint disease (DJD). Characterized by joint pain or stiffness, degenerative arthritis typically occurs in weight-bearing joints such as the hips and knees, but can also show up in hands, fingers, and feet. While it normally affects people over the age of forty-five, retired hockey star Wayne Gretzky was diagnosed with osteoarthritis of the shoulder at age thirty-eight. Ways of treating degenerative arthritis include taking anti-inflammatories, applying heat to the affected area, having a couple of days of rest, taking cortisone injections, moderate working of the joints, and, in severe cases, surgery. Some anecdotal evidence suggests dietary supplements such as chondroitin sulfate and glucosamine (two compounds found in healthy joints), and methyl-sulfonyl-methane have limited positive results, although they're as yet scientifically unproven. A recent controlled study showed glucosamine chondroitin sulfate to be the first treatment that actually slows the cause of degenerative arthritis, but other studies will be needed to confirm this.

A Prevention Plan for General Arthritis and Osteoporosis

• 1,200 to 1,500 mg per day of calcium (from food or supplements) to replace what's being lost to the aging process.

• 400 to 800 IU a day of vitamin D might aid in cartilage synthesis and repair.

• Establish an exercise regimen that includes some type of weightbearing exercise to build strength and improve the stability of joints, which reduces "wear and tear." Stretching exercises—and to a lesser degree aerobic exercise—also help, because they keep muscles loose (tight muscles aggravate affected joints by drawing everything closer together).

Muscles, Tendons, and Ligaments—
Dynamic Teammates

The nearly 650 muscles in the human body are made up of slender cells called fibers that can work independently or collectively. They range in size from the tiny muscles that make your eyelids blink to the massive groups that raise your legs. Muscles are nourished and maintained by the blood stream and convert your body's chemical energy into mechanical energy.

Tendons and ligaments are a little different from muscles. Both are relatively avascular, meaning their supply of blood is relatively scarce, and both are connective tissues (the tendons connect muscles to bone, ligaments bind joint bones together and connect bones and cartilage).

For muscles, tendons, and ligaments (all called dynamic tissues), their life is one continual battle with gravity. Watch a group of twenty-somethings play volleyball, and you'll see that the resilient, stretchy tissue many of us had at that age resists gravity very well. Now, look in the mirror and you'll know the natural tendency is for muscle, tendon, and ligament tissue to shrink and tighten as it ages, while skin and its underlying connective tissue loosen.

Even if you're in good shape, you know that your muscles can be stiff in the morning, feel good when they're warmed up, and then stiffen up later. This cyclical phenomenon reflects the fact that a stiff or tight muscle is actually a weak muscle. The tightening is usually a result of microscopic tears of muscle fibers caused by taking the muscle beyond where it wants to go. The injured muscle tightens up as a way of splinting itself to protect against further harm.

This muscle characteristic has surprised many men who have pulled or torn a muscle and said, "What happened, I didn't do anything unusual?" The answer is simple: As we age, our muscles are naturally constricting or shrinking, so what once was "normal" movement for you in your twenties or even thirties can now be abnormal if your body isn't properly prepared with stretching and strengthening.

This is why you can sometimes hurt your back simply by bending down to pick up a pencil, or why softball can be such a surprisingly dangerous sport for our age group. Quick sprints around the bases or taking off from a standing stop can cause problems if your muscles, tendons, and ligaments aren't properly warmed and stretched to handle what you want them to do.

The key word is *relative:* As you get older, the limits of how far you can take your muscles changes—even on a day-to-day or hour-by-hour basis. You know this is true if you try to do a thorough stretch immediately after getting out of bed. It can be hard to do—you can even hurt yourself stretching at the wrong time. In fact, some sports-medicine doctors suggest you get the most benefit from stretching after your regular routine of walking, jogging, or exercising, rather than before.

But stretching is only part of the equation—strengthening also has to occur for muscles to fully develop and be able to protect against injuries.

Strong and stretchable muscles not only help prevent injuries, they are the key to greater stamina as well. Scientifically, we can improve our cardiac output (heart efficiency) maybe 10 to 20 percent, and our wind (oxygen use) by 30 to 40 percent, but the increase we can achieve in muscle conditioning and growth can be off the charts.

Exercising Your Muscles Can:

- **Improve their internal efficiency.** We cannot greatly increase the amount of oxygen to muscles, but exercise stimulates certain chemical changes that increase the efficiency of our body's use of oxygen.

- **Slow muscle mass loss.** In the thirties you begin to lose muscle mass—some say a third- to a half-pound a decade. Exercise retards that and builds strength and stretchability in what you retain. In this case, "use it or lose it" is surprisingly accurate.

- **Buff you up.** No doubt about it, even a little muscle looks better than no muscle at all—just ask your partner.

While muscles reap the largest gains from exercise, tendons and ligaments can be strengthened with use. But strengthening must be done properly or damage may occur. Doctors worry more about damage to tendons, ligaments, and joints than to muscles. They know that muscles, unlike tendons and ligaments, have a greater ability to be rejuvenated, primarily because they have access to the body's nourishing blood supply.

Cartilage, Bursae, and Joints—
Protecting Them Now Extends Their Playing Careers

Cartilage keeps your bones from rubbing together. It is tough connective tissue that has no nerves, no blood supply, and is nourished via synovial, or joint, fluid. If your cartilage is severely damaged or worn out, there's little that can be done at present besides joint replacement (primarily of the knee or hip), although culturing and growing new cartilage is being studied.

Bursae are pouch-shaped membranous structures that allow the skin over your joints to move freely. The most obvious bursae are those protecting your elbow and knee. A hit or jarring impact can cause a bursa to swell up and become painful—a condition called bursitis.

The Musculoskeletal System

Joints (like cartilage and bursae) aren't as resilient as muscles or as able to rejuvenate, because they have only limited access to the body's nourishing blood supply. This makes them more of a concern as we get older. While most men under sixty usually don't need to worry about joint replacements, they can see signs of joint instability and wear and tear from years of overuse, misuse, or under-use. That's why the decade of the fifties should be a time of protecting and nurturing whatever level of joint integrity and cartilage remains.

How to Maintain Joints and Cartilage

- Avoid jarring, impact-prone activities, such as heavy-duty downhill mogul skiing.

- Moderately use your joints, while being careful not to overuse or misuse them. This helps to spread the nourishing synovial fluid over the entire surface of the cartilage.

- Integrate weight-bearing exercises into your routine to stimulate cartilage development—cartilage, to a certain degree, can remake or remodel itself.

Don't worry about wearing out your joints. Running, weight lifting, and other physical activities should all be fine—if done properly—and can make up a complete exercise program.

WHERE AND HOW PROBLEMS OCCUR, TREATMENT OPTIONS, AND PREVENTIVE MEASURES

The Spine

Ever since mankind decided that walking on two feet was better than rambling around on all fours, the human spine has been trying to adjust. To date, it still has a way to go. The evidence: Back pain is the third most common reason to see a doctor, behind only sore throats and colds.

The spine, or backbone, is comprised of thirty-three bones called vertebrae that stack up to form a firm, flexible column running from the base of the skull down to the pelvis. Science has grouped these bones into categories.

Five Categories of Vertebrae

1. **Cervical.** The first seven, starting from the top, make up the neck region.

2. Thoracic. The next twelve make up the chest region.

3. Lumbar. The next five form the lower back.

4. & 5. Sacrum and Coccyx. The last nine at the base of the spine fuse together by adulthood and form the sacrum, a bone between the hips and the coccyx, the tailbone.

Each vertebra contains an opening, and together these openings form a hollow canal that runs nearly the length of the spine. Inside this canal is the spinal cord, a major part of the central nervous system that contains vital nerves. These nerves branch off from the spine and reach nearly every part of the body, acting as communications links between the brain and body. Cushioning the vertebrae—so bone doesn't rub against bone—are round, flat, gelatinous tissues called discs.

In such an intricate setup it's rather surprising there aren't even more spine problems than there are. The chest region of the spine seldom experiences problems (it's less movable than other parts of the spine, so it's less prone to wear and tear), but that's not true for the neck and lower back portions, which can suffer everything from neck and back arthritis (serious, but mostly found in older individuals) to muscle strains and herniated (ruptured) discs.

Most of the spinal ailments we face in our fifties are soft-tissue-related—muscle strains, pulls, and tears—though there may be some disc problems and the development of spurs, which are small arthritic protrusions of bone in the wrong places. Most of these problems can be treated with a couple of days of rest, use of heat and ice on the affected area, physical therapy (prescribed by a doctor), and a carefully planned fitness program. Rarely is surgery required.

Medical science can't actually prove conclusively that medical intervention for acute back strain, or even some disc problems, makes a substantial difference—the fact is, many backs heal by themselves. A physician can certainly evaluate you to make sure it's not something worse than a strain and prescribe physical therapy or a good exercise program, but this is an area where the active involvement of the "owner" pays off handsomely. In fact, of all lower back problems our age group faces, only 20 percent require a physician's intervention—we can handle close to 80 percent ourselves.

An acute back strain, though, should be seen as a major wake-up call that you need to begin regular maintenance (a physical fitness program) to help your back become as strong and as flexible as it can be. And any back pain should be taken seriously. It could simply be a weekend warrior's reward of tired, strained muscles, or it could be something more serious, such as a ruptured disc. With

The Musculoskeletal System

the first, you can handle the situation yourself; with the second, a doctor's help is needed.

So how do you know when you should see a physician and when you should let time and rest try to heal a back problem?

Determining if Your Back Needs Professional Care

• **Severity.** If you can't stand the pain or you're immobilized, you need to see a licensed professional, whether you think it's a muscle strain or a disc problem.

• **Radiating Pain.** If the pain goes into your buttocks, legs, arms, or hands, you don't have to rush to the doctor if the pain's not severe, but if it persists, see a doctor soon.

• **Loss of Function.** If, along with the back pain, you lose bowel control or have trouble emptying your bladder (urinary retention and/or hesitancy), go to a doctor quickly. While urinary hesitancy can be caused by a disc pressing on a nerve, it can also be caused by the use of muscle relaxants and some antihistamines (see chapter 4 for urinary details). Any kind of muscle weakness in an extremity should also warrant a trip to the doctor.

• **No Improvement.** If you try working out your back problems on your own, expect positive results in one to three months. If you don't see an improvement within that time, see a doctor.

The Neck

While we might think of our necks as something only to shave or massage, it does serve some serious functions (beyond keeping you from losing your head). Basically, the neck is the communications and supply link between the body and head, channeling nerve impulses and blood between the two via the spinal cord, four arteries, and associated veins. Supporting all this are tendons, ligaments, muscles, and the first seven vertebrae (cervical vertebrae) of the spinal column.

Most neck problems—such as a stiff or sore neck—are muscle related and usually caused by stress and/or fatigue. A little rest, the taking of over-the-counter (OTC) anti-inflammatories, the application of heat, and a massage—self-given or administrated by someone else—does wonders to resolve such problems.

Two other neck ailments aren't so easily resolved: neck arthritis (not detailed in this book, because it normally affects much older men), and a herniated, or ruptured, disc—something that many fifties males will have to face.

HERNIATED DISC IN THE NECK

As shock absorbers of the spine, discs are little, flattened, donut-shaped cushioning tissues with a gelatinous center. They keep the spine's individual vertebrae from grinding together. Under certain conditions—repeated motion, injury, heredity, smoking, obesity, bad lifting mechanics, or just plain bad luck—they sometimes bulge and trap a nerve or nerve root. This is called a herniated, ruptured, or slipped disc. Both a bulging and a ruptured disc can produce irritation, inflammation, and pain (sometimes quite severe) along the course of the impinged nerve, much as a severed phone wire causes problems far down the line from the initial break. In humans this means that a nerve being pinched by a disc in the neck can cause pain as far away as the hand or fingers. Pain can also be right at the disc location, but not always.

Treatment/Prevention—Because disc pain can be far away from the actual ruptured disc, it can fool a person into believing there's nothing wrong with their neck. And when there is pain at the disc location, many times the pain feels like "normal" stress-related muscle soreness. That's why it's important to see a doctor, who will be able to determine the real source of your pain. In fact, the location of the pain can give a doctor the precise location of the disc problem. For example, pain extending down to the thumb and first finger, especially when accompanied by weakness, can indicate a problem with the disc that lies between the sixth and seventh cervical vertebrae.

Once the herniated disc has been precisely identified—typically by an MRI (magnetic resonance imaging) scan—usually the best course of action is to first do nothing drastic (such as surgery). The doctor will explain that many times the situation resolves itself within four to six weeks through a combination of personal and doctor-prescribed actions. They include:

- **A short period of rest**—two days, normally.

- **Taking anti-inflammatories**—either OTC or prescribed by your doctor for pain.

- **Physical therapy**—as prescribed by your physician to teach you how to properly exercise, stretch, and strengthen the muscles around the affected area during the period of rest and recuperation.

If, along with the pain, there are more serious symptoms, such as loss of any neurological functions (loss of strength or feeling, or numbness developing) and/or loss of bowel/bladder control, then surgery is usually required. Normally, surgery either removes any offending disc tissue that is pinching the nerve or pares away any bone that might be in the way. The surgeon may also fuse one vertebra to another to ensure that you don't end up with an unstable back, which is a source of chronic pain and disability. While fusion seems like an extreme procedure, it ultimately doesn't change the way the back feels to the recuperated patient.

An interesting side note to back surgery is that five years down the road, looking at people who have had surgery and those who haven't, you can't see much difference between them—that's why surgery is done only when serious symptoms are present.

If you are able to resolve disc problems without surgery, once the pain is gone there are some simple rules you should follow.

Taking Pressure off Your Discs

• Keep your back as straight as possible at all times.

• When lifting, bend your knees, keep your back straight, and lift with your legs.

• When standing for a long time, try to slightly elevate one leg periodically.

• When sitting for long periods of time, elevate your feet so your knees are higher than your hips.

• When sleeping, flip over on your back. Sleeping on your stomach puts unnecessary pressure on the spinal column.

The Mid and Lower Back

The midback, or chest region of your back, is comprised of the twelve thoracic vertebrae (explained earlier). Seldom does this portion of the back cause any problems.

The lower back, on the other hand, is another story. Made up of five lumbar vertebrae (explained earlier), the lower back is one of the few body parts that has caused consistent human misery ever since man first learned how to whine.

GENERAL LOWER BACK PAIN

In our age group, after years of benign neglect and abuse, the lower back starts exacting revenge. While most of us perceive ourselves as still young and strong eighteen-year-olds, our bodies—and specifically the lower back—are ready at a moment's notice to tell us the reality of the situation. We have to remember our real age and that what was once easily within our back's range of motion and strength is probably not anymore.

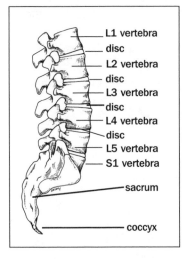

L1 vertebra
disc
L2 vertebra
disc
L3 vertebra
disc
L4 vertebra
disc
L5 vertebra
S1 vertebra
sacrum
coccyx

What Makes Your Lower Back Hurt

• Sleeping wrong

• Sitting wrong

• Bending and picking up something at a wrong angle

• Overuse (too many sit-ups, mixing concrete for a patio, hauling gravel for the drive)

• Problem with a lower-back disc (explained in the next section)

Treatment/Prevention—Typically, most lower back injuries are self-limiting—they hurt so much you won't be able to do anything even if you want to—and go away within a couple of days. That's because they are typically muscle related, involving strained, pulled, or fatigued muscles. Initially, you should apply ice; then later, apply heat to the affected area to help control inflammation and to aid in the healing process. Take OTC anti-inflammatories for pain and to reduce swelling. Rest for no longer than two days. Try to avoid re-injury. As soon as the pain allows, begin a little stretching. (It should be noted that the prescribing of muscle relaxants—basically tranquilizers—has been commonly used for this ailment, and patients still ask for them, but Gordon believes the cost in drowsiness is way too high for most people to pay.)

If the pain persists beyond a few days, see a doctor.

HERNIATED DISC IN THE LOWER BACK

A key point in understanding this problem is that the mobile parts of your back (the neck and lower back) put lots of stress, strain, and pressure on the discs, which can lead to wear and tear, and a herniated, or ruptured disc. In the case of the lower back, the discs that usually have the most problems are the last two (between the fourth and fifth lumbar vertebrae; and between the lumbar fifth and sacrum first vertebrae), because that's the area that is most impacted by all our bending, twisting, and turning.

The Musculoskeletal System

As with a herniated disc in the neck, a problem disc in the lower back can pinch a nerve that creates pain far from the injured disc. In this case, the pain can be in the back of the hip, can run down your leg, and can even generate a strip of numbness or tingling down the leg. Sometimes, there can be muscle weakness and, in severe cases (that must be handled immediately), a loss or change in bladder and bowel functions.

Treatment/Prevention. If there is loss of bladder or bowel functions with a herniated disc, the patient has little choice but surgery. It's a serious situation that needs to be taken care of immediately. Most other cases of ruptured disc give patients the luxury of dealing with it conservatively (nonsurgically). Because the pain of a herniated disc can be similar to a muscle strain or pull, it's important that lower back pain be checked out by a physician. For most cases, the treatment of choice is limited rest (no more than two days), application of ice to the affected area to control inflammation and to numb the pain (heat can be applied later to loosen up the area and to aid in the healing process), the taking of OTC anti-inflammatories for pain and to reduce inflammation, and, if your doctor prescribes it, physical therapy to show you how to properly exercise the muscles around the disc. (Because treatment for a herniated disc in the lower back is similar to the treatment for one in the neck, see the previous section, "Herniated Disc in the Neck," for additional details.)

Shoulders

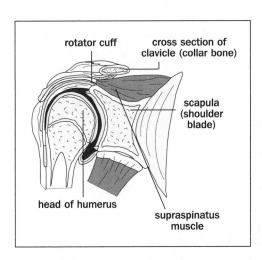

This is a biggie for fifties males, partly because it's such a complicated joint and partly because of a potentially dangerous recipe—you're still relatively active, while your shoulder has been weakened by years of overuse and abuse. The soft tissues (muscles, tendons, and ligaments) are becoming a bit tattered and have a greater chance of injury than ever before.

The shoulder is where the humerus (upper arm bone), the scapula (shoulder blade bone), and the clavicle (collarbone) come together in a ball-and-socket joint that's held together by numerous muscles, ligaments, and tendons. At the end of your upper arm bone is the relatively large ball portion of the joint that fits into the relatively small socket. Because the ball is so big in relation to the socket—like a golf ball is to a tee—your arm has a wide range of motion. This is both good and bad—good because you can do everything from throw a baseball to scratch your own back; bad because such a wide range of motion means there's a greater probability that something will happen to one or more of the component parts, especially as you get older.

The spot that causes the most problems for fifties males is an area within the joint called the rotator cuff. Comprised of four tendons and a bursa, the cuff rotates through a small area that barely has enough room for it. Much of the rotatory motion of the shoulder is handled by this aptly named area.

Common Causes of Shoulder Problems

• Muscle strain or overuse

• Tendinitis (inflammation or overuse of a tendon)

• Bursitis (swelling of the pouch-like covering of joints, called a bursa)

• Bone spur (a small protrusion) within the joint

The first three problems can be caused by taking the shoulder beyond where it wants to be, or working at activities where strength is needed above the shoulder, such as drywalling or painting the ceiling. Bone spurs are brought on by arthritis.

A common denominator for all shoulder ailments is pain, in a variety of forms and kinds. One example is radiating pain, which plagues many fifties males. It's a shooting pain along the back of the shoulder that seems to come and go with various motions or movements. The pain can travel beyond the shoulder to the forearm and into the hand and fingers and can include weakness and numbness along the arm and hand. While radiating pain seems to come from the shoulder, in fact, most times it comes from a herniated (ruptured) disc (see the disc sections in this chapter), neck arthritis (see the neck section in this chapter), or a bone spur in the neck (see the neck section).

Such ambiguity is a common theme in shoulder problems. The specific ailments aren't easily defined, are rarely distinct, and can plague patients in various combinations. Symptoms for different problems can be similar or can overlap so much that a patient simply can't tell the difference between ailments.

All of this makes a doctor's diagnosis a must for any shoulder problem. A physician, aided by a physical exam, X rays, and maybe even an MRI scan, can pinpoint the culprit.

STRAINS, TEARS, AND BONE SPURS

Usually injury or chronic overuse causes strains or tears in a rotator-cuff tendon, while bone spurs (small protrusions) in the shoulder joint are brought on by arthritis and can form at any time. Normally, with all three of these there's no pain when the joint's not in use. When there is pain, the shoulder will be achy, with sharp pain sometimes occurring when extending the arm, such as when putting on your coat, reaching into the back seat for your briefcase, taking your suitcase off the airport carousel, scratching your back, or even, in extreme cases, simply combing your hair. It's a safe bet that if you can't raise your arm above your shoulder, you've probably strained or torn a rotator-cuff tendon, or have a bone spur—only your doctor will be able to tell you which one it is.

Treatment/Prevention—There are several gradations of treatment for a strain: applying heat to the strained area, taking OTC anti-inflammatories for pain and to reduce inflammation, having a doctor inject cortisone into the joint to relieve pain and inflammation, and having physical therapy to slowly rebuild the shoulder's range of motion. If these fail, or if a tear seems likely, the doctor will probably get a scan of the joint using an MRI machine, followed by arthroscopic surgery (using a tiny tubelike device through a small incision) to determine exactly what's wrong. If you have a bone spur, arthroscopic surgery can remove it. Such surgery can also generally clean up the frayed or roughened edges of the joint, which will make the joint feel and work better but does add to its eventual degeneration.

BURSITIS

An inflamed bursa, or bursitis, over the rotator cuff usually comes from a jarring impact, multiple impacts, or intense overuse. The swollen bursa affects the motion of the rotator cuff, causing any shoulder motion to be intensely painful. Additionally, any kind of pressure—such as sleeping on it—can be painful and the pain will increase the longer the pressure is on the shoulder.

Treatment/Prevention. You can apply heat to the affected area and take OTC anti-inflammatories for pain and to reduce inflammation. The doctor could also administer a cortisone injection into the joint to relieve pain and reduce inflammation, and ultimately, if all else fails, could prescribe surgical trimming of the bursa.

TENDINITIS

Strain or injury can bring on tendinitis (inflammation) of the bicipital tendon along the front of the shoulder or along any of the four tendons of the rotator cuff. If you automatically roll over on your back or side at night, and the shoulder pain wakes you up, it's probably tendinitis. Because tendinitis pain is brought on by applying pressure, it feels similar to bursitis pain. Clinically, it can be hard to tell the difference.

TREATING MUSCULOSKELETAL PAIN
(UNDERSTANDING RICE)

Most musculoskeletal problems can be treated "conservatively" (without surgery), and many aches, pains, and strains of muscles, tendons, ligaments, bursae, and joints can be handled by yourself. If you're sure of the cause of the pain (too much weekend yard work, sliding into home plate, tripping while jogging, pushing your exercise routine a little too far, or even too much hunching over a computer screen), you can normally deal with the situation yourself.

Many times, all it takes for relief is the tried and true RICE treatment.

R—for Rest. A couple of days' rest is all that is needed—or wanted. While rest initially kick-starts healing, too much rest (more than two days) can only weaken muscles, create mechanical problems for the spine and joints, and prolong rehabilitation.

I—for Ice. When you apply ice to the affected area, blood vessels become restricted, which retards inflammation, and the numbing that occurs reduces the pain. Later, when the ice is removed, it stimulates the body to automatically re-warm the cold area, which effectively triggers increased blood flow. This means that the injured area gets more than normal amounts of nourishment and several chemical components that act as damage-control agents—all of which speed recovery.

Because of ice's two-fold value, it's the treatment of choice for pain over heat (which only increases the blood flow and aids flexibility).

C—for Compression. Commonly known as pressure, compression can be applied to the injured area usually through the use of a strip of elastic cloth (such as an Ace bandage). This helps to keep swelling under control.

E—for Elevation. Simply putting the hurt area higher than your heart (such as propping up a sore ankle when you're lying down) reduces swelling, which can become so excessive that it slows healing.

Last, but not least, you can take OTC anti-inflammatories to reduce pain and swelling. In worst-case scenarios, the diseased joint can be replaced by an artificial joint, but that is usually considered only if the joint is severely damaged (typically from a major injury).

Treatment/Prevention. You can apply heat to the area, take a couple of days of rest, and take OTC anti-inflammatories for pain and inflammation. If there's no improvement in a few weeks, a doctor might give you a cortisone injection into the affected area to help relieve the pain and reduce the inflammation.

DEGENERATIVE ARTHRITIS

While this can be a contributor to shoulder problems for some men in their fifties, it doesn't normally show itself fully until much later in life, usually the seventies.

Treatment/Prevention. There is no known cure for degenerative arthritis, although the symptoms—most notably pain, stiffness, and swelling—can be lessened with the use of ice or heat on the area, the taking of OTC anti-inflammatories, and light exercise to keep the joint as loose and mobile as possible. In worst-case scenarios, shoulder-joint replacement can be done, but it's usually considered only if the joint is severely damaged (typically from a major injury).

The Chest

Good news here. Within the musculoskeletal realm the chest is not a big problem area at this age. If there is a problem, it usually involves the cartilage and muscles that attach the ribs to the sternum, or breastbone. (See chapter 3 for other chest-related problems.)

Chest Pain

The chest cartilage and muscles can become inflamed and painful when they're strained or torn, but that's normally something that only happens with injury or severe overuse. Such a strain or tear causes pain, sometimes quite localized and severe.

If the pain is from the musculoskeletal system, there's not much to worry about. However, any pain in the chest area should be taken seriously, because it might be signaling a heart attack (see chapter 3 for heart details). If the pain comes only with bending, twisting, directly pushing on the area, or lying down, then it's probably muscle or cartilage pain.

Any other type of chest pain warrants an immediate trip to the doctor.

Treatment/Prevention. A couple of days' rest, use of ice or heat on the affected area, the taking of OTC anti-inflammatories for pain, and possibly getting a physician administered cortisone injection into the painful spot should do it. Limiting activities for at least a week is also a good idea.

The Arms

Known to doctors as the upper extremity, the arm is comprised of the upper arm (humerus), forearm (ulna and radius), and the wrist (carpus). While the arm might seem rather straightforward, it contains complicated and impressive joints (the elbow and wrist), and a tremendously intricate coalition of bones, muscles, tendons, and ligaments in the hand.

Happily, few major problems occur in the arm and its component parts.

Elbows

The largest number of complaints regarding the elbow involve the tendon and ligaments that attach the forearm to the bone of the elbow. To find those, simply grip hard—you can feel the muscle contract where it attaches to the bone; under the muscle are the tendons and ligaments.

TENNIS AND GOLF ELBOW (TENDINITIS)

You don't have to be a tennis player or a golfer to be afflicted with this ailment, associated with sharp and usually localized pain. It can be brought on by anything that includes a power grip, an extended arm, and a twisting motion that rotates the arm at the elbow. Using a hammer or screwdriver or even gardening can bring it on, as can a too-small or too-large tennis racquet handle (which affects your grip). If the soreness is on the upper outside part of the elbow, it's probably tennis elbow; if the pain is on the inside of the joint, it's what many refer to as golf elbow, because it afflicts golfers. Both are forms of tendinitis and both can be so painful that even shaking hands hurts.

Treatment/Prevention. Take OTC anti-inflammatories for pain and inflammation, change the motion that's been causing the pain, limit activity until the pain lessens, and apply ice to the joint after use to reduce pain and control swelling. A tennis elbow strap that compresses the forearm muscle just below the elbow can help with the condition or be used as a preventive measure. The strap works because it changes the angle at which a twisting force hits the tendon fibers, thus spreading out the effect to a greater number of fibers. Another option is to take a lesson from a golf or tennis pro who can show you the correct way to swing—which will probably help your tendinitis and might even improve your score.

BURSITIS

Landing hard on your elbow, continually hitting it, or contracting a severe case of gout can cause inflamation and swelling of the elbow bursa (the pouch covering the joint). Pain can be severe and swelling quite noticeable.

Treatment/Prevention. For injury-related bursitis, it's best, initially, to avoid surgery or other invasive medical procedures. Instead, try restricting movement, applying ice or heat to the joint to reduce inflammation, and taking OTC anti-inflammatories for pain and inflammation. Sometimes it can help to have your doctor use a syringe to draw (aspirate) the fluid from the bursa. In severe cases—where there's recurring injury—the bursa can be removed without much effect on normal functioning.

For gout-related bursitis, treatment includes change of lifestyle and eating habits, as well as the taking of OTC anti-inflammatories for pain and inflammation. (See the gout section in this chapter for details.)

Wrists and Hands

If you're in a situation where you begin to fall down, your body's automatic reaction is to throw out an arm to break the fall or cushion the landing.

That's logical—it's only natural to sacrifice a lowly hand, wrist, or arm for the possible protection of more important body parts, although your hand, wrist, and arm might see things a little differently. Those poor guys take the brunt of most falls. In fact, they end up dealing with so many falls that doctors call the resulting injuries FOOSHs (Fall On Outstretched Hand).

These FOOSHs are the most common source of wrist and hand problems for men in our age group. Next on the scale is probably arthritis, in parts of the hand or wrist. Carpenters, plumbers, and others who use their wrists a lot find their overuse can lead to arthritis. Beyond arthritis is carpal tunnel syndrome, which is the pinching of a nerve in the wrist area that results in pain, tingling, numbness, and/or muscle weakness. Causes can include arthritis and repetitive motions, such as prolonged typing. Carpal tunnel is a frequent cause of work-related disability. It can be prevented by frequent work breaks to stretch the wrists and hands and by close attention to workplace "ergonomics," the physical relationship between people and equipment.

RADIATING PAIN

A type of shooting pain in the upper arm and shoulder (see this chapter's shoulder section), forearm, wrist, or even the fingers can be a common problem. Most often this is brought on by a compressed nerve in the neck due to arthritis or disc disease. The location of the pain can actually pinpoint where the problem is in the neck (see the neck section). The pain can also be caused by an overdeveloped forearm (common in carpenters), where the Popeye-like muscle is causing pressure on a nerve in the forearm.

Treatment/Prevention. Take OTC anti-inflammatories for pain, apply ice and heat to the area to reduce inflammation, and try stretching the muscles around the pinched nerve. A change in activities can also help. For severe cases, surgery may be required to clear the obstruction from the nerve's path.

ARTHRITIS

Wrist arthritis, specifically in the bones of the wrist and at the base of the thumb, is fairly common for men in their fifties, possibly the price we pay for having the opposable thumb. (Finger arthritis is less prevalent in men than in women.) The pain from wrist arthritis can come on like the flicking of a switch—one day your wrist is fine, the next day it hurts in an achy way and it stays with you from then on. While there usually isn't pain when not using the wrist and hand, gripping something or putting pressure on the joint can be painful, as when shaking hands, rolling over in bed, unscrewing a jar, writing, or even in certain sexual positions where you're using your wrists to brace yourself.

Treatment/Prevention. Avoid activities that aggravate or worsen the problem, take OTC anti-inflammatories for pain and inflammation, apply ice or heat to the affected area, and try a stretching and strengthening home physical-therapy program. Little things, like changing to thick-barreled pens with minimal drag, help to alleviate pain while writing. Surgery may help in severe cases.

The Legs

The leg, extending from the hip down to the foot, is not only a thing of beauty when attached to someone we love, but a highly complex support and transportation system for the rest of the body. Involving numerous groups of muscles, tendons and ligaments, the leg also contains the critical hip, knee and ankle joints—some of the most complicated in the entire body.

Hips

A ball and socket joint that's relatively simple in design, the hip joint nonetheless bears some of the greatest stress and strain of any joint. As we stride through our day, putting serious pressure on the joint (especially if we're overweight), we also use the hips as heavy-duty fulcrums for lifting, moving, turning, and twisting.

The Musculoskeletal System

The biggest manifestation of hip problems is pain, pure and simple. It's usually an achy type of soreness, often with weight-bearing movement. Many people, though, think that soreness in the buttocks is caused by hip problems, when, in fact, that pain usually comes from back or disc problems. Hip joint soreness is felt in the crease between your thigh and lower abdomen that forms when you sit, or the pain can also radiate to the front side of the knee.

HIP AREA PAIN

Muscle problems around the hip joints can occur, including hip rotator strain, hernias, and pain in the buttocks, groin, and the hip joint's bursa. If you can't lie on your hip without it hurting, it's probably bursitis. If you have pain in your buttocks, calves, or back of the thighs while walking, but it stops or is relieved by rest, then you might have claudication, a lack of proper blood supply to exercising muscles that's caused by hardening of the arteries (see chapter 3 for artery details).

Treatment/Prevention. Take a couple of days' rest, use heat on the affected area, take OTC anti-inflammatories for pain and inflammation, sometimes a doctor administered cortisone injection into the problem area is needed, and try a stretching and strengthening exercise program.

DEGENERATIVE ARTHRITIS

A major problem for people in their sixties and seventies, degenerative arthritis can initially manifest itself in our age group. Pain and soreness will come with weight-bearing activities, such as jogging or walking, especially on hilly surfaces. Many golfers notice it as they climb in and out of sand traps, scramble through underbrush, or hoof it up and down bunkers.

While a formal diagnosis can't be done without X rays (which would show loss of joint space and/or loss of cartilage), experienced doctors can usually identify the problem in an office visit. The doctor will check for the joint's range of motion, especially rotation (the foot turning with the knee stationary). Diminished range of motion is common in sufferers, although many won't have noticed because it comes on gradually.

Treatment/Prevention. While there is no cure for degenerative arthritis, typical treatments include taking OTC anti-inflammatories for pain, and modifying activity, such as shifting from jogging to non-joint-impact exercises like bicycling or swimming. For severe cases, which mostly appear in older age groups, hip replacement is the most common treatment.

UNDERSTANDING OVER-THE-COUNTER AND PRESCRIPTION PAIN RELIEVERS

The majority of pain medications are NSAIDs (Nonselective Nonsteroidal Anti-Inflammatory Drugs), commonly referred to as anti-inflammatories. NSAIDs work by restraining the two normal processes of inflammation that are called COX-1 and COX-2. COX-1 protects the stomach lining from the stomach's powerful digestive juices; COX-2 brings inflammation chemicals to areas of injury. When NSAIDs are used that do inhibit COX-1, the stomach lining is open to being affected by its own digestive juices—causing, in some cases, stomach upset, gastrointestinal bleeding, and ulcers. NSAIDS can also cause kidney and liver problems when used for an extended period of time.c

While some NSAIDs are still by prescription only, many are now available over-the-counter (OTC). These OTC anti-inflammatories include such drugs as aspirin, ibuprofen (name brands include Advil, Motrin, and Nuprin), and naproxen sodium (brand name Aleve)—all of which inhibit both COX-1 and COX-2. These drugs can be very successful at treating pain, but even though they're OTC drugs they can still affect your stomach and cause kidney damage with extended use.

Acetaminophen (brand name Tylenol) is a painkiller (not an NSAID) that does not cause stomach problems, but it can harm the liver after long-term use or overdose, and can even cause death.

What are safe, maximum daily doses for these drugs?

Check with your own doctor, but generally: aspirin, six to eight 325 mg tablets per day; ibuprofen, 200-400 mg four times per day; naproxen sodium, 200 to 500 mg two times a day; and acetaminophen, under 4000 mg (divided into at least four doses) per day. None should be taken on a daily basis for longer than three months without talking to a doctor. And never take aspirin while taking ibuprofen or Naproxen sodium; although you can take acetaminophen with ibuprofen.

In 1999 a new class of prescription NSAIDs was introduced called COX-2 Inhibitors (brand names Celebrex and Vioxx). Because they restrain only COX-2, not COX-1, they have fewer stomach side effects, but can still cause kidney damage. They are available by prescription only and have been a real godsend to those people whose stomachs couldn't tolerate anti-inflammatories.

Another good new drug that doesn't affect your stomach is meloxicam (brand name Mobic). While not a COX-2 inhibitor, it has been confused for one because it's been marketed as not upsetting your stomach.

The Musculoskeletal System

Calves and Thighs

Because the calves and thighs are used so often—no matter how much we actually exercise—they're generally in better physical shape than other parts of our aging bodies. And they rarely give us many problems beyond strained, pulled, or torn muscles.

The one exception is if you experience pain when walking—especially uphill—that disappears when you stop. While this might simply indicate you're out of shape, it might also be a sign of claudication, a serious blood vessel problem (see chapter 3 for details).

LEG CRAMPS

At some point in our lives, everyone's probably felt that quick tightening of a leg muscle that signifies a cramp. We also know how painful they can be. The number one cause of muscle cramping is dehydration.

Treatment/Prevention. Proper intake of water (six to eight, eight-ounce glasses a day) usually cures the problem. A good stretching program can help prevent nighttime leg cramps.

SHIN SPLINTS

It hasn't been that easy for medicine to figure out what these are, although sufferers certainly feel them. Basically, shin splints are microscopic tears in the muscles and connective tissue of the foot flexors, which are the muscles that run down the front of the leg between the knee and ankle. Injuries come from overuse, from pushing off, from running on a hard surface, and from running more than your body is ready for. They can also develop from a too-rapid increase in the intensity and/or duration of your exercise program.

Treatment/Prevention. Change what you're doing that's caused the problem, rest for a couple of days, take OTC anti-inflammatories for pain, and apply heat to the affected area. As far as prevention is concerned, you should remember not to try to squeeze too much mileage out of your sneakers, whether it be on the tennis court, jogging track, or basketball court. Athletic shoes actually break down internally quicker than the tread wears out, thus leaving the wearer open to injury because of nonsupportive shoes. Even mall walkers should be watchful of this situation. Running shoes are usually good for 300 to 400 miles before needing replacement and are often better for walking than so-called "walking" shoes (better cushioning, better support, and more padding around the Achilles tendon).

HAMSTRINGS

Starting in the back of the buttocks, the hamstring is actually a group of muscles that attaches to the bone you sit on, extends down the back of the legs, and fastens in several places behind the knee. Your two hamstrings provide much of the propulsion for running, walking, and climbing.

Many sprinters get a pulled, strained, or torn hamstring as they suddenly extend it beyond its normal range. If the hamstring is not ready for a sudden movement or a quick acceleration beyond its normal limits, it can be strained or torn. Both situations cause pain and a feeling of tightness in the lower buttock area. Hamstring tightness not only limits your walking ability (you'll be hobbling around for a few weeks if it's torn or severely strained), but can also aggravate a lower back problem.

More and more men find that their hamstrings aren't as forgiving as they were during their teenage years. An important point to remember is that your fifties is no time to be sprinting—whether it be darting across a busy street or dashing around the bases at the company softball game—unless properly warmed up first.

Treatment/Prevention. Rest for a couple of days, take OTC anti-inflammatories for pain, apply heat to the affected area, and sometimes compression (a pressure bandage) to help prevent re-injury by keeping you from taking the hamstring too far again is needed. Critical to prevention is a good stretching program, because a tight muscle is a weak muscle, more prone to being strained or torn than a properly stretched one.

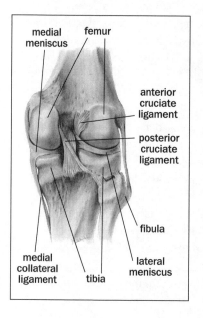

medial meniscus
femur
anterior cruciate ligament
posterior cruciate ligament
fibula
medial collateral ligament
tibia
lateral meniscus

Knees

The knees are somewhat unique in the musculoskeletal realm because in the fifties they can exhibit all three of the common causes of pain:

• **Injury**

• **Chronic overuse**

• **Degeneration**

For men in their fifties, the elbow sees more overuse, the wrist more degeneration, the shoulder more overuse and injury, and the lower back more injury and degeneration—but the knee gets all three, and in about equal measure.

The Musculoskeletal System

Like the hips, the knees are weight-bearing joints that take an incredible pounding. It's no wonder hips and knees are the two most commonly replaced joints in the body. Although knee replacement doesn't normally happen to men in their fifties (it's more likely when they're in their sixties and seventies), physicians are starting to see more and more problems with these joints in our age group.

Common sense says it's either because of past injuries, accidents, or overuse (not much you can do about those now), or because men are trying to maintain the same level of activity they once enjoyed without preparing their aging bodies. Basically, you're staying as active as you were in your twenties, while your knee joints are thirty years older. Here's when you can significantly help your knees by properly warming them up and stretching them before putting them through their paces.

If we leave out major injuries such as big falls, cuts, or large-caliber bullet wounds, most knee injuries befalling men in their fifties come from twisting falls or quick-impact sports accidents. These are generally called soft-tissue injuries, meaning the nonbony part of the knee has been hurt.

The various knee tears outlined below are classified by varying degrees of severity: one through four, with four being a complete tear. They're all treated with less medically invasive procedures today than they were only a few years ago. Many can be treated without surgery. Those requiring surgery can usually be done arthroscopically (a tiny tubelike device is inserted through a small incision), which is less invasive to the joint and leads to shorter recovery times.

One of the best ways to help your knee is to strengthen the muscle groups, tendons, and ligaments that surround and support the knee. This is especially true of the quadriceps, the four-part muscle group that makes up the muscular front of the thigh. While this muscle group is responsible for extending the knee, it also keeps the knee from wobbling. Most people don't realize activities like hiking and running do little to improve these muscles.

How to Strengthen Your Leg's Quadricep Muscles

• Bicycling

• Certain kinds of weight lifting with your knee

• Half-squats

• Wall sits (See chapter 8 for exercise details.)

THE MENISCUS

Helping sideways stability of the knee are two wedge-shaped pieces of cartilage called menisci that sit between the thigh bone and the shin bone. One is medial (on the inside of the knee) and the other is lateral (on the outside). Either can be torn when you get a hit from the side or a twisting kind of blow or fall. The tear causes pain, sometimes sharp, and sometimes instability of the knee, but you can usually still walk. Occasionally, "locking" of the knee in one position can occur if the torn fragment of the meniscus becomes lodged in the joint itself. Swelling within a day or two can be fairly significant, surrounding the entire knee. Because the pain and swelling can be acute—sufferers will be limping around and hurting—most will go see their doctor. If the situation improves in two weeks, then it probably was not a torn meniscus, but rather a strain. Early on, it's hard to distinguish between the two, because both create similar pain and swelling.

Treatment/Prevention. In the case of a strain, treatment includes taking OTC anti-inflammatories for pain and inflammation, and decreasing activity until the pain allows for the start of a flexibility and re-strengthening exercise program. In the case of a tear, surgery is warranted, and it's a relatively easy procedure with an arthroscope. Rehabilitation and recovery time is minimal—you'll be back to doing normal things within two to four weeks. A good knee brace, used judiciously (so the knee doesn't get weaker by relying on the brace), can go a long way toward preventing an injury or re-injury.

THE MCL AND LCL LIGAMENTS

These two ligaments (the medial collateral and lateral collateral) help attach the thigh bone to the lower leg, with the medial on the inside of the leg and the lateral on the outside. This gives the knee its sideways stability. A blow from the side or a twisting movement will damage these ligaments—especially in active men who are taking their joints and muscles beyond where they want to go. When a tear occurs, it usually means immediate and fairly severe pain, to the point where the knee doesn't feel secure when you try to walk on it.

If You Tear an MCL Or LCL Ligament

• You're not going to ski down the rest of the slope; you'll be riding in the ski patrol sled.

• The knee will still hurt when not in use, like a toothache.

• If you move it, it's really going to hurt.

• Swelling will be quick and involves fluid or blood in the knee joint.

• You'll want to get to the doctor right away.

The Musculoskeletal System

Treatment/Prevention. For less severe injuries, treatment may include some modified immobilization with a Velcro knee immobilizer, maybe crutches for a while, and taking the usual OTC anti-inflammatories for pain and swelling. Years ago, people who had torn the ligament completely were placed in a major cast that kept the knee immobilized to help the ligament heal. Unfortunately, a negative side effect was that surrounding muscles critical to knee stabilization wasted away, making overall recovery time much longer. Today, after surgery for the more severe cases, the treatment is about the same as with less severe injuries, but also includes prescribed physical therapy to keep the muscles strong so they do their part to shrink recovery time.

THE ACL AND PCL LIGAMENTS

If you hear someone's "blown" their knee, it usually means they've torn one of these ligaments (the anterior cruciate and posterior cruciate ligaments), which crisscross under the knee cap, attach the thigh to the lower leg, and give the joint its front, back, and rotatory stability.

An ACL injury is the most common and usually happens with a slipping-backward kind of slow twisting motion. Snow and water skiers who lose their balance backward and try to recover can injure these ligaments. You can even do it falling backward off a stool. The less common PCL injury usually occurs when landing hard on the knee—that's why it's a particular ailment of long jumpers. Both come with lots of knee instability and a fair amount of swelling.

Treatment/Prevention. Not long ago, there wasn't a good technique for repairing ACL and PCL ligaments, but that wasn't too bad, because repairing either of them wasn't really required for nonactive people. Athletes—professional or weekend—usually need the ligaments repaired, although retired football quarterback John Elway, who won two Super Bowls, did respectably well despite missing one since high school. Because the knee's unstable without an ACL, those who don't have them need to use an antirotation brace to protect the knee.

With the advent of arthroscopy, there is now a way of transplanting a piece of another tendon to replace the ligament—most commonly the ACL. Such surgery is followed by extensive rehabilitation that can take from six to twelve months.

TENDINITIS

Overuse of the knee is what causes tendinitis. It can occur in the tendons on both sides of the knee (although almost always to the lateral, or outside, tendon), as well as in the tendon directly in front of the knee (the thick cord that attaches the knee to the shin). Front tendon problems are more likely to occur with a shock or jarring impact.

Causes of Knee Tendinitis

• Kneeling on hard surfaces for long periods of time.

• Stepping up one's running schedule without proper stretching and strengthening.

• Running on an uneven surface—such as a severely banked indoor track—or on a small-diameter track.

Treatment/Prevention. Stretching the tendon properly, applying heat to the affected area, changing the activity that created the tendinitis, taking OTC anti-inflammatories for pain, and possibly a doctor administered cortisone injection into the injured tendon will usually do the trick. If the tendinitis has been caused by running on a banked or small-diameter running track, reversing direction periodically will help prevent the problem. Tendinitis is definitely an ailment that initially can be treated at home. If, however, the tendon doesn't seem to improve in two to four weeks, go see your doctor.

BURSITIS

Also an overuse problem, bursitis is seen in people constantly working on their knees, such as carpet layers or gardeners. Others who can get it include the weekend warrior doing a job that continually impacts his knees in ways he's not used to. The pain will be sharp and easily localized, and the swelling over the kneecap may be associated with redness.

Treatment/Prevention. Try a couple of days of rest, taking OTC anti-inflammatories for pain and swelling, applying heat to the affected area, avoiding re-injury. Very rarely, a doctor administered cortisone injection into the bursa is needed.

DEGENERATIVE ARTHRITIS

Also known as osteoarthritis (OA) or degenerative joint disease (DJD), degenerative arthritis is the wearing away of cartilage so that it doesn't replace itself. In part it's related to:

• Age

• Obesity

The Musculoskeletal System

• Overuse

• Underuse

• What the joint does and how it does it

• Injury or surgery, which can mean a greater chance of getting it later in life

How do we tell the difference between degenerative arthritis and overuse?

Overuse is more acute than degenerative arthritis, tends to be activity related, and can be cured.

Degenerative arthritis is chronic and progressive and we don't have any drugs that arrest the course of it. A tremendously disabling disease, it has no known cure. While its ravaging effects aren't usually seen in men until they've reached their sixties or seventies, men in their fifties can experience the first symptoms. Those include pain, stiffness in the morning, and sometimes swelling. Pain is of the toothachy kind and is hard to pinpoint—it feels like it's in the center of the knee. The pain will also be there when the joint is not in use and will increase with weight bearing and going up and down hills or stairs. Inflammation, which appears to be a symptom, not a cause, of the disease, may or may not be significant.

While both doctors and patients can suspect degenerative arthritis—and usually they're right—the only way to make a definitive diagnosis is with X rays.

Treatment/Prevention. Changing the activity that created the problem, taking OTC anti-inflammatories for pain, and use of heat on the affected area are sometimes helpful. Wherever possible, avoid repeated stress or impact to the knee. Strengthening and stretching of the soft tissues around the knee are important, because they'll help stabilize the knee and probably reduce pain. In severe cases, you may not be able to walk, you may not be able to run very much, but you can do other things—like bicycling, swimming, pool walking, and strengthening exercises. Weight loss can also help by reducing pressure on the knee.

A stop-gap measure—a way of buying time in a worn-out joint to postpone the inevitable knee replacement—is to have a "debridement" through arthroscopic surgery (a tiny tubelike device inserted through a small incision). This procedure removes loose pieces of cartilage or bone that shouldn't be there, although by doing so the surgeon may also create more damage.

If your cartilage is truly gone, there is a synthetic lubricant, Synvisc. It's a thick fluid that's poorly absorbed by the body so it stays in the joint for a while and provides lubrication. Simply injected into the joint, Synvisc doesn't cure anything, but it sometimes gives temporary relief.

Unfortunately, it's also expensive, and insurance companies may not cover it.

Cortisone injections (by a doctor) into the joint can also reduce arthritic knee pain.

The ultimate treatment for degenerative arthritis of the knee is knee replacement surgery.

UNDERSTANDING CORTISONE INJECTIONS

One treatment of last resort for musculoskeletal problems—especially for inflammation that won't go away—is an injection of cortisone directly into the affected joint, muscle, tendon, or ligament. While the shot itself can be quite painful, the results can be quick and dramatic—the inflammation will subside and the pain will diminish rapidly. This will allow the patient to begin, or resume, exercise programs that aid in recuperation and recovery.

So why is cortisone used sparingly?

Doctors are reluctant to prescribe it because cortisone is a part of the corticosteroid family of hormones that can have numerous side effects. When used locally, as with an injection into a tendon, cortisone side effects can include:

- Increased susceptibility to infection

- Weakening of the tendon

- Acceleration of cartilage deterioration

Outside of the musculoskeletal arena, when cortisone is used systemically (in the whole body)—as with pills, intravenously, or by an injection into the patient's rear end—side effects (other than a sore butt) include increased susceptibility to infection, fluid retention, peptic ulcers, emotional changes, raised blood pressure, and acceleration of osteoporosis.

The Ankles

Think about standing in place and maneuvering 200 pounds through a wide arc of movement—all at lightening speed and with complete fluidity.

That's what your ankles (if you weigh 200 pounds) do every day. A pretty incredible feat (pun intended). With such a job to do—day in, day out for seventy plus years—it's no wonder that the ankle is an extremely complicated joint, and so far no mechanical device has yet been devised that can mimic what it does.

Even though the ankle is complicated, it doesn't usually have major break-downs. For our age group the biggest concern is injury, notably ankle sprains and fractures. In older age groups the threat of degenerative arthritis to the ankle is very real, especially if there has been previous injury.

When You Should Seek Help for An Ankle Injury

- If you can't walk on it or bear weight

- If there's excessive swelling

- If you tap on the ankle bone, and it's very painful—which indicates it might be broken

SPRAINS

The most common ankle ailment for men in our age group is a sprain, and it can happen nearly any time or place, especially if you're out of shape. Step off a curb wrong, or miss a step—a quick snap here, a fast fold there—and you'll be hobbling for at least a week.

Strictly speaking, a sprain is the tearing of ligament fibers from a mechanical distortion, typically an inversion of the foot where the ankle buckles to the outside and the foot flips up inside. This stretches and puts all the pressure on the outside of the ankle joint. Swelling and pain are the quick results.

Sprains exist in four grades, one is barely an injury, while four leaves the ankle so unstable that it often requires surgery. Ironically, a four may not hurt as much as a one, because a torn ligament (a four) doesn't usually have as much bleeding and swelling as a sprain (a one). Re-sprains hurt a lot, but you get over them fairly quickly.

Treatment/Prevention. If it's a mild to moderate strain, follow RICE (take a couple of days' rest, apply ice and compression, and elevate the ankle—see the RICE sidebar in this chapter for greater detail). Walk as soon as it's reasonably comfortable to do so. Take OTC anti-inflammatories for pain and to reduce inflammation. With most mild to moderate sprains you'll usually be back to walking within a few days and maybe back to your sport or your previous activity within a week or two. Biking, with movements that are low impact and easy on joints, can be done almost right away.

More severe sprains will feel better with immobilization, often with an air cast (a flexible plastic sleeve inflated to the desired pressure). A severe sprain may continue to hurt and swell for up to a year.

Ankle rehab at home will help you recover from your injury or avoid the next by strengthening and providing flexibility for the foot muscles.

Five Good Ankle Exercises

1. **Pick up marbles with your toes,** which stretches the intrinsic muscles of the foot.

2. **With your heel stationary, pull a towel toward you with your toes,** basically using your foot as a claw. If you weigh the towel down with a book it gives the muscles a better workout.

3. **While standing up, put your toes on the edge of a stair step and gently go down with the heel to below where the toes are.** Brace yourself and go up and down, up and down.

4. **Sit down, stretch out your leg, hook a towel around your toes, then push your toes down, sideways, and back.**

WHAT'S WITH SWELLING?— UNDERSTANDING INFLAMMATION

Many men are horrified when a part of their body becomes inflamed or swells up after an insignificant injury, cut or scrape. In most cases, they shouldn't be.

Inflammation is a tissue response to irritation or injury, characterized by pain, swelling, redness, and heat. It's the process by which healing begins—white blood cells and a cascade of chemicals rush to the area and stimulate such important processes as clotting and tissue repair. This is how fractures rebind, skin reseals, tendons reattach, and infections are fought off.

The degree of swelling is based on how much blood is available. Cartilage, which receives little blood, won't swell up as much as a muscle or ligament, which receives more.

So why does swelling have to be so painful?

That, too, is good. Pain ensures the person won't use, or abuse, the affected area.

But if swelling is so good, why apply ice to retard it?

Sometimes the body overreacts with unnecessary excessive swelling, so ice and/or heat, OTC anti-inflammatories, and sometimes compression are used to lessen the inflammation. (See the RICE sidebar in this chapter for other details.)

5. Write your name on the floor with your big toe.

FRACTURES

Fractures of the ankle are not as common as sprains. Depending on the severity, immobilization may be required as well as surgical placement of internal screws and plates to stabilize the ankle. Once the ankle has returned to full strength, the hardware can usually be removed.

Treatment/Prevention. A displaced fracture (an obvious deformity of the foot or ankle) requires prompt orthopedic attention, often involving surgery. A non-displaced fracture requires immobilization, usually with a splint until the swelling subsides, later with a cast for up to six weeks.

The Feet

Think about how many times your feet hit the floor every day; how many times they cushion you from shocks, falls, and sudden missteps. They take a tremendous beating throughout your life. It's no wonder, then, that nearly every guy in his sixth decade has feet that hurt in some way or another, whether it's their toes, arches, heels, or soles.

A critical element for proper foot care is picking the right shoes.

General Guidelines for Picking Shoes

- The instep must be wide enough

- There should be a thumb space between your big toe and the end of the shoe

- The ball of your foot should be at the widest part of the shoe

- Your heel should never be able to slip out of its proper place

- If need be, go with a shoe that's a little too large rather than one that's too small

- Fit shoes to your larger foot (yes, your feet probably aren't the same size). If one foot has a bunion, accommodate the bunion.

• Have enough room in the toe box to allow descent—such as walking, running, or skiing— without your nails bumping up against the front of the shoe

• Try on shoes at the end of the day, when your feet are largest

• Uncomfortable shoes in the store will stay that way, even with "breaking in"

If you know you're going to overuse your feet—let's say you're taking a backpacking trip where you'll carry a lot of weight on your back—you should consider adding padded insoles to your shoes.

Added socks also help. The best combination is a polypropylene inner sock (so your feet can sweat and "breathe" properly) and an outer sock of wool (a good, resilient material).

Foot health also means skin health, including blister prevention. Generally, you need to keep your feet dry, wear the correct socks and properly fitted shoes. A good way of keeping your feet dry—while also solving the problem of foot odor—is to spray an aluminum-containing anti-perspirant directly on your feet. It will help keep your feet dry, which can prevent chafing.

While dry feet are important, overly dry feet can cause skin breakdown or cracking as well. Regular use of moisturizers on your feet can solve that problem.

ACHILLES TENDINITIS

An inflammation of the famous tendon at the back of the heel, this condition usually strikes runners or serious walkers and is brought on by one of the three components of overuse: change in activity, change in the individual, or change in footgear. Remember, footgear should match the activity.

Treatment/Prevention. Apply heat, try stretching, take OTC anti-inflammatories for pain, and sometimes a doctor will recommend immobilizing the tendon with a rigid or flexible orthopedic device to give the tendon a chance to heal. Never, or almost never, are cortisone injections prescribed, because there's a chance they could weaken the tendon. If a weak tendon ruptures, there's usually no alternative but surgery.

ARCHES

Your arches are made up of connective tissue that holds the foot in its bowstring-like configuration. Their primary purpose is to cushion the foot bones. When you have fallen arches, it means that the connective tissue has lost its strength. The condition usually happens over a period of time and is thought to be familial (inherited). The pain associated with fallen arches can be moderate to severe and is localized to the bottom of your foot.

Treatment/Prevention. You probably can't prevent fallen arches, although you can provide external support. A good place for most people to start is to experiment themselves. Buy over-the-counter shoe inserts and see if they give enough support to keep your feet from hurting. If they don't, you'll probably need to see a podiatrist for a custom fitting.

ATHLETE'S FOOT

Who among us males hasn't had athlete's foot? It would be a surprise if more than a handful said they hadn't. The condition usually starts between the toes with a fungus that can later be replaced by bacteria.

Treatment/Prevention. The scourge of active men everywhere, athlete's foot can now be treated very effectively with nonprescription antifungal preparations. They work well. While those little tubes of cream are somewhat expensive, remember that if you can get any over-the-counter drug that actually does something, it's probably worth a premium.

BUNIONS

A kind of deformity of the big toe joint, a bunion is a bony protrusion of the outside of the joint. Probable causes include congenital predisposition and wear and tear. Bunion pain is right in the joint and usually hurts with use.

Treatment/Prevention. Apply heat to the affected area, take OTC anti-inflammatories for pain, do foot massages, and use proper foot wear. Surgery is a last resort option (more often required in women than in men). You should try to get by without surgery for as long as possible—surgery is done too often and the results can vary greatly. Unfortunately, there's not much that can be done for those who have had surgery and are still having problems.

DEGENERATIVE ARTHRITIS

The first real signs and symptoms of arthritis of the feet are common in fifties males, most notably in the big toe joint. The pain is similar to other arthritis pain, dull and achy and aggravated by use.

Treatment/Prevention. Take OTC anti-inflammatories for pain, use heat on the affected area, and make sure your shoes have an adequate toe box and cushioning. Sturdy shoes with relatively stiff soles can help. Surgery (joint replacement) is sometimes required.

GOUT

Many people think gout went the way of sixteenth-century French royalty who endured the painful ailment while resting silk-stockinged legs on satin pillows. While pampered aristocrats are now hard to find, gout is still very much with us, striking more and more men in their fifth decade.

Gout Risk Factors

• **Being male**—gout affects ten times more men than women.

• **Family history**—probably the largest factor.

• **Too much alcohol and protein-rich foods**—which allows uric acid to accumulate in certain body parts.

If you have all these risk factors, you might as well dust off the satin pillow; you're probably going to get gout sometime after forty.

Scientifically speaking, gout occurs when uric acid, a byproduct of protein metabolism, accumulates in the blood and joints—most notably the big toe and the elbow. In certain situations—such as too high a concentration in the blood or very slight blood cooling that can take place in a joint distant from the center of the body—the uric acid transforms from a liquid into crystals, much like dissolved salt or sugar can crystalize. Inflammation and pain can be so severe that even a thin bed sheet on the affected joint can cause trouble. Gout's long-term effects can include joint destruction and kidney stones.

Treatment/Prevention. An acute attack or flare up is usually treated by taking OTC anti-inflammatories for pain, which are quite effective. In severe cases, the very strong pain-and-inflammation prescription drug indomethacin (Indocin) can be used for short periods of time, although possible side effects limit long-term use. For long-term use, there are drugs that maintain reduced levels of uric acid, but sufferers should consider lifestyle changes such as losing weight, cutting down on alcohol consumption, and reducing the intake of protein-rich foods (most notably game and organ meat, and shellfish).

The Musculoskeletal System

MORTON'S NEUROMA

A traumatic growth of the nerves between the second and third, and third and fourth toes, Morton's is fairly common in runners or in people with arthritis in their feet. The condition is tender and painful—it feels like someone put a toothpick in there and is rolling it around. There's no particular age predisposition; anyone can get it.

Treatment/Prevention. Proper footgear and padding the area to avoid squeezing the ball of the foot usually does the trick. If that doesn't work, surgery is the final option.

PLANTAR FASCIITIS

Common among fifties men, this is a condition where the connective tissue that holds the arch, particularly where it connects to the heel bone, is strained or torn. The pain can be severe and feel like a stone bruise. It's especially painful just when you get out of bed, but once you get a little flexibility going, it doesn't hurt as much. It's usually associated with walking and running and caused by one of the three components of overuse. Some people find it happens when they suddenly go from wearing shoes to walking barefoot on a beach.

Treatment/Prevention. OTC anti-inflammatories for pain, application of ice to the area, massage, stretching of the foot via the exercises mentioned earlier, padding the foot, and possible doctor administered cortisone injections can all help.

PLANTAR WARTS

Their name is worse than the problem. These are simply warts that appear on the bottom (plantar) surface of your feet. Our age group is just as prone to getting them as anyone else. The warts themselves don't cause pain, but the calluses that build up over the warts can really hurt. Such a situation can feel like pebbles in your shoe.

Treatment/Prevention. There are a variety of remedies, including acid plasters, liquid nitrogen, and lasers to erode or burn off the warts. Care must be taken so a scar isn't left behind; the scar might get a callus that will cause pain of its own.

It should be mentioned that, given enough time, warts do go away spontaneously. People don't have warts for their entire lives; they do disappear. So temper the urge to do something quickly with the knowledge that they're not permanent.

TOENAILS

Two basic problems are ingrown nails, which can be very painful, and toenail fungus, where a fungus invades the nail bed and nail, turning it dark and ugly.

Treatment/Prevention. For ingrown nails, you can sometimes nudge the skin back over the growing nail or put a small wad of cotton between the skin and nail edge to avoid the problem. With a full-blown ingrown nail, a little outpatient snipping and clipping by the physician might be necessary. Prevention is to always trim your nails straight across, not in a curve.

Toenail fungus used to be almost untreatable, because we didn't have safe drugs that could penetrate into the nail and nail bed to reach the reservoir of fungal organisms. Now, there are two prescription drugs that are effective: Sporonox and Lamisil. Unfortunately, they have three- to six-month treatment times and are expensive. Because the fungus is mostly a cosmetic concern, not a functional problem, it's your choice as to whether or not you want to go through the treatment.

REAL LIFE TALES

Number One: Exercise—Who's Got the Time?

Bill is a sales representative who works hard and is constantly on the go. He finds it difficult to make time for exercise and rarely thinks a lot about what he's grabbing for a meal. He's overweight by 10 to 15 pounds and is battling elevated cholesterol and blood pressure. In terms of physical condition, he's probably a five or six out of ten.

Shortly after his fiftieth birthday, Bill started getting lower back pains. Most times they were a kind of dull ache, but sometimes they got pretty bad. There were some mornings he'd wake up hurting worse than when he went to sleep. He hoped the pain would go away, but it didn't, so after a few weeks he went to see a doctor. He was told to take it easy for a while, take ibuprofen (an anti-inflammatory) for pain, apply heat and ice to the painful areas at the end of the day, and do some exercises to strengthen the back muscles. He did a few things—especially taking the ibuprofen—but he kept thinking that with his busy schedule he didn't have the time to do anything else.

When the pain still didn't go away, the next option was physical therapy. Bill was shown what exercises to do that might alleviate the pain. He did them for a few days, but most times he forgot. With his lower back still hurting, he was given an MRI scan of his back. The test found that Bill had the beginnings of degenerative arthritis of the back and degenerative disc disease, both of which were putting pressure on some of his spinal nerves, causing the pain.

The Musculoskeletal System

Surgery was getting to be a real option. As a last result before that, though, the doctor suggested Bill see an anesthesiologist for a cortisone shot into the affected area. That would temporarily relieve the pain so he could start exercising, which might give some relief. Once again, though, Bill just didn't find the time to make the appointment.

This was partially because as a volunteer for the Boy Scouts, Bill left home to attend a summer camp in New Mexico. During his stay there, he had to participate in a two-week, ninety-mile wilderness trek. The first few days of the hike were everything he had expected—constant pain so bad he could hardly sleep. After a while, though, as he got into better shape and shed some weight, the pain started going away. By the end of the trip, Bill had not only lost thirteen pounds, but the lower back pain as well.

When he returned home, a checkup revealed that there was nothing wrong with him and that he was probably now a seven or eight on the fitness scale. Bill's newly strengthened and stretched back muscles were giving the spine good enough support that the nerves were no longer being pinched. Bill was warned, though, that he needed to find some kind of physical outlet to help him stay in good shape, or the weight—and the pain—would come back.

Bill likes how he feels and how he looks now, and vows to stay in shape, but there's a little voice still inside his head that's whispering: "Who's got the time?"

Number Two: A Correct Diagnosis Requires All the Information

As a fifty-six-year-old who's relatively fit, Sam tries to eat right, exercises a bit, and is justifiably proud that eight years ago he kicked a two-pack-a-day, thirty-year smoking habit.

He's also a service technician, who's constantly getting in and out of his car, going up and down stairs, and carrying his tools wherever the job takes him. Sam knows his feet take a beating every day, so he wasn't too surprised when one of his heels started hurting. Probably just a strain, he thought. The pain was pretty bad when he got out of bed in the morning, then faded a little after he walked around for a while. But it never fully went away, and every morning it was as intense as the day before. After a few weeks of suffering, he went to a doctor.

He was assigned an intern (a newly graduated physician supervised by an experienced doctor), who asked lots of questions—some of which Sam didn't think had anything to do with his feet. Nevertheless, the diagnosis was that Sam had plantar fasciitis, or sore heel, where the muscles of the arch that attach to the heel have been strained or torn. He was given an anti-inflammatory (ibuprofen) for the pain, shown some foot exercises, and told that rest and strengthening would probably take care of the problem.

A few weeks later, though, the pain was still there and Sam went back to see the same intern. This time, after more seemingly irrelevant questions, Sam admitted he hadn't had an erection in a few years. The intern didn't seem to think this was important and told Sam to continue taking the anti-inflammatories and doing the exercises.

On a third visit, with the prodding of more questions, Sam remembered that the pain didn't just stay in his heel but sometimes traveled up into his calf, especially when walking up hill. The calf pain would disappear as soon as he stopped walking.

The intern got excited and told him it could be claudication, which means insufficient blood flow to the legs and feet, due, in most cases, to blocked arteries. It's a condition that smokers get, even after they've stopped smoking. If it was claudication, then the pulses in Sam's feet should be barely perceptible, if at all. In Sam's case, however, the foot pulses were fine; the intern was stumped, and Sam was definitely getting frustrated.

The intern then called in his supervisor, who questioned Sam extensively. Sam still couldn't understand why the doctors needed to know so much, but answered all the questions truthfully and even admitted again to a lack of erections. The supervising doctor told him that the lack of erections all but proved his problem was claudication—lack of erections in this case shows that blood flow is restricted. As for Sam's good foot pulses, they were, in this case, a red herring.

After Sam visited a vascular surgeon, claudication was confirmed. He was told that with any luck the pain in his legs—and his lack of erections—could be taken care of through surgery (which it was).

Today, Sam is a happier, healthier man—and ready to answer any doctor's questions, no matter how irrelevant they might seem.

Number Three: Good Pre-Habilitation Means Quicker Rehabilitation

As a high school physical education teacher, Peter is in excellent physical condition. He does not look or act like an average fifty-six-year-old. He's also tough and stoic, rarely complaining about pain or other problems—preferring to work them out on his own through exercise programs he develops himself.

Quite suddenly, Peter developed shoulder pain. At first he thought it was just a strain from an overly zealous workout. But the pain also brought with it numbness and the sensation of pins and needles all up and down his arm. At times, it felt as if his arm was dead, lacking in any strength or feeling. The weakness in his arm seemed to progress as every day passed. After three weeks of trying to exercise through the problem, he finally gave up and went to a doctor.

Because of Peter's superb conditioning, the rather dramatic localization of symptoms, and the quick onset of weakness in the arm, he received a full work up faster than most people do. This included an MRI scan of his neck and a visit to a neurosurgeon.

Peter was surprised to find that the problem didn't stem from the shoulder—where the pain had started—but from a ruptured disc in his neck. There was no pain right at the ruptured disc, but the rupture was putting pressure on nerves, which, in turn, caused the problems in his shoulder and arm. He was told that because of the rapidly progressing arm weakness and the fact that he hadn't responded to nonsurgical treatments (his exercising), he needed surgery at once.

Ten days after successful surgery, Peter told his doctor and surgeon that he was off on his annual survival trip into the mountains with just a map, compass, and a few essentials. Both physicians told him he shouldn't go, but for Peter the trip was an important psychological journey. He went and everything turned out okay.

Later, during a routine checkup, Peter had questions about what had caused the disc to rupture in the first place. He was assured that in some cases, no matter what a person does, things do go wrong—and, in his case, that no matter what he did, surgery was necessary to resolve the problem. The good news, though, was that his excellent physical conditioning before surgery (called pre-habilitation) had ensured a quicker rehabilitation.

KNOWING WHAT YOU PUT IN YOUR MOUTH— A DRUG CHART

NAME	EXPLANATION AND USE	POSSIBLE SIDE EFFECTS
NSAIDS[a]		
Aspirin[b]	Previously for mild inflammation and pain. Was once the mainstay of treating rheumatoid arthritis. Now more for prevention of inappropriate blood clotting (heart attack, stroke prevention) for which it's effective in remarkably low doses.	Ulcers, kidney damage, hearing loss.
Acetaminophen (Tylenol)	Useful as a minor pain reliever with no anti-inflammatory effects. Not likely to adversely affect the stomach. Often combined with narcotic pain relievers such as codeine and its derivatives.	Very toxic to the liver in high doses (such as over-doses). Can cause death.

NAME	EXPLANATION AND USE	POSSIBLE SIDE EFFECTS
NSAIDS[a]		
Phenylbutazone (Butazolidine)	One of the strongest for pain and inflammation available, but seldom used because of side effects.	Ulcers, bone marrow suppression.
Indomethacin (Indocin)	One of the strongest for pain and inflammation available. Good for acute gout, arthritis, and migraines. Not used as much anymore for long periods or time (has been replaced by less toxic drugs). Still very useful because of its strength for episodic pain relief that involves inflammation.	Ulcers, headaches, kidney damage.
Ibuprofen (Motrin, Advil, Nuprin, etc.)	Most commonly used of NSAIDs. For minor pain, irritation, inflammation. Good benefit to risk ratio. Much less toxic than Indocin, so safe enough to be sold over the counter.	Ulcers, kidney damage.
Naproxen (Naprosyn, Aleve, etc.)	Longer acting than ibuprofen, so doses less frequently. Safe enough to be sold over the counter and used for long periods.	Ulcers, kidney damage.
Meloxicam (Mobic)	This newest of the NSAIDs is by prescription only. Longer lasting than most (once daily dose). Reputed to be more "stomach friendly" than its fellow NSAIDs.	Ulcers, kidney damage.

NAME	EXPLANATION AND USE	POSSIBLE SIDE EFFECTS
COX-2 INHIBITORS[c]		
Celecoxib (Celebrex)	May be more effective with relieving pain and reducing inflammation with fewer gastric side effects.	Kidney damage.
Rofecoxib (Vioxx)	May be more effective with relieving pain and reducing inflammation with fewer gastric side effects.	Kidney damage.

Note: By no means is this a complete listing of all available drugs. It does, however, contain the most likely drugs you'll encounter, with a few other drugs mentioned for historical perspective.

a. Nonselective Nonsteroidal Anti-Inflammatory Drugs—which inhibit both phases of inflammation (COX 1 and COX 2). COX 1 helps to protect the stomach lining, so that's why NSAIDs can cause stomach upset and ulcers.

b. Never used for anyone under 18.

c. New class of NSAIDs that are more selective than the older drugs, because they only inhibit one phase of inflammation (COX-2), not the other (COX-1). Because of this, they less commonly cause stomach upset or ulcers.

THE GOOD NEWS

• The musculoskeletal system is the key to general health. Overall health is, in large part, due to how physically fit you are, which is dictated by how well you exercise, which is dependent on the fitness of your musculoskeletal system. We can improve our heart output by 10 to 20 percent, and our wind (oxygen use) by 30 to 40 percent, but our musculoskeletal system has the capability of being improved by triple digits—especially in the fifties decade.

• You can slow the loss of muscle mass that begins in your thirties and build greater strength and stretchability with a well-planned exercise program.

- Muscle health improves with exercise and so can the more inert structures—bones, tendons, ligaments, cartilage—which can then handle greater pressure, stress, and tension.

- Inflammation is normally a good thing—it's the process by which the affected tissues draw to themselves all the forces necessary to begin healing.

- The effects of degenerative arthritis (which has no known cure) can be lessened by stretching and strengthening the muscles around affected joints.

- Many musculoskeletal ailments can now be treated "conservatively"—without surgery.

- Prolonged immobilization is rarely used because it creates its own problems and extends rehabilitation time.

- Arthroscopic surgery (use of a tubelike device inserted through a small incision) makes surgery much less invasive, with less recovery time.

- Celebrex and Vioxx—neither of which cause much gastrointestinal upset (a common side effect of some pain medications)—were released in early 1999, bringing about a major step forward in the fight against musculoskeletal aches and pain.

- A proper exercise program can help some people with proven structural damage to joints and discs avoid surgery and greatly improve their situation.

- Some major knee problems—and many other musculoskeletal ailments—are no longer disabling because of better medical knowledge and surgical advances.

3: THE CARDIO-VASCULAR AND RESPIRATORY NETWORKS

An Unbeatable Delivery System

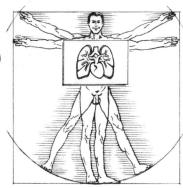

BACKGROUND BASICS

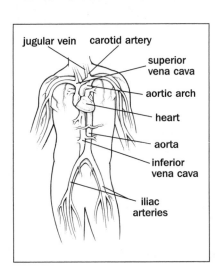

jugular vein   carotid artery
superior vena cava
aortic arch
heart
aorta
inferior vena cava
iliac arteries

During high school biology class, sometime between the frog dissections and sex ed talks, most of us probably heard—though it didn't sink in—that the heart and lungs are an incredible delivery system for oxygen, nutrients, and other elements. Unlike UPS and Federal Express, however, this network is so vital and so critical to our bodies that only a few minutes' interruption can cause major disabilities or death.

Now, some forty years beyond those biology classes, we're starting to sit up and take notice—if only because the heart and lungs are starting to draw our attention. We're getting winded after reaching only first base, our chest goes through some heavy-duty heart-pounding just doing a little snow shoveling, and we sometimes can't shake that winter cough for a month or more.

What's going on?

There's no denying that age is having its effect. Even if you're fit and healthy, by the time you're fifty your respiratory system has diminished by about 25 percent from its peak in your twenties. The heart should still be good and strong, but the all-important arteries might be starting to clog or harden, which will have a serious impact on your heart and the rest of your body.

Sound bad?

Take heart (pun intended)—counterbalancing all the bad news is a tremendous amount of good news. In fact, there's more good news attached to this chapter than to any other in this book. You only need to take a historical look at the end result of heart attacks and strokes to see just how far we've come in a very short period of time. Back one or two generations ago, quite a few people in their fifties died every year from heart attack and stroke (the sudden disruption of blood flow to the brain) or were permanently disabled. While, unfortunately, there are some in our age group who still die from heart attacks, death by stroke in the fifties decade is nearly unheard of anymore. The near eradication of stroke in the fifties decade is one of science's great success stories, and one that will someday encompass heart attacks as well.

Overall, the battle is being won on two fronts: (1) The total number of heart attacks and strokes is shrinking; and (2) When a heart attack or stroke does occur, more people are surviving and doing so with less long-term damage or disability. All this good news is a direct result of something we don't see often enough—science merging perfectly with public action.

How We're Winning against Heart Attack and Stroke

- Development of highly effective drugs to regulate blood pressure and cholesterol levels (major contributing factors in both heart attack and stroke).

- Public awareness of the importance of good blood pressure and cholesterol, and how diet and fitness play a role in maintaining both.

- Personal awareness of the importance of not ignoring chest pains, of taking an aspirin at the first sign of a heart attack or stroke (see the aspirin sidebar in this chapter), and of seeking immediate medical attention at the onset of any suspected attack.

- Development of highly effective drugs that, if given soon after a heart attack or stroke, may nearly eliminate potentially permanent damage.

Fifties Men and the Heart—
Pay Attention Guys, You're in the
Critical Heart Decade

You only have one heart.

Redundancy, as we all know well, is the hallmark of most of the human body. Two arms, two legs, two eyes, ears, lungs, kidneys, testicles. And what doesn't come in pairs, like the liver, has the ability (albeit limited) to regenerate itself. But you only have one heart—and one brain—indicating just how important and life sustaining the heart and brain are. (Yeah, it's true you only have one penis, but, contrary to what you might think, you really could live without it.)

Why Fifties Men Should Pay Attention to Their Hearts

- Almost twice as many men die from heart disease as from all types of cancer.

- Heart disease is the leading cause of death in Americans, according to the American Heart Association.

- Coronary artery disease—*the* leading cause of heart attacks in everyone—is particularly prevalent in fifties males.

- Simply by being male and over forty-five, you automatically have "earned" two risk factors for having a heart attack.

- Heart disease is the second leading cause of death in fifties males (after cancer).

- Approximately 25 percent of all heart attacks are "silent," with no discernable symptoms.

- About 40 percent of all heart attacks still end in death, according to the American Heart Association.

Even though the incidence of heart attack is not highest in fifties males (that's later on), traditionally, this is the decade in which the medical community worries about it most, because more "useful" life can be lost than in the fifties than in later decade.

Are you paying attention now?

Doctors certainly are: They know that there is a major difference between an eighty-year-old man dying of a heart attack and a fifty-four-year-old man dying from one. That's what is meant by the term "useful" life—generally speaking (and putting aside all moral judgments), a man in his fifties who dies from a heart attack loses more potential, or "useful," life than does the man in his eighties. Knowing this, doctors are constantly on the lookout for those with the most risk factors.

Risk Factors For Heart Disease

- Maleness

- Age (beyond forty-five)

- Heredity

- Smoking

- High blood pressure

- High cholesterol

- Obesity

- Diabetes mellitus (where the pancreas has decreased or stopped secreting insulin)

- Nonactive lifestyle

The good news is that, besides age, gender, and heredity, you can directly affect all other risk factors, sometimes to a tremendous degree. And concerning heredity, there are definitely extenuating circumstances you should consider. First, in most cases, heredity plays only a 30 percent role in your overall health. Second, the family members who did die from heart attack probably didn't take care of themselves (through diet and exercise), which leads to the third, most important point: You can't change the heredity cards you were dealt, but you can certainly change the way you play those cards. You can choose not to smoke, watch your diet, and exercise. On the other hand, it's a sure bet that if you choose to ignore your risk factors, and your father died of a heart attack at fifty, there's a strong probability you'll suffer a heart attack around that age, too.

There's no need for that, though, if you only use science and a little personal effort.

How It All Works—
Without the Delivery of Raw Materials by
the Heart and Lungs, Nothing Can Happen

To fully understand how the system can break down, a rudimentary understanding of how it works is necessary. Here's a quick overview of how your body gets its "fuel" (oxygen and nutrients). It all begins with a simple breath by your:

Lungs—When your chest wall and diaphragm move, they cause your chest cavity to enlarge, which creates air pressure in the lungs that is lower than the atmospheric pressure outside your body. As a result, air (which contains oxygen) automatically rushes in through your nose and/or mouth to equalize the inner and outer pressure. The oxygen then moves quickly deep into the intricate and extensive airways (bronchial tubes) of the lungs, finally ending up in the:

Alveoli—tiny sac-like chambers that are bordered by a very thin permeable membrane. On the other side of the membrane are tiny blood vessels (capillaries) that are part of the body's circulation system. It is here where oxygen is transferred from the alveoli to the capillaries for transportation throughout the body. At the same time, carbon dioxide (a waste product of cells) is transferred from the capillaries to the alveoli for its exit journey through your nose and mouth. The transfer and transportation of both oxygen and carbon dioxide could not be done without:

Hemoglobin—A compound in your red blood cells that not only makes your blood red, but also has the ability to bond with, and then release, at just the right time, oxygen. Once the hemoglobin has attached itself to oxygen, it heads into the circulatory system, flowing into the:

Pulmonary Veins—which lead directly to the heart. (This is the only place where oxygenated blood is carried by veins; by definition, veins carry blood to the heart; arteries carry blood away from the heart.) The blood from the lungs enters the heart in the **left atrium**, a small upper chamber of the heart, before it then flows through the **mitral valve** into the:

Left Ventricle—the powerhouse of the heart. This is the organ's biggest muscle, the major pumping chamber of the heart, and the one that dominates the entire image of the heart. It's what pushes the blood from your head to your toes. The journey begins when the blood is pumped from the left ventricle into the **aorta**, the major trunk line out of the heart from which all arteries (other than the pulmonary) branch off. The order in which the arteries break away from the aorta shows a definite hierarchy of importance. First to branch off are the:

Coronary Arteries—three of which, with their tributaries, feed the heart muscle with life-sustaining oxygen. Next to branch off are the:

Arteries to the Brain—Because the brain is so important, there are four of these: Two are in the back of the neck, called **vertebral arteries**, and two in the front, called **carotid arteries** (not the two superficial ones that you can see and feel; they're the veins known as "jugular veins").

Remaining Arteries—From this point on, the blood flow has no real hierarchy as it spreads out to the entire body's muscles, tissues, and organs. The blood, traveling in smaller and smaller arteries, ends up in tiny capillaries at its various destinations. At this point, what takes place is:

Oxygen Transport—which is another way of saying there is a transfer of oxygen from the lungs to a specific destination, as well as a pick up of carbon dioxide (a waste product of cells) for ultimate transport back to the lungs. While this is being done, there is also:

Delivery and Pickup—meaning the delivery of nutrients that have been carried by the blood from the digestive tract and liver, and the pickup of waste products by the blood for transport to the kidneys and/or liver. The waste-laden blood now moves from the capillaries into the:

Veins—which, ultimately, return the blood to the heart by a process called **venous return** (aided, in part, by muscle movements of the arms and legs). When it reaches the heart, the blood enters the **right atrium** (a little anteroom) before flowing through the **tricuspid valve** into the **right ventricle**, which pumps the

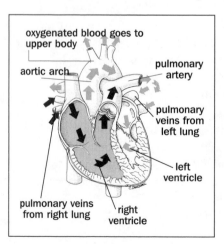

oxygenated blood goes to upper body

aortic arch

pulmonary artery

pulmonary veins from left lung

left ventricle

pulmonary veins from right lung

right ventricle

blood a short distance over to the lungs. At this point, the blood flows into capillaries for the drop-off of carbon dioxide and the pickup of oxygen—which begins the process all over again.

Understanding Blood Vessels—
They're the Key to the Whole Ball Game

The entire heart and circulatory network comes down to one simple, yet highly important, statement: *A strong heart with bad blood vessels is a bad heart.*

We all know that our circulatory system is made up of a pump (the heart) and a delivery network (the blood vessels). Your blood vessels include arteries, veins, and capillaries, with the arteries being the major players. Altogether, the blood vessels make up a closed circulation system that's like a tree whose tiniest twigs are connected to its tiniest roots: The heart pumps blood rich in nutrients and oxygen into the trunk, or arteries, where it travels out into the smallest capillaries, or twigs, before flowing back to veins, or roots, that lead back to the heart.

All this means that if your blood vessels (most notably the arteries) are weak, damaged, or clogged, the delivery of life-sustaining oxygen and nutrients is jeopardized, restricted, or in severe cases interrupted (meaning heart attack or stroke). Interruption of blood flow to organs other than the heart or brain occur less commonly, but when that does happen, the heart and brain are often involved as well.

What all this means is that the old cliché about a chain being only as strong as its weakest link is definitely true in this case. The entire circulatory system is only as strong as its weakest blood vessel. If any blood vessels are "bad," in effect the heart is "bad" as well, regardless of how strong or healthy the heart really is.

The primary reason why blood vessels are the weak link is that they are constantly and repeatedly being affected by various other forces:

• **Blood Pressure.** The sheer force of blood being pumped through the network has a tremendous impact on blood vessels.

• **Control Signals.** Numerous other organs and systems, such as the brain and kidneys, help regulate the entire network through various electrical and chemical signals that impact the blood vessels.

• **Substances.** Elements such as cholesterol, salt, and nicotine can have drastic and dramatically negative impacts on blood vessels.

With those kinds of forces constantly buffeting the blood vessels, it's no surprise that they can weaken or break down, especially after fifty years or more of work.

In fact, there are three specific problems, or diseases, that are a direct result of all this blood vessel-body interaction:

1. Hypertension, or high blood pressure.

2. Arteriosclerosis, or "hardening" of the arteries (loss of flexibility of artery walls).

3. Atherosclerosis, or clogging of the arteries (also known as coronary artery disease when affecting the coronary arteries).

In many cases the three can be interrelated and/or one can help cause another. Any of the three can also cause a host of ailments (such as blood clots and aneurysms) that ultimately lead to a heart attack or stroke—although in the early stages, all three are surprisingly symptomless.

The good news is that science—in just the last fifty years—has developed highly effective drugs that can combat blood vessel diseases. Coupling those drugs with active participation in a good diet, exercise, not smoking, and taking the drugs as prescribed can translate into a tremendous reduction in the risk of heart attack and stroke.

WHERE AND HOW PROBLEMS OCCUR, TREATMENT OPTIONS, AND PREVENTIVE MEASURES

SECTION ONE: THE HEART AND BLOOD VESSELS

Your heart is a truly incredible organ, if for no other reason than how others treat it: Poets have sung its praises; young and old have felt it break; ancient priests have ripped it from living human sacrifices; and warriors have devoured it from their vanquished foes to gain strength.

What's all the fuss about?

Even in our highly enlightened, technologically-oriented day, the heart is still one dazzling piece of machinery. Just look at the stats. Your heart pumps about 2,000 gallons of blood through your body in an average day. By the time you've reached fifty, it will have struck two billion beats. All of that will have been done without resting (other than between beats) and—in normal, healthy people—without much, if any, complaining.

Only about the size of a balled-up fist (five inches long by about three inches wide), the heart is a rounded cone that weighs about ten to twelve ounces in healthy, adult males. The heartbeat that we all know and love is stimulated by elec-

The Cardiovascular and Respiratory Networks

trical signals that travel through special neuro-conductive tissues that spread the impulse throughout the heart muscle on an almost instantaneous basis. This is why an EKG, or electrocardiogram, which measures your heart's electrical activity, is used to see how healthy your heart is (and to see if you've suffered a heart attack).

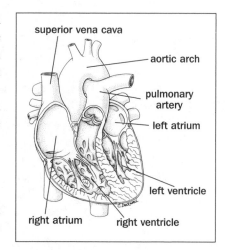

The Heart's Four Chambers

- **Right atrium**—a small anteroom that receives de-oxygenated blood from the veins and passes it on to the:

- **Right ventricle**—which only has to pump the blood a short distance to the lungs for a fresh supply of oxygen. The newly oxygenated blood then flows into the:

- **Left Atrium**—another small anteroom that receives the blood and passes it on to the:

- **Left Ventricle**—which has the huge job of pumping the blood out to the entire body.

From these job descriptions, it's obvious the left ventricle is the powerhouse of the heart—it's the dominant muscle that does most of the work. Thick-walled and muscular, it's most of what you see in pictures or diagrams of the heart. When the left ventricle pumps, it does an amazing thing—it forces blood through the elaborate network of arteries, all the way into the tiniest capillaries of your fingers and toes, then through the extensive network of veins back to the heart.

That pumping action needs to be—and is—tremendous. It also puts pressure on the walls of the arteries, which creates our blood pressure (see the following section for details) as well as a regular, rhythmic beating of the arteries, which is our pulse. For adult males, the average resting pulse should be between sixty and eighty beats a minute. Physical conditioning has a lot to do with pulse rate—a couch potato's poorly exercised heart needs to pump more beats a minute (maybe 90 or 100 at rest), while an athlete's well-conditioned heart is so efficient that it beats less (sometimes as low as the forties or fifties at rest).

The Blood Vessels

As to the blood vessels themselves, many people think of them as simply a system of pipes that allows the blood to flow. That's just as erroneous as thinking our bones are like the static framework of a building. If we did have nonresponsive, rigid "pipes" instead of arteries and veins, any kind of action on the part of the body would drastically affect the flow of blood to particular areas. This would mean that we tough, hardy men would faint every time we stood up quickly, we probably couldn't exercise without passing out, and we'd definitely stop thinking the moment our penises got all the blood for an erec—ah, wait a minute.

Penis-brain jokes aside, arteries and veins are actually active participants in the circulatory system.

The arteries are strong, dynamic tissues that are made up of thick, resilient muscle. They need to be thick-walled and muscular because they have to withstand the continual pounding and pressure of the heart pumping blood through them. They absorb this pressure shock and cushion it, then contract a little to help push the blood along.

Additionally, networks of arteries can be selectively constricted to redirect, or "shunt," blood to where it's needed most. That's how more blood can get sent to your muscles when you're exercising; and how more blood is diverted to your digestive tract when you're eating.

While the veins are much more passive than arteries, they do have a small amount of wall movement and do react to surrounding muscle contractions—both of which aid blood flow back to the heart in a process referred to as venous return. Additionally, one-way valves within the larger veins ensure that blood does not flow backward on its long return passage from your toes to your heart. These long veins and their valves are basically the price we pay for standing upright—we wouldn't need them if we were still using our knuckles as training wheels.

The All-Important Blood Vessel Lining

Inside both arteries and veins is an extremely important and special lining called the endothelium. It's made up of flat cells that are very smooth, so that blood, with all its extra baggage of either oxygen and nutrients or carbon dioxide and waste products, can slide through unrestricted. This non-stick endothelium is especially necessary in the arteries, because their walls are constantly expanding or contracting in reaction to various control signals that aid circulation.

When it's all said and done, arteries are much more important than veins. This is because they do more, are ordered around by more organs and systems, and—as a result—have more areas in which breakdowns or problems are possible.

Blood Pressure

Ever since circulation was first vaguely understood in the 1600s, doctors have known that the human body must maintain a certain blood pressure to stay alive. In fact, for most of this century, blood pressure has been regarded by most of the medical profession as an important gauge of a person's current—and long-term—general health.

While medical science has taken huge diagnostic steps in the last fifty years, creating vastly more sophisticated tests and gauges, blood pressure remains a critical early warning signal in the fight against an array of heart and circulatory diseases. And it's still measured in the same way as when our great-grandparents were around: A sphygmomanometer (that black Velcro tourniquet we've all seen) is wrapped around your upper arm and then inflated. This compresses your arm's artery so that blood stops flowing. As the cuff's pressure is slowly released, a stethoscope is used to hear when your blood starts to pulse through the artery again. As most of you already know, there are two numbers in the blood pressure equation.

What the Numbers Mean

- **Systolic pressure** is the top number. It's measured when the first pulse is heard returning to the artery. This reflects the force of your blood at its strongest, when the powerful left ventricle is squeezing off a beat.

- **Diastolic pressure** is the bottom number. It's measured just after the last blood sound is heard in the stethoscope. This represents the force of your blood between beats, when your heart is relaxing and expanding in preparation for the next beat.

Much can be learned or deduced from each number, as well as the relationship between the two. For many years it was thought that the diastolic pressure was the more important figure, because it represented the minimum pressure on the arteries all the time. Now, we realize that both numbers are equally important. As to the relationship between the numbers—a substantial distance between the two numbers can be an indicator of such ailments as hardening of the arteries.

While optimum blood pressure is 120 over 80, it's unusual for someone to have that actual measurement. More importantly, the "normal" range of good blood pressure is approximately 120 to 129 for systolic pressure and 80 to 84 for diastolic pressure. Thinking of blood pressure in terms of a range rather than specific numbers is best, because blood pressure can vary with numerous factors.

Factors that Can Affect Blood Pressure

- Age

- Sex

- General health of the arteries

- General health of the heart

- Force of the heart muscle contraction

- Emotional state

- Exercise and level of general fitness

- Drugs, both commonplace (caffeine and decongestants) and less so (amphetamines, cocaine, anabolic steroids)

- Nicotine (in all types of tobacco products, both smoked and smokeless)

For years, it was thought that high blood pressure (hypertension) was just part of the aging process. Today, we know that is not the case. Because high blood pressure can strike at any age, and is associated with a higher risk of "vascular catastrophes" (strokes, heart attacks), it must be controlled regardless of age.

Complicating the entire issue of blood pressure are the facts that we have only one heart and no way stations along the circulatory tract. This means that maintaining blood pressure is an incredibly complicated procedure that takes a tremendous amount of coordination among various parties. To orchestrate this symphony of circulation there are numerous influences.

Blood Pressure Influences

The Kidneys. These are your body's volume-control mechanism, controlling how much fluid balance and sodium (salt) are in the body. The amount of fluid in the blood has a direct impact on blood pressure—more fluid increases blood pressure, less fluid decreases it. The amount of salt also impacts the amount of fluid—the more salt the kidneys detect in the body, the more water the kidneys will retain to dilute the salt. The kidneys also function as glands, producing hormones (renin and angiotensin) that have a major effect on blood pressure levels and arterial health.

The Central Nervous System. With anxiety or stress, the central nervous system can stimulate the famous "fight or flight" reflex we all have. This reflex constricts blood vessels, which sends blood pressure up. One of the major elements in this reflex is adrenaline (also called epinephrine), part of a group of powerful hormones produced by the adrenal gland that can cause increased breathing, heart, and metabolic rates—all of which create higher blood pressure.

The Heart. Receiving control signals or messages from other parts of the body—including the brain, autonomic nervous system, kidneys, adrenal glands, and even the arteries—the heart can pump harder and/or faster, thus causing increased blood pressure.

The Arteries. If they have lost some of their flexibility and are becoming rigid or "hard" (arteriosclerosis), blood pressure will rise.

Angiotensin. This hormone, produced by the kidneys, causes arteries to constrict, which raises blood pressure.

All of these influences are in some way or another necessary for the body to respond to emergencies, such as injury, illness, fright, or stress. Unfortunately, if their effects (increased heart rate and/or increased blood pressure) are sustained over too long a period of time, they can permanently damage the structure and function of the arterial walls—making permanent hypertension, heart attacks, and strokes more likely.

With all these influences, it's no wonder that numerous problems can arise.

Hypertension (High Blood Pressure)

Strictly speaking, hypertension is merely the condition of blood pressure being persistently above 140 over 90. Unfortunately, that simple definition hides an insidious disease. That kind of blood pressure puts a tremendous amount of pressure on the entire system, especially the arteries. If that pressure is maintained for an extended period of time it will damage the arteries, which can lead to one or both of the two major catastrophic results of hypertension: heart attack or stroke.

Hypertension can be caused by emotional stress or disorders of the kidneys, the adrenal gland, or the thyroid. In the most common form—called essential hypertension— the specific cause is unknown or hard to pinpoint.

Contributing Factors to Hypertension

• **Obesity**—which puts added pressure on the heart to pump harder.

• **Hypercholesterolemia**—which means higher-than-normal cholesterol levels. These elevated levels can block the arteries, reduce their flexibility, and create higher blood pressure (see the following cholesterol section for details).

• **High salt levels**—which result, because of kidney action, in more fluid in the blood. Increased fluid generates higher blood pressure.

• **Family history**—if your parents had high blood pressure, you're likely to have it also.

At some stage or other, we all have short, quick bouts of high blood pressure—when we get excited, when we exercise heavily, when we get stressed at work. These are perfectly natural and a part of the general human response to life. Problems only arise when these bouts of elevated blood pressure become sustained and persistent. That's when it becomes hypertension. And that's when the possibility of artery damage begins.

Compounding the problem is the fact that hypertension quickly becomes the proverbial vicious cycle—the pounding that the arteries take from a higher-than-normal blood pressure damages them, and damaged arteries, in turn, raise blood pressure.

As if that wasn't bad enough, hypertension rarely shows any symptoms in the majority of people. This has earned it the infamous title of "silent killer" because, in the past, many victims weren't even aware that they had high blood pressure until they had a heart attack or stroke.

How Hypertension Is Diagnosed

Blood pressure measurement is the primary way. Because blood pressure readings can fluctuate, they are usually taken several times at varying intervals to get an accurate assessment. Once that is done, your blood pressure is plugged into a relatively standardized set of figures that indicate if you have a problem or not.

BLOOD PRESSURE LEVELS		
Level	**Systolic**	**Diastolic**
Ideal	120 or less	80 or less
Normal	120-129	80–84
High normal	130-139	85–89
Stage 1 hypertension	140-159	90–99
Stage 2 hypertension	160-179	100–109
Stage 3 hypertension	180-209	110-119
Stage 4 hypertension	more than 210	more than 120

The Cardiovascular and Respiratory Networks

Anyone with blood pressure persistently above 140 over 90 should be treated, while those with figures only slightly lower are good candidates for treatment as well. Doctors strive to keep patients as far below those numbers as possible without causing side effects and without an unreasonable number of medications.

Because blood pressure goes up during exercise—but should never increase beyond a certain point—a different set of measurements apply for blood pressure checked during exercise: A fit person, exercising as close to his maximum as possible, will probably have a blood pressure range around 180 or 190 over 90. If, however, that athlete has 230 over 110, that's too high, even for someone who exercises, and it should be treated.

While blood pressure should not ideally be affected by age—a fit ninety-year-old man can have as healthy a blood pressure reading as a fifty-year-old—in today's world that is not the general rule. In fact, hypertension can hit those in their twenties, thirties, and forties, and is quite common in fifties men.

The effects of hypertension are directly related to how high the blood pressure is and how long it's been high. People with readings consistently in the 140s over the 90s will have a significantly increased risk of heart attack and stroke over a period of a couple of decades. This is especially true for men, and for African-American men in particular. Those with very high readings of 240 over 120 could conceivably see problems occurring within days, weeks, or months.

Even though hypertension is dubbed the silent killer, there are still many people who believe that elevated blood pressure can cause numerous symptoms. That's rarely the case. It is usually only after other associated problems occur in the arteries, kidneys, brain, eyes, or elsewhere that symptoms show themselves. By the time symptoms show up, the person is potentially in serious trouble.

Possible Hypertension Symptoms

- Headaches

- Rapid and strong beating of the heart

- Flushed face

- Blurry vision

- Labored breathing after moderate exertion

- Fatigue

- Ringing or buzzing in the ears

- Dizziness and spinning (vertigo)

It should be stressed that, contrary to what many believe, "uncomplicated" blood pressure (meaning it hasn't, as yet, created complications in other parts of the body) *does not* cause dizziness, headaches, fatigue, nose bleeds, or facial flushing.

Treatment/Prevention. Because high blood pressure is such a dangerous disease, it's critical that it be brought under control as quickly as possible. This means that the best initial treatment is the use of drugs, which are highly effective. Once blood pressure has returned to an acceptable level, patient-based treatments—such as improving diet, exercising, and learning how to handle stress—can be discussed with a doctor.

Regarding blood-pressure drugs, there are numerous and excellent groups available to maintain a lower, healthier blood pressure.

Three Main Classes of Blood Pressure Drugs

Diuretics—which act on the kidneys to make them pass more water and salt in the urine so that the liquid volume of blood is reduced. This brings down the pressure.

Beta Blockers—which interfere with the hormone and nervous control of the heart (blocking adrenaline), which slows the heart and causes it to beat less forcefully. This brings down the pressure.

Vasodilators—which act on the arteries themselves to relax and expand them. This brings down the pressure. Within the vasodilators are three other groups of drugs: alpha adrenergic blockers (alpha blockers), calcium channel blockers (CCB), and angiotensin-converting enzyme inhibitors (ACE inhibitors). The alpha blockers, which work by relaxing smooth muscle, such as those found in arteries and the urinary tract, have been more or less replaced by other blood pressure drugs, but continue to be used for urinary tract problems. (See the drug chart in this chapter for greater details about blood pressure drugs.)

Because each of the various groups of drugs works on different aspects of blood pressure, some are better suited for various people than others—African-Americans and women seem to respond better to diuretics, while younger men usually respond better to ACEs and CCBs.

In some cases, the drugs themselves create other problems (e.g., diuretics can cause an imbalance of salt and potassium) that, in turn, are handled by other drugs—meaning that some blood pressure treatments involve a combination of drugs.

Lastly, it should be noted that in some cases the drug treatment may, initially, cause the patient to feel worse until his system has readjusted to normal blood pressure. These temporary symptoms might include weakness, lack of energy, depression, and the feeling of dizziness when standing up.

While all this might sound complicated and somewhat daunting, the reality is that blood pressure drug treatments are relatively unobtrusive to the average lifestyle, and the good they do is immeasurable.

Prevention and/or Early Detection Methods for Hypertension

A blood pressure check by a health care professional at least yearly.

Adequate rest—restorative sleep is one of the best ways of fighting stress, tension, and anxiety, all of which can lead to raised blood pressure.

DON'T FOOL YOURSELF—
WHITE COAT HYPERTENSION

Blood pressure (BP) can be affected by stress and tension. Because of this, some people believe their high BP levels at the doctor's office are due only to their anxiety about seeing a doctor. This is known as "white coat hypertension"—the doctor, with his white lab coat, actually causes the patient's blood pressure to rise abnormally. More and more patients are bringing in BP readings taken at home, at the supermarket, or at the drug store that are consistently lower than those taken in the doctor's office. To them, these readings prove they don't have hypertension.

Why white coat hypertension is a somewhat bogus concept:

- People with hypertension can have normal readings some of the time, because BP does fluctuate with numerous variables.
- Doctors can't take the liberty of ignoring BP readings the patient doesn't like.
- Each and every reading (good or bad) can, in fact, be valid, which still means you have hypertension, because you have some readings that are high.
- People who have blood pressure that rises over the anxiety of visiting a doctor will more than likely have elevated BP in many other everyday situations. This means that the low BP reading taken in the quiet of the home is more likely to be the less representative than the one taken at the doctor's office.

A final, critical note: *Leaving hypertension untreated is as dangerous as playing Russian roulette—with all chambers loaded.*

A diet low in salt and fat to control the intake of chemicals that can cause blood pressure to rise, to prevent a rise in cholesterol (which can lead to blocked arteries; see the next section on cholesterol for details), and to prevent obesity, which puts a strain on the heart and may lead to hypertension.

An exercise program—which directly helps to lower blood pressure, but also helps to lower it indirectly by decreasing stress, tension, and anxiety.

An eye exam—the retina of the eye is the only place on the human body where arteries are directly visible, so they can be a good indicator of arterial health.

Cholesterol

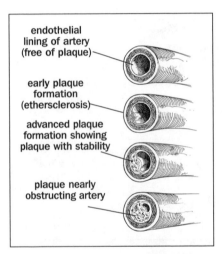

endothelial
lining of artery
(free of plaque)

early plaque
formation
(ethersclerosis)

advanced plaque
formation showing
plaque with stability

plaque nearly
obstructing artery

For the past fifteen or twenty years, cholesterol has been one of the major buzz words in heart and circulatory health (spoken in the same breath as blood pressure and smoking). You can't shop at a store, eat at a restaurant, read the paper, or watch a health-related TV show without the word cholesterol popping up numerous times.

Does it deserve all this attention?

You bet. Cholesterol is the main element in the substance that collects on arterial walls in the artery-clogging disease atherosclerosis. Research has found those with a high level of cholesterol in their blood have a greater risk of heart disease (the number one killer in the world) than those with a low cholesterol level. Additionally, cholesterol can cause the formation of gallstones.

Back in the mid 1960s, before it was fully understood how big a role cholesterol plays in blood vessel health, Gordon had a medical school professor, Dr. Pothoff, who taught a preventive medicine class. A standing joke involved his peculiar demand that all his students know their cholesterol levels. After class the students would imitate what they thought were his rantings and ravings about the importance of cholesterol in circulatory health. Little did they know that thirty-plus years later all doctors would be giving the same speeches to their patients and demanding they know their cholesterol levels. This is especially true for fifties male patients—who are particularly susceptible to the negative impact of high cholesterol levels.

The Cardiovascular and Respiratory Networks

As with many other substances in our bodies, cholesterol has that two-steps-forward-one-step-back quality: There is a good reason for cholesterol, and in the right amounts it is essential for a healthy life, but in excessive quantities it can be harmful, even lethal.

What Is Cholesterol?

Cholesterol is a complex chemical, a waxy, fat-like substance that is produced in the liver and is widespread in the body—most notably in bile, the brain, blood, adrenal glands, and nervous tissue. Primary responsibilities of cholesterol include:

• Aiding in the formation and/or repair of cell membranes.

• Helping in the breakdown of fatty acids in the digestive tract.

• Contributing to the maintenance of nerve cell health and function.

• Contributing to the production of certain hormones, bile acids, and vitamin D.

While cholesterol is present in some foods, it is also a substance the body can manufacture. If the raw materials for cholesterol production are available in abundance, high cholesterol levels are likely to result. These raw materials are present in certain foods, most notably all animal fats, milk products, and eggs. Especially bad are saturated fats (those that are solid at room temperature), which our bodies convert into cholesterol. Basically, our bodies produce cholesterol based upon the amount of saturated fat in our systems—meaning that the cholesterol count of what we're eating is not as important in raising our blood cholesterol as the amounts of saturated fats we eat.

Once cholesterol is in the body, it travels through the blood stream, hitching a ride with carriers called lipoproteins, which are a combination of fats and proteins. They give rise to the names of the two kinds of cholesterol, which, with an additional substance, the medical community now monitors:

• **LDL (low-density lipoproteins) or "bad" cholesterol**—meaning low protein/high cholesterol content. LDL transports lipids (energy reserves) to muscles and to fat stores. The LDL cholesterol that's not used by the cells or stored continues to circulate through the blood, often sticking to arterial walls. This clogging of the arteries (atherosclerosis) is what can ultimately lead to heart attack and/or stroke. Memory tip: The L of LDL can stand for "lousy."

- **HDL (high-density lipoproteins) or "good" cholesterol**—meaning high protein/low cholesterol content. HDL gets the halo, because it travels through the blood vessels picking up LDL cholesterol that's unused by the cells and returning it to the liver for processing. Memory tip: The H of HDL can stand for "healthy."

- **Triglycerides**—not actually related to cholesterol, although many times mentioned along with it, triglycerides are actually fats that are chemically different from cholesterol, but they can affect your cholesterol levels and increase your risk of heart disease. They are produced by the liver, but are also found in animal fats and plant oils. A major difference from cholesterol is that triglycerides don't stick to artery walls. They do, however, reflect your risk of numerous diseases, including heart disease and diabetes mellitus. A normal triglycerides level is 200 mg and lower, with borderline high being 200 to 400 mg.

How Cholesterol Is Measured

Gauging your total cholesterol level is done via a simple blood test to determine how much cholesterol is in your blood. There are three established or standard readings:

- **Desirable**—less than 200 mg per deciliter. You're doing well; keep up what you're doing.

- **Borderline high**—between 200 and 239 mg. You're entering potentially dangerous territory here—you now have twice as high a risk of heart attack as the guy in the desirable range.

- **High**—above 240 mg. You're in for some major lifestyle changes and some cholesterol-lowering drugs; if not, better get that cardiac care insurance up to date.

Some interesting factors about total cholesterol involves the town of Framingham, Mass. Since 1948 all the men in the town have been monitored to help scientists determine the risk factors for heart disease and stroke. So far, not one of the men with a total cholesterol level under 150 mg has died of a heart attack. Additionally, the Framingham Heart Study has found that heart attack rates rise 2 percent for each 1 percent increase in blood cholesterol over 200 mg. These are pretty impressive and meaningful findings as they relate to cholesterol.

While the total cholesterol count is important, a better, more accurate reflection of cholesterol appears when the total count is broken down into LDL and HDL

The Cardiovascular and Respiratory Networks

levels. This is done through a blood test after you've fasted for twelve hours (be very good about this—even a cup of coffee with milk can screw up the results).

Once your LDL and HDL numbers are established, here are some guidelines to remember: The best case scenario is to have high HDL and low LDL; conversely, it's bad to have high LDL and low HDL. If your total cholesterol count is high because of high HDL, you have little to be concerned about. In fact, your HDL should be as high as you can achieve—it's the LDL count that's critical.

What the Cholesterol Numbers Mean

Ideally, a man in his fifties should have less than 200 mg of total cholesterol, with less than 100 mg of LDL and more than 40 mg of HDL. Those figures change as risk factors are added, and for those who have already suffered one heart attack, the standard is very strict: the LDL level should be below 80 and the total cholesterol count should be less than 160.

When looking at cholesterol figures, the total count is *not* the simple adding together of LDL and HDL, although there is a rough correlation. Doctors not only look at the individual LDL, HDL, and total count, but at a ratio of HDL to the total as well. While the average of that ratio for the general population is between five and six, that's actually way too high (a ratio of six might mean an HDL of 50 and a total count 300, which is unacceptable). A desirable ratio is more like 4.5 or less.

The American Heart Association's National Cholesterol Education Program has created recommendations for LDL levels and total cholesterol levels, as follows:

Recommended Cholesterol Levels

LDL Cholesterol—
Primary Target of Therapy

Less than 100	Optimal
100-129	Near Optimal/Above Optimal
130-159	Borderline High
160-189	High
More than 190	Very High

Total Cholesterol

Less than 200	Desirable
200-239	Borderline High
More than 240	High

Cholesterol levels vary with age, sex, heredity, race, hormone production, and even occupation, and are thought to depend mainly on the amount manufactured in the body rather than what is actually consumed.

The good news in all this is that we can directly affect our cholesterol level, both through medication and through active participation in diet and exercise. And, because there is both good and bad cholesterol, there are numerous ways to positively affect cholesterol levels: (1) Increase your HDL only; (2) Decrease your LDL only; or (3) Increase your HDL while decreasing your LDL, which doubles the benefits. (See the treatment/prevention section of hypercholesterolemia, below, and chapter 8 for details on affecting cholesterol levels.)

Hypercholesterolemia

Higher than normal levels of cholesterol is what hypercholesterolemia means. The condition is associated with clogged arteries (atherosclerosis) and other cardiovascular diseases. For those who have high cholesterol primarily because of genetics, the condition is called familial hypercholesterolemia.

What are the symptoms of higher than normal levels of cholesterol?

As with high blood pressure, there are no symptoms. That's the problem with both ailments, they can sneak up on anyone.

Because there is a strong genetic predisposition to developing high cholesterol in some people, anyone over the age of twenty should have his cholesterol checked. From age fifty on, it should be checked at least once a year. One point to keep in mind: Years ago, cholesterol was one of the elements checked with nearly every blood test done. Now, however, due to changes in health-care financing (in this case, *negative* changes) that is not always the case, so it might be necessary to ask your doctor to check your cholesterol.

Treatment/Prevention. Once it has been determined that you have higher than normal cholesterol levels, what can be done?

A lot. A good diet, low in cholesterol and fats—especially saturated fats—is a must (see chapter 8 for diet details). The American Heart Association recommends less than 300 mg of cholesterol from food daily—that's about the same as three or four large eggs a week. If you already have heart disease, that figure drops to 200 mg a day. Reportedly, the average guy already has one strike against him, because he consumes approximately 450 mg of cholesterol a day.

The Cardiovascular and Respiratory Networks

How to Take Charge of Your Cholesterol Levels

- Limit your fat intake to about 30 percent of your daily calories.

- Eat fewer fat calories as a way of losing any excess weight, because fat has twice as many calories per gram as either carbohydrates or proteins.

- Eat more fruits, vegetables, and fiber, while replacing saturated fats with monounsaturated fats (generally, those that are liquid at room temperature). A high fiber diet would probably help lower cholesterol counts.

- Exercise—especially aerobically—for at least twenty minutes at a time. Regular aerobic exercise has been shown to raise HDL. In fact, the more intense the exercise, the higher the level of HDL (check with your doctor before launching into any new exercise program).

While exercise definitely helps your cholesterol stats, you should know that it will take a few months of solid exercise for you to reach your best results, and all the good results will disappear quickly if you stop your exercise routine.

One of the biggest problems in limiting cholesterol and fat intake is that fat tastes so good. There's nothing better than a greasy burger and fries, or a slab of fat-marbled steak. To compound the taste dilemma, fat actually takes longer to digest than other foods, so it gives you that warm, satisfied feeling after you've eaten it. There's no quick-fix for these two problems regarding fat—it just takes some good old-fashioned self-control. If you are having trouble with self-control, go talk to your doctor, who does have other ways of helping you.

On a happier note, moderate drinking has been shown to increase the level of good HDL cholesterol (see the drinking sidebar in this chapter for details).

For some unfortunate few, doing all of the above still doesn't bring cholesterol levels within healthy ranges. For these—and for people having difficulty following self-regulated activities—there are medications that can be highly successful. These include two drug categories: (1) Bile acid sequestrants, which lower cholesterol by reducing the amount of fat absorbed by the body; and (2) HMG CoA reductase inhibitors (known as "statins"), which inhibit the enzyme HMG CoA and interfere with the natural process of cholesterol making (see the drug chart in this chapter for details).

The overriding thought to remember here is that the control of high cholesterol, like that of high blood pressure, is now very firmly in the grasp of medical science. It only takes knowing that you have the condition to put the wheels in motion to improve, if not cure, the condition.

BOTTOMS UP
DRINKING AS PART OF GOOD HEALTH

When it comes to alcohol, the medical community talks about the French Paradox—despite smoking, drinking wine, and eating rich foods, the French have a lower risk of heart attack than Americans. It was believed that an element in red wine restricted blood clotting, which prevented heart attacks. But then another study showed white wine was better than red. Harvard Medical School reported that wine, beer, and hard liquor all do a similar job. Another study showed that simple grape juice has the same benefits as red wine.

In general, it's now believed that moderate drinking—meaning one to two drinks a day—decreases your risk of death compared to teetotalers by:

- Restricting blood clotting, which reduces the risk of both heart attack and stroke.

- Lowering stress levels, which reduces the risk of heart attack.

- Increasing the "good" HDL cholesterol, which carries away the artery-clogging LDL cholesterol. A Harvard study showed an average increase of 17 percent in HDL, which translates into a 40 percent reduction in heart disease risk.

What constitutes a drink? Twelve ounces of beer, five ounces of wine, or one-and-a-half ounces of hard liquor. Should everyone drink? No. Those who never started should not start now—10 percent of all drinkers cannot control their consumption. But moderate drinkers should know they are not harming themselves and are probably helping their overall health.

A final warning: Any number of drinks over two a day actually increases your chance of accidents and death over those of teetotalers.

Cardiovascular Problems

Because of the complex nature and relationship of the heart and circulatory system (most notably the arteries), the breakdowns that can occur are numerous and varied. In fact, it is basically impossible to pinpoint one single, identifiable cause for many heart and circulatory problems. That's because there can be numerous causes for many conditions; a lot of causes for just a single condition; diseases in and of themselves can cause other diseases; and, most times, there is an overlapping of causes and effects.

The Cardiovascular and Respiratory Networks

Overall, it's a pretty confusing situation. To make matters a little more complicated, terms such as heart disease, cardiovascular disease, coronary heart disease, and coronary artery disease can and do cover a broad spectrum of heart and circulatory problems, and in some cases are interchangeable names for the same problems.

Just keep in mind that the primary problem in all the various common cardiovascular ailments is restricted flow of blood through the arteries. On the one hand, restricted blood flow can be caused by numerous factors and elements. On the other hand, restricted blood flow can cause numerous other problems. Generally speaking, the following is a quick, three-step ailment summary that shows a little of the complicated web of interrelationships that usually exists among the various problems. (Details of each of the following items are given under their own heading in this chapter.)

Two Instigators of Heart and Circulatory Problems

- **Hypertension** (persistent high blood pressure)

- **Hypercholesterolemia** (higher-than-normal amounts of cholesterol in the body)

Can Lead To

- **Arteriosclerosis** ("hardening" of the arteries)

- **Atherosclerosis** (clogging of the arteries that's also referred to as coronary artery disease when it affects the heart's arteries)

All Four of Which Can Ultimately Lead, Separately or in Combination, To

- **Heart Attack** (interruption of normal blood flow to the heart muscle; also known as myocardial infarction)

- **Stroke** (interruption of normal blood flow to the brain; also called a cerebrovascular accident or brain attack)

- **Kidney Failure**

- **Aneurysms** (ballooning out of a blood vessel)

- **Leg Pain** (Claudication)

One of the few certainties in this entire complicated equation is that smoking has a tremendous detrimental effect on both the heart and blood vessels and, therefore, is a contributing factor to all of the above-mentioned ailments (see the smoking section in chapter 8 for details).

Arteriosclerosis (Hardening of the Arteries)

This term describes a number of conditions in which fatty deposits and minerals, called plaque, collect in the arteries. This causes the arteries to become rigid and inflexible, which, in turn, leads to restricted blood flow. While the condition can occur in all the arteries, it is most dangerous when occuring in the arteries that supply blood to the brain and heart. If the condition gets bad enough, it can lead to a stroke (see the stroke section of this chapter for details) or heart attack.

Because you can't feel the buildup of plaque in your blood vessels, symptoms of arteriosclerosis are rarely felt. Early detection is possible, though, due to the fact that the causes of arteriosclerosis are hypertension (high blood pressure) and hypercholesterolemia (too much cholesterol in the system)—meaning regular checkups of your blood pressure and cholesterol levels are critical.

Mostly known to affect the elderly and those with hypertension, arteriosclerosis is not as prevalent a condition in fifties men as are other cardiovascular diseases. Additionally, because the term arteriosclerosis is somewhat imprecise, it is being used less and less by the medical community. Instead, doctors talk more about atherosclerosis (clogged arteries), which is the most common form of arteriosclerosis.

Treatment/Prevention. In many cases, treatment for arteriosclerosis is the same as for high blood pressure: drugs (diuretics, beta blockers, or vasodilators), exercise, and proper diet to control salt intake and the build up of LDL, or "bad" cholesterol.

Prevention includes exercise, a healthy diet low in fats and salt, an aspirin a day (see the aspirin sidebar in this chapter), and daily intake of antioxidants like vitamins C (250-500 mg) and E (100-400 IUs).

Atherosclerosis (Clogging of the Arteries) and Angina

Atherosclerosis is a form of arterial degeneration that is the number one killer in the Western world. It's responsible for about half of all deaths in Western countries. In the United States, more than 950,000 people die of it each year. And as developing countries begin to adopt more Westernized lifestyles (primarily cigarette smoking and consuming a greater proportion of total calories from animal sources) atherosclerosis incidence is increasing rapidly.

The Cardiovascular and Respiratory Networks

If there is a disease that uniquely strikes men in their fifties, it is atherosclerosis. This is when the disease reveals to many men that it has already caused significant havoc in their circulatory system. Happily, today most of those fifties men afflicted do not die in their fifties. But still, approximately 10 percent of all deaths from atherosclerosis are in men fifty to sixty years old.

Scientifically speaking, atherosclerosis is where the walls of your arteries become thick and irregular due to the accumulation of cholesterol, fats, and other substances (all called plaque). In laymen's terms: clogged arteries. Although most arteries are affected, it's the coronary arteries, which supply the heart muscle with blood, that are most at risk. This is why the condition is also known as coronary artery disease. Additionally, though, the arteries to the brain can often be affected. In its most severe manifestations, atherosclerosis can cause heart attack (if blockage is in the heart arteries) or stroke (if blockage is in the brain arteries).

Researchers have shown that atherosclerosis begins to clog arteries even in children—autopsies of young soldiers during the Korean War proved this—and progresses as we age. Heredity seems to play a role in those who are susceptible, as does being male. In this case, it's definitely better to be a woman than a man. Because a woman's estrogen has the unique ability to keep her arteries generally free and clear of plaque, she is naturally "protected" from clogged arteries up until menopause (although with an increase in women smokers and an increase in their overall stress levels, the difference between men and women, when it comes to the incidence of coronary artery disease, is shrinking all the time). Men could take estrogen to protect themselves from atherosclerosis, but then they'd develop breasts—not a very desirable side effect.

As with other cardiovascular illnesses, atherosclerosis rarely has symptoms in its early stages. High blood pressure and high cholesterol may lead to a diagnosis, but many people first find out that they have atherosclerosis when they get angina pectoris.

Angina Pectoris

Angina, as it's most commonly called, is pain in the chest that can come on any time a heart with narrowed coronary arteries is called upon to pump more vigorously than usual. In a healthy heart and arteries, when the heart needs to pump harder and/or faster, blood flow increases to the heart muscle, bringing necessary oxygen and nutrients. In a circulatory system with atherosclerosis, where blood flow is restricted, when the heart muscle begins to pump harder, it needs more oxygen then it gets. That oxygen deprivation causes the chest pain that is angina.

Because angina causes pain—but usually not life-threatening heart attacks—it is the primary warning sign of coronary heart disease. It's a wake-up call not to be ignored.

91

Common Descriptions of Angina Pain

- Feels heavy, suffocating, strangulating, or pressure-like in nature

- Starts under the breastbone, or on the left side of the chest

- Spreads to other parts of the body, such as the throat, neck and jaw, the left shoulder, and the arm

- Occasionally extends to the right side of the chest (but seldom is exclusively right-sided)

Specific conditions can bring on an angina episode or attack. These include stress, a heavy meal, emotional excitement, cold weather, and exercise—even so slight as climbing stairs. Rarely does angina occur at night; if it does, it lasts longer than five minutes but less than thirty. Be aware that an episode of more than fifteen minutes could indicate you're having a heart attack. Conversely, it should be noted that the symptoms of angina can be similar to those of heartburn, indigestion, and gas, although the symptoms of these three conditions usually go away quickly after simple over-the-counter antacids are taken. If they do not, call your doctor or 911 immediately.

Other Signs of Coronary Heart Disease
(Besides Angina and/or a Heart Attack)

- Shortness of breath—more than just being a little winded as we get older.

- Dizziness and fainting spells—which can also indicate other ailments (such as hypertension and ear infections).

- Nausea and generalized sweating.

- Extreme fatigue that has no obvious cause.

- A dry, hacking cough (a very rare sign).

- Swelling in the legs, feet, ankles, or abdominal area.

The only conclusive way to know if you have atherosclerosis and/or angina is through a physical exam and an EKG (electrocardiogram), which measures your heart's electrical activity. The EKG is good at telling doctors if heart muscle damage has already occurred and if there are any rhythm disturbances, but it has little ability to predict what's going to happen next. You can also have a stress test, in which an EKG is used while you're on a treadmill, often combined with additional imaging tests, such as a heart scan or an echocardiogram. Or you can have the more invasive angiography test, in which dye is injected into your blood and then X rays are taken. All of these will indicate just how blocked your arteries are.

Treatment/Prevention. Once blockage in your arteries has been found, treatment can involve three elements: self-care, medications, and possible surgery.

Self-care means implementing lifestyle changes that will make a huge difference in your cardiac health.

Seven Primary Self-Care Treatments for Clogged Arteries

• Don't smoke

• Exercise

• If overweight, lose the extra pounds

• Eat a well-balanced diet that's low in salt

• Have your blood pressure checked regularly

• Remain calm in stressful or tense situations

• Know your cholesterol level and be actively involved in its control

As for medications, they may not resolve the problem of plaque build-up in your arteries, but they do attack the problem by reducing blood pressure, slowing down your heart rate, enlarging your blood vessels, and reducing the workload of your heart. Drugs include beta blockers to slow your heartbeat, vasodilators to relax your arteries and increase blood flow, calcium channel blockers to help open up your arteries, and ACE inhibitors to reduce your heart's workload. (See the drug chart at the end of this chapter for details.)

If nonsurgical measures aren't working, there are several surgical options available.

Surgical Options for Clogged Arteries

• **Bypass surgery,** in which the clogged portion of the artery is bypassed using a grafted piece of leg vein or implantation of a healthy artery from the chest wall, so that blood flow is restored to the heart muscle.

- **Angioplasty,** in which a tiny balloon is inflated inside the artery, right at the clog, so that the plaque is flattened against the arterial wall and blood flow is restored. Occasionally, a rotary blade inserted into the artery shaves away some of the arterial blockage in a procedure called atherectomy.

- **Stenting,** in which a tubular mesh is placed inside the clogged artery to keep it open.

Balloon angioplasty, stent placement, and atherectomy are much less traumatic and severe than bypass surgery, because they're done as part of a cardiac catheterization, which involves a tiny tube inserted through a leg artery, local anesthesia, and conscious sedation; bypass surgery requires general anesthesia, the opening of the chest, and use of a heart-lung machine.

Prevention of atherosclerosis involves the active participation of the individual. Although science has already shown that atherosclerosis begins to take hold at a very early age, the disease is not inevitable. With the above-mentioned lifestyle changes, you can usually ward off atherosclerosis and its painful effects for most of your life.

Heart Attack

If we're really honest with ourselves, this entire chapter—with all of its definitions, explanations, symptoms, causes, and effects—all comes down to this two-word phrase: heart attack.

Why do those words strike such fear into most of us?

The stats tell a lot of the story: While there is close to a 90 percent chance of survival after a heart attack (if no complications develop), 23 percent of previous heart attack victims will have another attack within six years, and fully 40 percent of all heart attacks do end in death.

Unfortunately, it's in the fifties decade when all these realities begin to hit home. We're no longer spring chickens, and, what's worse, we're finding out we don't to live forever. A heart attack is one of the biggest reminders of that in fifties men.

What exactly is this frightening beast?

Known to doctors as a myocardial infarction (MI), a heart attack takes place when a blockage or clot (a coronary thrombosis) occurs in one or more of your coronary arteries, which supply oxygen and nutrient rich blood to the heart muscle. As a result of the clot, the blood flow is either severely restricted or completely cut off, which leads to the sudden disruption in the heartbeat. Depending on how long and how severe the attack is, it can then lead to damaged heart tissue (known as an infarction) and/or death. That's a heart attack.

The Cardiovascular and Respiratory Networks

How Do You Get an Artery Blockage in the First Place?

As we've seen, contributing factors include hypertension (high blood pressure), hypercholesterolemia (too much cholesterol in the blood stream), arteriosclerosis (hardening of the arteries), and atherosclerosis (clogging of the arteries). Many times, an actual heart attack occurs when plaque (cholesterol, fats, and other substances), which has collected on artery walls, narrowing the blood flow, suddenly crack, or ulcerate, and combine with clot formation to create a sudden blockage.

When a heart attack does strike, it can come in a broad range of ways. On the lowest end of the scale, a heart attack can be so small it's hardly felt (called a "silent" heart attack), with the outward symptoms passing so quickly that the whole experience is dismissed as just another case of indigestion, heart burn, or angina. But be warned, just as a spark can cause a forest fire, so too a "small" heart attack can cause death. On the highest end of the scale, a heart attack can be so massive that the victim is dead before his face hits the soup bowl. Most heart attacks fall somewhere between these two extremes.

Possible Signs You're Having a Heart Attack

- Any pain, from the navel to the ears, but typically, in front and not caused by anything in particular, *might* be an indication of a heart attack.

- Chest-area pain that lasts longer than fifteen minutes or is not affected by antacids or angina medicine such as nitroglycerin. Remember, indigestion pain usually goes away once you get up, walk around a bit, and take an antacid. So if the pain hasn't faded soon after taking action for indigestion, it could quite possibly mean you're having a heart attack.

- In severe cases, pain that is so crushing that it takes your breath away, feels like someone is standing on your chest, or like a tight band around the chest. Normally, it starts in the chest and radiates out into the left arm, back, or shoulder. Sometimes the pain crosses to the other side of the body.

- A cold and clammy sweat.

- Nausea and/or vomiting.

- Shortness of breath.

If you experience any of those symptoms, especially in concert, you should call 911 or have them checked out by a physician.

One of the biggest problems with first-time heart attack sufferers—especially those in their fifties—is denial: "I can't be having a heart attack!" "I'm too young!" "It's only indigestion." "The pain will pass soon; then I'll be okay."

Unfortunately, this is the worst time to take a positive, upbeat approach to a problem—where's that negative, cynical outlook that many fifties males are famous for? In this case, it's actually healthy to assume the worst initially, because time is of the essence—it's been shown that half the people who die from a heart attack do so because the heart arrests within three to four hours of onset—meaning, of course, that the faster you receive proper medical care, the better.

What Happens When a Heart Attack Strikes

By way of illustration, the following is a step-by-step outline of what might happen. It starts in bed because that's where many heart attacks happen. They often occur in the wee hours of morning (2 to 5 A.M.), when adrenaline starts pumping into the system to prepare the body for the coming day, which increases the workload of the heart. This means that you will have gone to sleep without any inkling of what's to come. Suddenly, you:

Wake up with a chest pain that feels like the old indigestion kicking in. Don't automatically think it's just from the heavy meal you ate a few hours ago. You're a little surprised to find you have a clammy sweat all over. You decide to:

Get up, take some antacid tablets with water and sit up in a chair for a few minutes to see if the symptoms go away. After about ten to fifteen minutes, you start to:

Worry, because the pain hasn't gone away. In fact, while it's still in your chest, it also seems to be spreading a little to your neck and right arm. You're thankful it's not your left arm, because you think it has to be your left arm to be a heart attack (a *wrong* assumption). After a few more minutes of sitting in the dark, contemplating your situation, you finally:

Commit to the fact that this is a heart attack. Now in quick succession you:

Take one aspirin of 325 mg.

The Cardiovascular and Respiratory Networks

Wake up your partner. You might need help sooner than you think.

Call 911, because this is no time to drive yourself or have your partner drive you to the hospital. Today's ambulances are, to a certain degree, mobile intensive-care units, and the paramedics are trained professionals. They can stabilize a situation that could be fatal if you decided to get yourself to the hospital.

Treatment/Prevention. When the paramedics arrive, they will immediately get you on oxygen, check your vital signs (pulse, breathing, physical appearance), and hook you up to some monitors to see what's happening. Assuming it is a heart attack, they'll be doing their job at the same time they're transporting you to a hospital emergency room.

The usual emergency room procedure is to rush you to the cardiac area, where the first priority will be to stabilize your condition.

Emergency Room Procedures for a Heart Attack

- Continue the oxygen, recheck your vital signs, and assess quickly your general status, including your heart rhythm.

- Draw blood and hook you up to an EKG machine (both used to diagnose the attack and its severity).

- Conduct blood tests for higher than normal enzyme levels (done several times over several hours), which will tell if there's been heart muscle damage.

- Administer clot-busting drugs, or thrombolytics, to break up the clot, restore blood flow, and prevent any further damage to the heart muscle. These drugs are much more effective when given within two hours of a heart attack. They will *not* be given if it's been more than six hours since the start of the heart attack, because by then the clot will have solidified so much that the drug will be ineffective and might even cause bleeding elsewhere.

- Administer a beta-blocker drug, which slows the heart and causes it to beat less forcefully.

- Give you pain killers, blood pressure medications, or other drugs, depending on your condition.

If your condition is that unstable, you might undergo a cardiac catheterization and angiogram, or "heart cath." This is a surgical technique where a tiny tube is inserted in the artery of your groin and fed all the way up into your blocked artery. At the site of blockage, either a balloon at the end of the tube is inflated to flatten the clot against the artery walls, or a "stent" (a woven piece of wire tube) is inserted. In either case the artery is reopened. While the procedure is going on, the cardiologist can also take blood samples and determine heart-chamber pressure.

In the most severe heart attacks, emergency heart bypass surgery is done, although this is happening less often as heart attack procedures improve. Heart bypass surgery is "open heart" surgery, where your chest is cracked open and where sections of blood vessels taken from your legs or chest wall are grafted around any blocked sections of the coronary arteries so that blood will flow freely to your heart again. Angioplasty techniques (see details below) have eliminated the need for some major open heart operations.

Once your condition has stabilized, it's time to begin the long and sometimes laborious process of finding out just what caused the attack and what needs to be done next. The first order of business is rest, which will relieve some of the stress that might have brought on the attack.

Depending on the severity of the attack and your physical condition, you might be in the hospital for only a few days, but during that time, expect a multitude of tests, exams, and procedures—all of which are designed to help you, although they might not seem like that at the time. Even after you've been released from the hospital, the tests will go on until the doctors have all the answers they need to determine what happens next.

Tests that Might Be Given after a Heart Attack

Angiography—This is a process by which dye is injected in your blood vessels and an X ray shows any blockages. From this, a determination is made whether or not the blockages would respond best to drug therapy or to angioplasty. If you did not have an emergency catheterization done when you were in the emergency room, then very soon after your condition is stabilized, you may have an angiography.

EKG—or electrocardiogram, is a graphic recording of the electrical activity of the heart. With it, doctors can detect abnormalities in the transmission of the cardiac impulse through the heart muscle, which can indicate various heart ailments. You will probably have numerous EKGs taken, starting at the onset of your attack and throughout the recuperation period.

The Cardiovascular and Respiratory Networks

Stress Test—the heart attack patient (or someone believed to have heart problems) walks on a treadmill while being hooked up to an EKG and monitored by medical staff. It is an excellent diagnostic tool that's administered under carefully controlled conditions. It will likely be repeated several times during your convalescence and at least yearly for an indefinite period of time. It may be combined with imaging studies such as a heart scan or an echocardiogram.

By using any one or more of these exams and procedures, the doctors will be able to tell how much—if any—permanent damage has been done to the heart muscle. The degree of permanent damage (from nearly nonexistent to severe) will dictate recovery time and what life will be like after the heart attack.

Life after a Heart Attack

If you have no permanent heart muscle damage and you turn your life around—meaning you stop smoking, lose weight, reduce stress, eat right, and exercise—then you have an excellent chance of making a full and complete recovery and being healthier than you were before the attack. The bottom line is that if you suffer a heart attack, you *will* have another unless you eliminate the risk factors that caused it.

If, however, you have lost some heart tissue, the amount and type lost will dictate how drastically your life *must* change (or you'll be revisiting the emergency room very soon). These can include major changes—changes that you might never have thought possible, such as quitting smoking or cutting fats from your diet, but that seem easier to handle once you've survived a heart attack.

In the no-heart-damage scenario, the patient walks out of the hospital with a "perfect" heart, although his arteries certainly aren't perfect; that's how he got the heart attack in the first place. In the damaged-heart scenario, the patient now has two strikes against him—an imperfect heart and bad arteries. In the first case, lifestyle changes are not absolutely necessary (although if they're not made, look out somewhere down the road); in the second case, lifestyle changes are mandatory.

In either case, turning your life around will make a world of difference. Unfortunately, as we all know from personal experience, human nature is such that people don't usually embrace change unless there are direct consequences associated with the changes. One of the few positive elements to a heart attack is that it's usually a sufficiently serious consequence to motivate change in people—there's something about counting the holes in the ceiling tiles of the coronary care unit that concentrates your mind on lifestyle changes.

One question that is usually on the minds of most male heart attack sufferers is: Will the excitement of sex bring on another heart attack? Check with your doctor, and definitely don't attempt sex the day after a heart attack, but, otherwise, having sex with your regular partner is usually fine. That can't always be said for sex as part of an affair—the additional stress and tension that's usually associated with having an affair can put an unreasonable burden on a post-heart-attack heart. (Another good example of how honesty with your doctor can be critical to your health.) An interesting statistic that might put the whole sex-after-a-heart-attack question into perspective: You have about a one in 50,000 chance of causing another heart attack by having sex—those are approximately the same odds of having another heart attack from getting out of bed in the morning.

Prevention of heart attacks involves some very straightforward changes—all of which should be fully discussed with your doctor before they're implemented.

Elements of Heart Attack Prevention

- A healthy diet low in fats and salt (see chapter8 for diet details).

- Possibly, medications to lower cholesterol and/or stabilize plaque.

- A complete exercise program that includes, aerobics, stretching, and strengthening (see chapter 8 for exercise details).

- An aspirin a day (see the aspirin sidebar in this chapter) reduces the chances of a second heart attack by 40 percent.

- The use of a beta-blocker drug—in a fairly small dose—to reduce the incidence of a second heart attack by 30 or 40 percent.

- Moderate drinking (see the drinking sidebar in this chapter).

- Reducing stress. This is critical. Somehow you must find a way to tame this unwanted beast in your life. That might mean yoga, relaxation therapy, maybe a mild antidepressant, or simply deep breathing whenever anything starts getting to you.

Prevention also includes avoiding certain heart attack-inducing activities. The leader by far is the exertion of snow shoveling, which attracts heart attacks like trailer parks attract tornadoes.

Why Snow-Shoveling Causes Heart Attacks

- Cold weather stimulates blood vessel constriction, which drives up blood pressure.

- Upper body exercise and contraction of muscles stimulates blood-vessel constriction, which drives up blood pressure.

CAN IT REALLY HELP?
AN ASPIRIN A DAY

Numerous studies show that most men over fifty—and definitely those who have had a heart attack—benefit from taking an aspirin a day (81 mg for healthy men as prevention; 325 mg for those with diagnosed heart disease). Taking 325 mg during a heart attack is tremendously helpful. Consult your doctor before starting a daily regimen, because the use of aspirin by healthy individuals for heart prevention is somewhat controversial and is not safe for everyone; some studies show an increase in the risk of stroke or bleeding with daily aspirin use.

For those who can—and should—take aspirin, it can be plain or buffered (to protect against stomach upset). Take it at the same time every day, preferably after a meal. Don't take it just before bedtime, because it might cause stomach upset or even an ulcer.

Benefits of taking an aspirin a day include:

- Reduction in the risk of both heart attack and stroke by preventing blood clots.

- Reduction in the risk of colon cancer.

- Possible prevention of cataracts.

An aspirin taken as soon as you think your chest pain is more than just indigestion will retard the already-started clotting process and quite possibly save your life. It works by inhibiting platelets (the tiny cells behind blood clotting). While clotting is good in most circumstances, in heart disease and heart attacks it can be fatal. The one aspirin taken during a heart attack keeps the clotting blood from totally solidifying, so that when you do reach the hospital the procedures you might undergo (drug therapy and angioplasty) will have the best possible chances of success.

- Muscle demands for more oxygen and nutrients stimulate extra heart pumping, which drives up blood pressure.

- The heart's workload is dramatically increased by this unfortunate sequence of events.

Put it all together, and it's ground zero for that tornado. You might keep this in mind the next time your neighbor's kid offers to shovel your walk—there are much better, healthier, safer ways to get your exercise.

Arrhythmia (Irregular Heartbeat)

At one time or another, we've all felt our heart shift gears, change speeds, or just flutter for a moment. These usually fleeting events are called arrhythmias—just a fancy word for your heart beating irregularly. Normal hearts can sometimes beat irregularly, often because of external situations (usually associated with "adrenaline rushes") such as seeing your soul mate for the first time, getting five out of six numbers in the lottery, or having a narrow miss on the highway. Stimulants such as caffeine and decongestants can also cause arrhythmias. The vast majority of these are harmless arrhythmias that are usually fleeting, have no symptoms, and disappear once the external stimulus has been removed—no harm, no foul.

There are other times, however, when an arrhythmia can have serious consequences, causing chest pain, lightheadedness, shortness of breath, or, in the worst case, a heart attack or stroke. These situations develop because the intricate flow of electrical impulses that stimulates the heart to beat properly has been disrupted. As a quick reminder, the heart has four chambers: the left atrium and right atrium, and the left ventricle and right ventricle. The two atria are like two small anterooms that don't have much pumping responsibility, while the larger right ventricle and the huge left ventricle do most of the pumping. Without a precise, coordinated set of electrical impulses to these four chambers, no pumping would take place.

Contributing Factors to Electrical Disruptions in the Heart

Age—the older we get the more likely an arrhythmia will occur. This is because our electrical pathways, or "wires," get a little frayed as we get older and can sometimes cause a kind of short circuit.

Coronary artery disease (clogging of the arteries)—in the process of damaging the heart muscle, it can also damage the heart's electrical system.

High blood pressure—can cause structural damage to the heart that affects the electrical flow as well.

Recreational drugs—such as cocaine and amphetamines can upset the electrical flow.

Other heart diseases—such as rheumatic heart disease and some other valve diseases.

Thyroid disease—both hyper- (overactivity of the thyroid) and hypo- (decreased activity of the thyroid) can create electrical disruptions.

Certain viral infections—can cause electrical disruptions.

The first three factors (age, coronary artery disease, and high blood pressure) can definitely be prevalent in many fifties men. This means there's a real potential for experiencing some sort of arrhythmia while in that age group. Bill Bradley, the ex-basketball player turned politician, is a perfect example of a healthy, fit fifties man who has had to deal with the problem off and on for many years.

The medical community has divided arrhythmias into three categories: fast, slow, and irregular (the latter can occur in combination: fast and irregular; slower and irregular, etc.). Each can have numerous causes, and each can come with or without symptoms.

Causes of fast heartbeat range from the perfectly normal and safe, to the dangerously abnormal and deadly.

Causes of Fast Heartbeat Arrhythmias

- **Exercise.** This generates a perfectly normal heart rhythm that happens to be fast for good reason—you're working out so your heart needs to beat faster to supply your muscles with oxygen and nutrients. It is only unacceptable—and dangerous—if your heart rate goes beyond 80 percent of your maximum rate (220 minus your age is your maximum heart rate; a rate that should *never* be reached).

- **Fever.** When you're sick and you have a fever, your heart beats faster, in part to help speed recovery. A slightly elevated heart rate while suffering a fever is normal.

- **Regular rhythm that's fast.** A heartbeat that's abnormal but regular and fast. It can come and go and is caused by an electrical short circuit that's usually congenital. Unless sustained for longer than a few minutes, it's usually nothing to worry about.

• **Atrial fibrillation.** The most common chronic arrhythmia is atrial fibrillation, in which the electrical impulses originating in the left atrium and right atrium are disrupted. This electrical disruption causes the atria to "quiver" rather than contract in the synchronized way that they're supposed to, which can lead to potential problems, such as:

   1. Blood can pool in the atria, which makes clots more likely to occur and increases the risk of stroke due to an embolism (a piece of a clot migrating to and blocking a blood vessel in the brain). An embolism can also travel to other locations and do damage.

   2. Reduction of the filling pressure from the atria to the two ventricles, which leads to reduced heart output (less blood at less pressure).

   3. Unorganized electrical impulses getting to the ventricles, which disrupts their critical pumping pattern (see the next item for details).

• **Ventricular tachycardia.** Almost always associated with coronary artery disease, ventricular tachycardia is basically the too-fast beating of the two ventricles. This can produce a heart rate in the range of 150 to 200 beats a minute. (The normal range is 60 to 100). It's a dangerous and unstable situation, because the heart is not only beating fast but pumping inefficiently. Sometimes ventricular tachycardia will simply stop, and your heart will return to a normal rhythm, but in many other cases it turns into ventricular fibrillation, a long name for cardiac arrest or "sudden cardiac death." Can you tell the difference? Don't bother trying to—both ventricular tachycardia and atrial fibrillation are serious enough that you should seek medical help if you feel their symptoms: chest pain, lightheadedness, and/or shortness of breath.

Causes of Too Slow Heartbeat Arrhythmias

• **Exercise.** Yep, the same as too-fast heart rates. In this case, very athletic people can have such an efficient heart and good muscles that their resting heart rate can be as low as in the 30s. In these cases, their heart rate is normal and safe.

• **Disease.** Specifically, hypothyroid disease can cause the heart to beat slowly. Treating the disease cures the heart-rate problem.

- **Drugs.** Beta blockers (see the drug chart in this chapter for details) can cause the heart rate to drop below normal. This can be handled with little difficulty.

- **Disruption in the electrical impulses.** If there is a disruption in the nerve pathways that carry the electrical impulses to the heart, the rate can slow. The disruption can come from age—the frayed wires problem—and from damage due to coronary artery disease or a heart infection. The condition can cause symptoms such as fatigue, an intolerance to exercise, and occasionally fainting. Sometimes the condition is permanent, other times it's intermittent. In cases where the condition does cause persistent symptoms, a permanent pacemaker implanted surgically is necessary to keep the heart beating at a normal rate. The most common ailment that demands a pacemaker is "sick sinus syndrome," which falls into this arrhythmia category. This is where there is loss of reliable production of a normal heartbeat, primarily because of age and/or damage from coronary artery disease.

Irregular Heartbeat Arrhythmias

The third and last category of arrhythmias is irregular heartbeat arrhythmia. The most common of this type are called premature heartbeats. Originating in either the atria or the ventricles, they usually come and go harmlessly. They are the surprised or love-struck heartbeats that we've all experienced. Less common but more dangerous are irregular heartbeats that lead to atrial fibrillation (see above).

From studying all the various kinds of arrythmias within the three categories, it's obvious that the two most potentially dangerous are atrial fibrillation and ventricular tachycardia. A word of warning: If you begin to feel symptoms such as a fluttering sensation in the chest or neck, chest pain, fatigue, and/or lightheadedness, don't spend time trying to decide which kind of arrhythmia you have. Severe arrhythmias should be treated as seriously as a heart attack (which might be right behind them), so medical attention should be sought immediately.

Treatment/Prevention. As mentioned before, minor arrhythmias caused by external situations or elements are usually not treated, because they take care of themselves quickly.

For atrial fibrillation, treatment usually involves drugs, which can control the heart rate and can sometimes cause the rhythm to revert to normal. It may be necessary, however, to use a defibrillator to electrically shock the heart back into its normal rhythm. Chronic atrial fibrillation requires the use of an anticoagulant (blood thinner) to reduce the higher risk of stroke associated with it.

For ventricular tachycardia, once the initial crisis has been handled with drugs, a defibrillator surgically implanted in the chest may be required.

While prevention of most arrhythmias is somewhat difficult because of their seemingly random onset, generally speaking, good heart-care measures—exercise, good diet, and monitoring and/or maintenance of blood pressure and cholesterol—are the best line of defense.

Stroke

Like a heart attack, a stroke is an interruption of blood flow, but a stroke is an interruption of blood to the brain, not the heart muscle. To help people understand stroke better, the National Stroke Association is promoting the term "brain attack" because of the condition's similarity to heart attack. The actual blood flow interruption occurs in one or more of the four arteries that feed the brain.

Possible Blood Flow Interruptions

Thrombus—a blood clot within an intact blood vessel. It's usually brought on by long-term buildup of fatty deposits (such as cholesterol) found in the diseases hypercholesterolemia (high cholesterol) and atherosclerosis (clogging of the arteries), and by the constant pounding that comes with hypertension (high blood pressure).

Embolus—also a blood clot, but one that has formed elsewhere in the body, broken away, and travels to the brain. Common sources of stroke-causing emboli are diseased carotid (neck) arteries and, sometimes, problems within the heart itself.

Hemorrhage—another name for a burst blood vessel—blood leaks out of the blood vessel and into the brain. Many times this can be due to an inherent weakness in a blood vessel, usually present from birth that suddenly pops (this falls into the "shit happens" category). The bursting can be aided, however, by such diseases as hypertension (high blood pressure), hypercholesterolemia (high cholesterol), and atherosclerosis (clogging of the arteries).

Strokes brought on by a thrombosis or an embolism are known as ischemic strokes. They account for 80 percent of all strokes. The other 20 percent are hemorrhagic strokes, caused by the bursting of a blood vessel in the brain.

No matter what the cause, the effects of a stroke can vary widely, with no two strokes being exactly alike. A mild stroke can leave few permanent or serious side effects. Many strokes, however, are not that forgiving. That's because your brain uses about 25 percent of the total oxygen your lungs take in, and that oxygen can only get to the brain via the blood, so any interruption—even for the shortest period of time—can have devastating results. Depending upon the degree of stroke and the part of the brain affected, the victim can permanently lose motion in parts of his body (usually on one side only) and the ability to speak. In the worst case, a stroke can kill.

Currently, stroke is the leading cause of disability in America, as well as the third leading cause of death (behind heart disease and cancer). According to the American Heart Association, 600,000 Americans suffer a new or another stroke every year.

American Heart Association Risk Factors for Stroke

- High blood pressure (as low as 130-139 systolic) is the most important risk factor associated with stroke

- High cholesterol levels

- Coronary artery disease

- Family history

- High red-blood-cell count (which encourages the development of clots)

- Recurring or chronic atrial fibrillation (see previous explanation)

- Cigarette smoking

- Lack of exercise

- Too much salt in the diet

- Excess weight

The good news is that a stroke is a very rare event in fifties men, although it is more prevalent in men than in women. Normally, in the healthy population, strokes are now confined to people in their seventies and beyond. This wasn't always the case. Until about forty years ago, stroke—along with heart attack—was a significant contributor to death in the sixth decade. But because of a better understanding of stroke, by both the medical community and the public, screenings (such as cholesterol and blood pressure checks) have become routine, drugs have been developed to stem arterial degeneration and to lower high blood pressure, and the public has become aware of how important diet, exercise, and non-smoking are to keeping arteries healthy.

In fact, pushing back stroke to the last few decades of life has been one of science's great success stories. Since the early 1960s, the incidence of stroke is down approximately 60 or 70 percent. Only two generations ago, most Americans would have had at least one parent or grandparent who had suffered a stroke in their fifties. Today, that just doesn't happen. Overall, in all age groups, the risk of dying from a stroke is now less than half of what it was only twenty years ago.

Treatment/Prevention. Once a stroke is suspected, call 911 immediately. Transport to an emergency room should be prompt. Within the first four hours, thrombolytic drugs (clot busters) may be able to reduce damage. A long convalescence is often required. Stroke rehab, including occupational therapy and sometimes speech therapy, can significantly reduce long-term disability.

Prevention, in this case, is critical. As usual, that includes a healthy diet low in fats and salt, a good exercise program, periodic checks of your cholesterol levels and blood pressure, and, if warranted, drugs to control either high blood pressure or high cholesterol levels. Smoking cessation is essential.

Kidney Failure

The incidence of kidney failure because of a deterioration or blockage in the renal arteries feeding the kidneys is very rare—especially in fifties men. Normally, other arteries, such as the heart or brain arteries, would show signs of deterioration and create symptoms long before the renal arteries would. This kind of kidney failure is usually a complication of high blood pressure and/or congestive heart failure due to coronary artery disease. All of the contributing factors and effects of hardening of the arteries and clogging of the arteries apply to renal artery deterioration (see chapter 4 for kidney details).

Treatment/Prevention. Treatment is the same as with any other arterial disease: Depending upon the patient, one of a number of drugs would be used to control blood pressure and/or lower cholesterol levels, while the patient would be encouraged to maintain a healthy diet low in fats, salt, potassium, and protein, and to begin a comprehensive exercise routine. Medical supervision to avoid the use of certain medications (including nonprescription drugs—especially NSAIDs) that may worsen kidney function is important.

Another treatment is dialysis, a medical procedure for filtering waste products from the blood of kidney-disease patients. Dialysis is used for buying time in the case of an individual who has irreversible kidney failure and is waiting for a kidney transplant.

Prevention is exactly the same as with other arterial diseases: healthy diet, good exercise routine, and meticulous control of high blood pressure.

The Cardiovascular and Respiratory Networks

Blood Clots and Aneurysms

Throughout this chapter's section on the heart and blood vessels, blood clots and aneurysms have been mentioned only as the immediate causes of heart attack and stroke. Because of their importance, and the very serious consequences they sometimes entail, they deserve their own section—although it should be noted that life-threatening blood clots and aneurysms are unusual.

BLOOD CLOTS

Scientifically speaking, a blood clot forms when blood turns from a liquid into a semisolid gelatinous mass. The mass is comprised of red and white blood cells, disc-shaped smaller elements called platelets, and an insoluble protein called fibrin. Normally, when the body senses that there has been a break or cut in any part of the circulatory system, blood clotting occurs as a way of repairing the damage and stopping the flow of blood. This, as we all know, is why we don't bleed to death when we get a paper cut.

Additionally, blood clotting can take place even in an intact blood vessel. In healthy blood vessels, the inner lining, or endothelium, is very smooth, allowing for easy and unrestricted flow of blood. If, however, the blood vessels begin to deteriorate—as a result of such ailments as hypertension (high blood pressure), hypercholesterolemia (high cholesterol), arteriosclerosis (hardening of the arteries), or atherosclerosis (clogging of the arteries)— that inner lining loses its smoothness and becomes rough, even jagged, in places.

The rough or sharp edges inside the blood vessel cause the blood to clot around those edges to try and smooth them out. As blood vessel deterioration continues, arterial narrowing occurs, becoming more obstructive to the normal flow of blood. At some point, at the site of the roughened, narrowed arterial wall, clotting may occur. The affected blood vessel will then go from being restricted to suddenly being completely blocked. If the sudden blockage takes place in a coronary (heart) artery, it results in a heart attack; if the blockage takes place in a brain artery, it results in a stroke, or brain attack.

There are two categories of blood clots that are defined by where they are located:

1. **Blood Clots in Arteries**—A blood clot in an artery is known as an arterial thrombus and usually occurs because of arteriosclerosis (hardening of the arteries). Such a clot causes problems by restricting or cutting off blood flow "downstream" from where it's lodged. This damming of blood flow can cause such serious problems as a heart attack (if the thrombus is in a heart artery)

or a stroke (if the thrombus is in a brain artery). Making matters worse, if a piece of an arterial thrombus breaks off and floats away, it's called an embolus. If an embolus ends up in the brain, it too can cause a stroke.

2. **Blood Clots in Veins**—A blood clot in a vein is called a venous thrombus. It can interrupt blood flow that's returning from the outer reaches of the body to the heart. Such a blood clot can cause swelling of a leg or an arm. Just like with arterial blood clots, a venous thrombus can have a piece break off and float away. The broken off piece is also called an embolus. If this venous embolus travels to the lungs, it becomes a pulmonary embolus, which can cause severe disability or even sudden death.

One of the most common causes of a pulmonary embolus in healthy individuals is prolonged sitting, such as on airplane flights longer than two to four hours, during which circulation in the legs is slowed or becomes restricted. It is important to try to stand up and walk around every hour or so during a flight or anytime you're sitting for long periods. If this is impossible, take a few minutes every hour or so to stretch out each leg, rotate the foot as much as possible, and/or clench and re-clench the foot, calf, and thigh muscles as a way of promoting circulation.

If, in the three or four days after the flight, your leg or foot swells up, and you feel a pain in any of your leg muscles (and you haven't been straining or exercising them), this might mean you have a clot in the veins of your leg. If the pain is in your calf and seems to get worse when you pull your toes back toward you, you should see a doctor immediately. In fact, any pain within any extremity (such as an arm) that is accompanied by swelling should be checked out.

The reason for concern is that if a piece of the blood clot breaks, forming an embolus (as mentioned previously), it can travel through your circulatory system and possibly lodge in your lungs (a pulmonary embolus) and cause severe disability or death. In some cases, death is nearly instantaneous—not such a bad way to go, but if you're only in your fifties, it means you'll miss out on a lot of good living.

ANEURYSMS

Besides blood clots, there are aneurysms. An aneurysm is a ballooning out of a blood vessel—usually the main artery called the aorta, but many times the brain arteries as well—due to a weakening of its walls. This weakness is usually caused by hypertension (high blood pressure), atherosclerosis (clogging of the arteries), or is congenital, but the weakness can also be caused by injury or even infection. Aortic aneurisms are strongly associated with cigarette smoking.

The Cardiovascular and Respiratory Networks

Aneurysms are dangerous when they rupture; escaping blood causes severe tissue damage and cell death in the affected area, resulting in a stroke (brain aneurysm) or severe blood loss (aortic aneurysm). In fact, a ruptured aneurysm can cause nearly instantaneous death. While a ruptured aneurysm happens much more often in people who are seventy and older, it isn't an unheard of event in fifties males.

Treatment/Prevention. For proven arterial blood clots, a range of treatments is available. If life- (or limb-) threatening, surgery can sometimes be done. If the situation is less grave, a "clot buster" drug can be given. For even less severe arterial clots, a blood-thinning drug is usually prescribed, with the recommendation not to do any strenuous exercise (which might dislodge the clot) for a week.

For clots in veins, hospitalization for five to seven days used to be the standard, but with newer forms of blood thinners, this has begun to change.

As to prevention of dangerous clots: Clots are one of the reasons why it is now recommended that most men over fifty take aspirin regularly. Aspirin helps to thin the blood, which protects against overzealous clotting (see the aspirin sidebar on page 101 for details).

An aneurysm that bursts in the wrong place often means death or severe disability, although, with prompt (usually surgical) intervention, the incidence of death or disability decreases.

As to prevention of aneurysms: Many people feel that a burst aneurysm falls into the category of "shit happens." Since an aneurysm is a weakness of a blood vessel wall that can't be felt until it bursts, there is a certain validity to this opinion. Generally speaking, though, trying to prevent or lessen the effects of high blood pressure and/or the clogging of arteries should go a long away toward decreasing your chances of a burst aneurysm.

Leg Pain (Claudication) and Varicose Veins

While most blood vessel ailments and diseases affect the upper half of the human body, there are two notable exceptions that take place in the body's lower half: claudication and varicose veins.

Claudication is a condition in which the muscles in your legs don't get enough oxygen and nutrients when called upon to function. This translates into leg pain and cramps when you exercise or walk, especially uphill, but disappears when you stop. (Leg pain or cramps that come on while at rest might simply mean dehydration, while a specific pain or sore spot in the calf muscle might be a strained muscle; a pinched nerve, as with a disc; or possibly a more serious blood clot, detailed previously.)

With claudication, the legs aren't getting enough fuel for exercise, because the blood flow feeding the legs is restricted due to narrowed arteries. Contributing factors can be high blood pressure, diabetes, high cholesterol, hardening of the arteries, and/or clogging of the arteries.

Another major contributing factor to claudication is smoking. Even if you stopped smoking many years before, claudication can still develop. (See the smoking section in chapter 8 for details.)

As for varicose veins, those swollen, tortured and twisted looking bulges that stick out from your legs mean that there are abnormalities or deterioration in the valves of your leg veins. Because the valves are not properly stopping backward blood flow, blood pools in certain areas and then swells the vein. Symptoms include pain, muscle cramps, and a feeling of heaviness in the legs. More prevalent in women than in men, varicose veins are also strongly linked to pregnancy, obesity, and congenitally weak valves.

Treatment/Prevention. Claudication usually requires a visit to a vascular surgeon, who will suggest one or more of the following treatments: stopping risk-factor behaviors (such as smoking), exercising, and/or undergoing balloon angioplasty or surgical bypass. For less severe cases, certain medications can marginally improve arterial circulation to the leg.

With varicose veins, elevating the legs and the use of elastic stockings can often help, but severe cases may require surgery to obliterate or remove the affected varicose veins.

Other Forms of Heart Disease

Besides the heart diseases mentioned above, there are other cardiovascular ailments. These include valvular heart disease, congestive heart failure (also called dropsy or edema), congenital heart defects, heartbeat irregularities, heart muscle diseases, and pericardial disease (the latter refers to the sac that protects the heart). All of these are so unusual in fifties men that they are only worth this quick mention. A triumph of modern medicine is the near elimination of heart-valve disease due to rheumatic fever (caused by a virulent strain of strep throat), because of the development of antibiotics.

SECTION TWO: THE RESPIRATORY SYSTEM

The respiratory tract is a set of organs, structures, and muscles that enable you to breathe. It is broken into two portions: the upper respiratory tract, which consists of the throat, the nose, and an extensive labyrinth of nasal passages, sinuses and airways; and the lower respiratory tract, which consists of the lungs.

The lungs are a pair of highly elastic and spongy organs made up of sections, or lobes (three in the right, two in the left), with the left lung being slightly smaller than the right so the heart can be accommodated. When we breathe—which is about every five seconds or nearly 17,000 times a day—air is fed to the lungs from the throat via two bronchial tubes (one for each lung). The bronchial tubes lead to smaller and smaller tubes (numbering nearly 250,000) that spiderweb out into the lungs until they end in tiny air sacs, or alveoli (numbering an incredible 300 million or so). The alveoli are where oxygen is transferred to the blood in exchange for the waste product carbon dioxide.

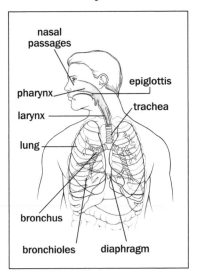

For the all important oxygen/carbon dioxide transfer to function properly, there must be a great deal of alveoli surface area. You'll be surprised at how much there is: If you could spread out all the alveoli in the healthy lungs of a young man, they would equal, incredibly, the size of a tennis court.

Why do we need such a large and extensive respiratory system? Why don't we just have blow holes in our chests?

The answer is that we're warm-blooded, land-dwelling mammals who need to maintain a narrow body temperature range (normally 96 to 100 degrees Fahrenheit) and a certain moisture level in our body's center, or core. Our internal organs and systems could not survive direct contact with most of what the outside world has to offer. That goes double for the lungs, which lie at the core of our bodies. Their intricate latticework of tiny air sacs would dry up like raisins if they came into direct contact with dry, hot desert air, while they'd probably flash-freeze the moment subzero arctic air hit them.

None of that happens because our extensive respiratory tract moderates and adjusts incoming air—both its temperature and moisture—before it reaches our lungs. As air enters your mouth and/or nose (the upper respiratory tract), it travels over and through warm, moist passageways that make the air more compatible with your inner body.

Simultaneously, the upper respiratory tract also protects our bodies from airborne pollutants, bacteria, and viruses that can cause illness, disease, and even death. The first line of defense is to trap irritants such as dust and microbes before they get very far into the respiratory system. This job is achieved in part by mucus, which contains antibodies to help fight infections; and cilia, tiny hairlike projections that line most walls of the respiratory system. The mucus and cilia work in concert: The mucus collars any foreign bodies, then the cilia, with their wavy action, move the now-contaminated mucus up into the throat where it's either swallowed or expelled by a cough, a sneeze or blowing of the nose. Even your nose hairs get into the act, snagging a lot of the larger air pollutants, then sending them packing through sneezing and nose blowing.

Because of the delicate nature of each element of the respiratory system, there are numerous ways it can break down. Of course, this isn't anything new—by the time we've reached our fifties, we've all experienced at least a few of these problems.

How Our Respiratory System Can Temporarily Fail

• Infections by bacteria and/or viruses can take place in the respiratory system.

• If the infection is in the upper respiratory tract, or has started there, it can be a common cold, sore throat, sinusitis, tonsillitis, strep throat, or influenza.

• Infections of the lower respiratory tract (the lungs) can mean bronchitis and pneumonia.

• Ailments such as the flu (influenza) can start in the upper respiratory tract but quickly spread into the lower tract.

• Respiratory problems not started by viral or bacterial infections include allergies (such as hay fever), asthma (also called reactive airways disease), emphysema, and chronic bronchitis—all four of which are known as obstructive lung diseases because they're associated with an obstruction of airflow when breathing out.

• Generally speaking, because numerous symptoms or effects of many respiratory illnesses are similar, the lines between them can blur. Some of the illnesses can happen at the same time (such as emphysema and chronic bronchitis) or can aid in the development of others (long-term allergies can lead eventually to emphysema), challenging the diagnostic skills of physicians.

Chronic lung diseases such as asthma, chronic bronchitis, and emphysema kill millions of people a year worldwide.

Amid the numerous and potentially deadly respiratory problems, there is some good news. When the lungs and respiratory system are healthy, they can last for a very long time. It is true that age does decrease the lungs' elasticity and capacity, but there is usually no need for healthy lungs—even those that have reached 100 and beyond—to require breathing aids such as extra oxygen. If you take care of your lungs, they'll keep working relatively well your entire life.

So, how should your lungs be performing in your fifties?

The Cardiovascular and Respiratory Networks

In terms of physical fitness, your lungs and respiratory system represent your "wind" or endurance. Whereas speed, quickness, and strength rely to a large degree on the musculoskeletal system—and therefore peak in the early to mid twenties—endurance continues on beyond that. Well into your thirties your lungs should still be working at nearly peak capacity. By the early forties, their elasticity and capacity will begin to diminish. By the time you've reached fifty, your lungs may be about 75 percent of what they were when you were thirty-five (with considerable individual variations, and taking smoking out of the equation).

For those who have never thought of themselves as athletic, or never consciously tried to stay in shape, there is good news related to your lungs. If, in your fifties, you "get religion" about fitness and maintain proper exercise routines (as well as good eating habits), you'll find that your endurance may be better than when you were in your thirties. While, strictly speaking, you cannot improve your lung capacity—the way your alveoli (tiny air sacs) transfer oxygen to the blood—you can improve breathing efficiency. This occurs when the newly conditioned muscles of your chest and diaphragm (the muscular partition that divides the chest from the abdomen) provide better inhaling and exhaling, while other newly conditioned muscles throughout your body utilize oxygen better. All of this translates into feeling better and having more endurance during physical exertion.

Lung Cancer

This is one of the most common forms of cancer and is explained in greater ßdetail in chapter 7. Suffice it to say here, however, that the number one cause of lung cancer is smoking (see the smoking section in chapter 8 for details), with other air pollutants such as asbestos and coal dust running distant seconds.

Treatment/Prevention. Treatment depends on the type of cancer, where it's located, and how far it's advanced, but it usually includes surgery, chemotherapy, and/or radiotherapy.

As to prevention, that's easy: Quit smoking, if you haven't already.

Emphysema and Chronic Bronchitis (Obstructive Lung Diseases)

Here is a perfect example of two different respiratory illnesses having similar effects.

Emphysema is a condition of the lungs in which the alveoli are continually overinflated, which ultimately leads to a breakdown of their walls and a decrease in their respiratory function. Causes include smoking, other airborne irritants, heredity, old age, and even other obstructive lung diseases (such as allergies and chronic bronchitis).

Chronic bronchitis, on the other hand, is the continual and long-term inflammation of the bronchial tubes. The inflammation will narrow the airway passages, cause spasm of the bronchial tubes, and increased production of mucus, which further narrows the pathways. Causes can include smoking, other airborne irritants, and recurrent infections—most notably bronchitis.

While the internal workings of emphysema and chronic bronchitis are different, the results are the same—shortness of breath that can range from mild to life-threatening and a cough that never goes away. With chronic bronchitis there is the additional problem of excess mucus production (the body's way of trying to lessen the inflammation). Rarely do doctors see a pure case of emphysema or a pure case of chronic bronchitis—usually it's some mixture of the two.

As both conditions worsen—becoming what's known as chronic obstructive lung disease (COLD) or chronic obstructive pulmonary disease (COPD)—the sufferer loses the ability to move air rapidly and, with the breakdown of the alveoli (those tiny air sacs), loses a huge amount of surface area needed to exchange oxygen. That tennis court of alveoli surface area is now about the size of a handball court.

Happily, men in their fifties who have never smoked or have quit more than fifteen years before have little risk of contracting either illness. Unfortunately, those who are still smoking or have only quit in recent years (see the smoking section in chapter 8 for details) can already be exhibiting some early signs of both respiratory conditions. Normally, though, it's in the sixties and seventies that these two killers begin taking their tolls.

Treatment/Prevention. There is no cure for emphysema or chronic bronchitis. Currently, the best that medicine can do is to: (1) slow or nearly stop the respiratory deterioration by removing the causes (smoking or other airborne pollutants); and (2) treat the symptoms. Shortness of breath in mild cases can be treated with hand-held spray inhalers to open bronchial tubes, while in severe cases full-time oxygen use might be necessary. Overproduction of mucus can be treated with hydration and mucus-thinning medication. Chronic infections can be treated with antibiotics (less often now than in the past), and chronic inflammation and spasm of the bronchial tubes are often treated with cortisone-like medications.

Before chronic bronchitis has set in, most cases of bronchitis are viral and, in nonsmokers, often clear up without much treatment. For smokers, however, antibiotics are usually required.

Prevention of both emphysema and chronic bronchitis involves general fitness as well as keeping air pollutants out of your respiratory system. If you are a smoker, remember—it's never too late to quit.

YOU'LL NEVER CONQUER THIS HILL:
HOW A TREADMILL TEST WORKS

A treadmill is a machine with an adjustable moving platform to simulate various kinds of walking and running—everything from strolling along a flat track to jogging up a steep hill. It can be set at such an extreme angle and speed that no person, no matter how physically fit, can "max" it out. It's a hill that's never going to be conquered.

Doctors use a treadmill to screen and test people under physically demanding conditions, because some ailments don't show themselves while a person is at rest. Those who are tested usually have a variety of risk factors for particular diseases, most notably heart disease. While the person is walking in a treadmill test, his vital signs (pulse, heart rate, blood pressure, breathing), as well as his heart's electrical activity (via EKG machine), can be monitored constantly by staff who are trained to handle any medical crisis that might occur.

A treadmill test is often combined with a heart scan that maps the circulation to the heart muscle or a limited echocardiogram that detects abnormal heart-wall movement that may occur when the heart muscle is not getting enough blood.

WHAT TREADMILLS TEST FOR:

Blood pressure—to see if it goes up too high when a person is exercising, which might indicate hypertension (high blood pressure) requiring treatment.

Diagnosis of Coronary Artery disease—in a person with chest pain of unknown cause, exercise-induced symptoms, EKG abnormalities, or other signs or symptoms of coronary artery disease.

Exercise Capacity—especially in someone with known heart disease or coronary artery disease.

Prognosis (prediction of what will come)—especially in someone with known heart disease or coronary artery disease.

Treatment assessment—especially post-heart attack, post-angioplasty, and post-cardiac surgery.

Screening—if you're in your fifties, have no symptoms, but have a number of cardiac risk factors (such as family history, cigarette smoking, hypertension, and high cholesterol), you might want to talk to your doctor about taking a treadmill test.

Asthma and Allergies

Because asthma and allergies usually rear their wheezing-and-stuffy-nosed heads long before the fifties, you probably already know if you suffer from either.

Asthma is a respiratory disorder that's characterized by periodic bouts of wheezing, coughing, overproduction of mucus, and difficulty breathing. All of this is caused by inflammation and/or spasm of the bronchial tubes, which, in turn, is initially brought on by infection, exercise, stress, or exposure to an allergen (any substance that can cause such a reaction). The World Health Organization reports that approximately 135 million people suffer from asthma.

An allergy is a hypersensitivity reaction to an allergen that, for most people, is basically harmless (e.g., animal hair, dust, and pollen). As most know, allergies are very common. Some reports say that more than 15 percent of the U.S. population suffers from some kind of allergy. Symptoms can vary widely, but most commonly they include overproduction of mucus (a stuffy or runny nose, or productive cough), inflammation and/or spasming of the bronchial tubes, itchy eyes, and skin rash.

•**Treatment/Prevention.** During an asthma or allergy attack, treating the symptoms is the first course of action. In the case of asthma this means use of a bronchial inhaler to open up the airways and corticosteroids to decrease the bronchial inflammation. Mild allergies are usually handled with over-the-counter antihistamines; more severe cases might need prescription antihistamines. For both ailments, staying clear of the offending substance (if known) is the best way of preventing attacks, as in not smoking.

Allergy shots to desensitize the individual to the offending substance are helpful for some. Chronic asthma requires long-term management with, among other measures, inhaled cortisone.

Common Cold, Flu, and Pneumonia

A cold is a minor viral infection of the nasal passages, and we all know its symptoms: runny nose, watery eyes, and sometimes a sore throat. A cure has so far eluded science, primarily because a cold is caused by any number of viruses, which are unaffected by antibiotics. More an inconvenience than a serious affliction, a cold shouldn't be taken too lightly by fifties males, especially smokers, because it always has the potential of spreading to the lungs and transforming into a serious illness, such as bronchitis, sinusitis, or pneumonia.

The Cardiovascular and Respiratory Networks

Influenza, or flu, is blamed for a variety of aches, pains, and general maladies. Scientifically speaking, it is an acute and contagious virus-caused infection of the entire respiratory system. As those who have had it know, the symptoms can come on like an out-of-control locomotive, laying you out as flat as those pennies we used to put on railroad tracks. They include cold symptoms as well as a headache, sore throat, fever, cough, muscle aches, and general fatigue.

For healthy men in their fifties, the flu is usually not much worse than a cold. For the very young, the elderly (seventies and beyond), those who smoke, or those with weakened immune systems, the flu—and complications such as bacterial pneumonia—can be devastating to the point of death. Some of our parents, and definitely our grandparents, can attest to this, because they lived through the 1918–1919 worldwide flu epidemic that killed more than twenty million people. The last major outbreak of flu in America was in 1968, and scientists are continually warning us that another is due anytime. Even in nonepidemic years, 15,000 to 20,000 people die in America of influenza.

Pneumonia, like the flu, is a respiratory infection caused by bacteria, a virus, or a complication of a cold or flu. With pneumonia, the lungs' alveoli (tiny air sacs) become inflamed; symptoms include headache, fever, chills, cough, chest pain, overproduction of mucus, and, in advanced cases, difficulty breathing and rapid pulse. Most healthy men will recover from a bout of pneumonia with outpatient treatment (usually with antibiotics), but sometimes more severe cases can require hospitalization.

Treatment/Prevention. Because colds are caused by viruses that aren't affected by antibiotics, treatment is symptomatic, meaning the symptoms are dealt with, not the cause. So the order of the day is to rest, take pain relievers, drink more fluids, and, in the case of flu, take fever reducers. A cold usually runs its course in three to five days, while the flu can take up to a full week to beat.

Influenza can be successfully treated if one of several antiviral drugs is taken during the first forty-eight hours. The same drugs, used after exposure in an unimmunized person, can actually prevent the flu.

As for cold prevention, there are a number of measures that can be taken—from staying fit, eating right, and frequently washing your hands (to lessen the possibility of catching some wayward viruses), to taking vitamin supplements such as vitamin C and trying popular (but not yet fully tested) over-the-counter products like echinacea and zinc lozenges, which reportedly help prevent catching a cold and cut its severity if you already have one.

Flu prevention is much simpler and more scientific—get a flu vaccination every autumn, a few weeks before flu season begins. While the medical community strongly recommends that the young, the elderly, and those with weakened immune systems get a flu shot every year, there is no reason why everyone shouldn't get one. Common sense makes a strong case for taking a shot that might prevent eight to ten days of feeling miserable—and, no, it is not scientifically possible to contract the flu from a flu shot, although there is a small chance you might experience a few slight symptoms the day after the shot. Getting a shot can also keep you from spreading influenza to other higher risk people—such as an elderly parent or young child.

As for pneumonia prevention, one important step is to stop any other respiratory illness in its tracks before it has a chance to develop into pneumonia. Additionally, there is a pneumonia shot that is a vaccine against the most common bacterial cause of pneumonia (pneumococcus). While the shot is advertised as a life-long prevention, it's probably wise to get a second one after five or six years, as a booster. Those who should get one include the elderly and those at risk for respiratory problems.

REAL LIFE TALES

Number One: Sometimes the Best Self-Help Still Doesn't Help Hypertension

Tony is fifty-six years old, an airline employee, and a marathon runner. He is one of the leanest, fittest people around. About fifteen years ago he decided to make sure he was as fit and healthy as he thought he was, so he went in for a complete physical.

Much to his and the doctor's surprise, he had hypertension, or high blood pressure. It measured 160 over 110, when the average range is 120-129 over 80-84.

Tony could not believe the findings. He felt great. He was running better than ever and he just knew, with a certainty that matches the "can-finish" attitude of marathon runners, that the blood pressure reading must be wrong.

After numerous follow-up readings, his blood pressure still remained too high to be ignored. The doctor told Tony about the dangers of constant hypertension—how it contributes to hardening of the arteries (arteriosclerosis), clogging of the arteries (atherosclerosis), and a greater risk of ultimately suffering a heart attack and stroke. The lack of symptoms, the doctor said, was normal with hypertension; that's why it's commonly referred to as the "silent killer."

With Tony still in disbelief, the doctor put him on a treadmill, where his vital signs were monitored as he exercised. This wasn't the normal procedure, but it was a definitive way to convince Tony he had hypertension that had to be treated. True to hypertension, Tony's blood pressure skyrocketed way past the normal high range expected when exercising. The test was worth it, because it got Tony to admit he had a problem that had to be treated.

The Cardiovascular and Respiratory Networks

Being the self-disciplined individual that he is, though, Tony wanted to know what he could do to control his hypertension. The doctor explained that the usual culprits weren't present in his case: He wasn't overweight, he didn't smoke, and he was conscious of how much salt he ate. There was nothing further he could do, short of medication, to help his condition.

In this case, Tony has a glitch or maladjustment in the interrelationship among the organs that regulate blood pressure, so that his blood pressure's "set point" isn't quite right. It's nothing that can be specifically identified, and even if science could nail down a cause, it probably wouldn't guide the doctor toward a specific treatment. Nevertheless, that kind of blood pressure demands that something be done.

Luckily for Tony, he lives in an age where there is a wide variety of medicines that can bring down high blood pressure. Only forty years ago, that wasn't the case. So, after a few trials with various drugs, Tony has ended up with a calcium channel blocker and a diuretic that are unobtrusive in his day-to-day life (see the drug chart in this chapter for details). They have lowered his blood pressure to about 130 over 80—not bad. The doctor could probably bring it down even lower with another drug, but Tony is at a point where adding another drug might not make sense for the added benefit—the side effects might become more intrusive than the benefits warrant.

Tony should be commended—not only for his healthy lifestyle, but for getting a physical even when he felt good. This one action—while initially causing some upheaval—has probably added *quality* years, if not decades, to his life.

Number Two: Nothing—Absolutely Nothing— Offsets Smoking

Harold is in his late fifties and very active as a rancher. On the fitness scale, he's probably about a seven or eight out of a possible ten. He's also a smoker and has been for his entire adult life.

Relatively early in his adult life, Harold was diagnosed with hypertension (high blood pressure). He fell right into lock step with the medical community over his high blood pressure, taking drugs to control it, exercising (jogging and handball), controlling his weight, watching what he ate, and coming in for periodic office visits. Unfortunately, though, he still smoked, despite an ongoing "discussion" with his doctor about its hazards. If he didn't smoke, all the positive things he was doing (exercising, eating right) would negate any long-term harm caused by hypertension. But because he smoked, his positive efforts to counteract hypertension were canceled out.

One day, during a routine office visit, Harold mentioned that he occasionally felt some "discomfort" or "pressure" in his chest when he exercised. When the doctor referred to this as chest "pain," Harold was quick to say it wasn't pain, just pressure. Harold was being a typical male in his fifties—if chest pain is acknowledged, that would mean the frightening possibility of a heart attack would have to be acknowledged, so many fifties males try to avoid the whole issue by simply believing the pain isn't really pain, just "pressure."

While most heart problems do not create a bring-you-to-your-knees kind of pain, they certainly do make their presence known with varying degrees of pain—something the doctor knew Harold probably was feeling. With little regard for semantics, the doctor had Harold undergo a resting EKG test, which would indicate whether or not he had already experienced a heart attack and/or if any permanent damage had been done. Happily, it was negative on both counts: The resting EKG was normal.

The next step was to get Harold on a treadmill to see what the EKG said while Harold's heart was under the strain of exercise. Immediately, it indicated that Harold's heart was not getting enough blood to function under the extra rigors of exercise, thus causing the pain. Harold had a condition called angina that's caused by blocked or clogged arteries to the heart. He underwent a cardiac catheterization that showed three-vessel coronary artery disease. Harold ended up having a triple coronary artery bypass so that blood could once again flow freely to the heart muscle.

Today, about eight years later, Harold is doing fine. He continues to take his hypertension medicine, continues to exercise, watches what he eats, and takes an aspirin (325 mg a day; see the aspirin sidebar in this chapter), as well as antioxidants like vitamin E (400 IU per day). Best of all, though, he stopped smoking.

All along, Harold had labored under the misconception that he was doing so many good, healthy activities that somehow, on the cosmic balance sheet, he was offsetting his smoking. While all the other things were good, they didn't offset the harm he was doing to himself by smoking. There is nothing—absolutely nothing—that will offset the harm smoking does.

In Harold's case, smoking is what brought his condition to what could have been a fatal crossroads. Happily, he was stopped before he went through that intersection. He knows that he's now getting further and further away from the danger of smoking and a heart attack; unfortunately, he also knows that it will be many years before he's safely distanced himself from the danger of smoking and cancer.

Number Three: Yeah, I'll Quit Smoking— Right after My First Heart Attack

Larry just turned fifty. He's a landscape contractor who's outside all the time, running from project to project, jumping into work in short, quick bursts as his crews require. It's a physically demanding and stressful job. As a result, Larry is lean and generally fit, although it's not aerobic fitness; it's more strength fitness— his muscles get more daily workout than his cardiovascular and respiratory systems do.

Larry is also a heavy smoker. He has smoked at least a pack a day since he was fifteen years old. Additionally, he has a bad family history of heart problems.

If Larry were on his own, he probably never would have gone to see a doctor— and he would probably be dead now. His wife nagged him for years to have a check up. A few years ago, in his late forties, he finally agreed. The physical found he had normal blood pressure, a normal EKG reading, and was generally normal, except for a high level of cholesterol. His count was about 240 with a ratio in the sixes (the average should be around 190 and with ratio of around 4.5).

The doctor treated Larry with drugs for his cholesterol, then gave him the routine lecture on how harmful smoking was, especially when combined with high cholesterol and a bad family history. Larry replied with his standard yeah-yeah-yeah speech and went back to work.

Over the course of the next few years, the doctor saw Larry only when he had a case of bronchitis. Each time, the doctor repeated his smoking warning. Larry's pat reply: "Yeah, doc, I intend to quit, but I just haven't gotten around to it yet."

The next time the doctor heard from Larry, he was in an emergency room—he had had a heart attack at fifty years old.

The day started when Larry went to one project site and began lending a hand by shoveling some dirt. Suddenly, he developed severe chest pain. His foreman told him to sit down. Larry sat under a tree and had a cigarette (making matters worse, because smoking restricts blood vessels). Luckily for Larry, his foreman gave him two aspirin and said he wanted to call 911. Larry didn't want an ambulance on the site, so he made a very bad decision—he drove himself to a hospital. Once again, luck was on Larry's side; he didn't suffer a fatal attack while driving, which would not only have killed him, but possibly hurt other people.

At the hospital, it was determined that Larry was in the middle of a fairly sizable heart attack. Because it was still less than six hours from the onset, he was given a clot-busting drug that helps prevent permanent damage to the heart muscle. Ultimately, he had to suffer through two separate heart catheterizations to unblock two coronary arteries.

Three times lucky, Larry ended up having no permanent heart muscle damage. This means that if he does everything right—takes medications, watches what he eats, does the correct kinds of exercise, and stops smoking—he should be able to return to a totally normal life.

So far, so good—he's even given up cigarettes. But because it's been less than six months since his heart attack, the jury's still out on how good Larry will be. He does have a better than average chance of staying on the straight and narrow, because he was seriously scared by the entire incident. And having to go back for a second catheterization (not something that's usual), gave him additional time to contemplate his condition.

He knows now that if he had stopped smoking years ago, the odds are great that none of this would ever have happened.

Number Four: I'm Too Fit to Have Heart Disease

Mister X is fifty-five, not overweight, has never been a smoker, and is in good physical shape. He hikes to the top of mountains, jogs nearly every day, does a proper amount of stretching, and enjoys a fair amount of strengthening work. He still relishes downhill skiing and, at times, attacks it like when he was in his twenties. He's a slight to moderate drinker and eats reasonably well.

What makes this real tale especially interesting is that Mister X is also a doctor. He's the kind of doctor who spends a fair bit of time trying to persuade many of his patients that stacking the odds of good health in their favor means changing a few personal habits—losing a few pounds, doing some physical activity each day, kicking the cigarette habit, maintaining normal cholesterol and blood pressure levels, and monitoring daily stress levels.

One of the points he continually makes to his patients is this: Being good in some situations doesn't allow one to be "bad" in others. He gives the example of a smoker who feels it's okay to continue the habit because he exercises and eats right. That, Doctor X tells his patients, is faulty logic that could land the person in serious trouble someday.

The only blip on Doctor X's personal radar screen of health is his cholesterol— 250 total, with LDL ("bad" cholesterol) at 160 and HDL ("good" cholesterol) at 70. (Ideals: less than 200 total; less than 130 LDL; more than 35 HDL). Many doctors would say Doctor X's cholesterol needs to be lowered with the help of relatively nonobtrusive drugs. Doctor X tells himself that his general lifestyle, coupled with his relatively high HDL level, offsets his high LDL and total levels.

Do you see where this is going?

One day Doctor X is climbing a mountain with friends. He suddenly notices a tightness or burning in his chest. When he slows down, the feeling eases; when he speeds up, it returns. After half-an-hour—just as he's thinking, "Could this really be . . . ?"—the pain disappears. He rejoins his friends and completes the strenuous sixteen-mile hike at substantial altitude with no further problems.

On the next weekend's hike, the same thing happens: a tightness in the chest that disappears after thirty minutes. This time he silences his own doubts with: "I'm too fit to have heart disease."

The clincher comes in the most unlikely of places—on vacation, no hike involved, down at sea level. As the relaxed and unsuspecting Doctor X picks up some suitcases, the chest pain comes a-calling. "Hey, doc," it calls out, "I won't be ignored."

Back home, Doctor X fails a treadmill stress test. He's got angina pectoris—chest pain caused by lack of oxygen to the heart muscle. Doctor X undergoes a heart catheterization—a surgical procedure where a tiny tube is inserted in a leg artery and threaded up to the heart. Two heart arteries are found to be clogged—one at 90 percent, the other at 95 percent. In some ways, this was a heart just waiting for an attack. Both arteries are fixed and returned to full flow.

A year later, Doctor X is doing fine. Now that he has heart disease, it's critical to control his cholesterol (the LDL needs to be 80 or less), which he's doing through a statin drug. He's also maintaining his exercise program and taking a daily aspirin, 400 IU of vitamin E, 800 micrograms of folic acid, and a multiple B complex. There will be quarterly cholesterol checks and yearly treadmill tests. He has improved his diet, which wasn't bad to be begin with, and is trying to moderate his stress (difficult for many doctors to do). He's lucky he didn't have a heart attack.

Three lessons Doctor X learned: (1) risk factors do count (in his case, high LDL, age, maleness, and stress); (2) good things can't offset bad things—each must be dealt with separately; and (3) don't ignore symptoms. Oh, by the way . . . Gordon is Doctor X.

KNOWING WHAT YOU PUT IN YOUR MOUTH— A DRUG CHART

Cholesterol Control Drugs

NAME	EXPLANATION AND USE	POSSIBLE SIDE EFFECTS
HMG-CoA reductase inhibitors (Statin drugs): **Atorvastatin(Lipitor)** **Pravastatin (Pravachol)** **Simvastatin (Zocor)** **Lovastatin (Mevacor) and others**	Acts on liver to reduce the amount of cholesterol it produces. State of the art for this purpose. Reduces total and "bad" cholesterol; reduces heart attacks and sudden cardiac death. Useful in known coronary artery disease as plaque stabilizer, seemingly independent of cholesterol lowering.	Liver damage (detectable, uncommon, and reversible); muscle damage, also reversible.
Fibrate drugs: **Gemfibrozil (Lopid)** **Fenofibrate (Tricor)**	Acts on liver to reduce triglyceride levels, desirable under certain circumstances to reduce cardiac events (heart attacks and sudden cardiac death). Milder effect on cholesterol. Less useful than statins, with which they can be (very cautiously) combined.	Same as statins.
Nicotinic acid (niacin) **Niaspan**	A vitamin that's used in drug level doses. Reduces total and "bad" cholesterol, and raises "good" cholesterol.	Side effects drastically limit usefulness of this drug. They include skin flushing (hot flashes) and liver damage.
Bile acid sequestrants (resins) **Cholestyramine (Questran)** **Colestipol (Colestid)**	Binds in the intestine to bile (which is very rich in cholesterol), thus preventing the reabsorption (and thus the recycling) of the bile. This reduces the total body quantity of cholesterol.	Bad taste or mouth feel, nausea, gas, and constipation limit the usefulness of this class of drug.

126

Blood Pressure Drugs

NAME	EXPLANATION AND USE	POSSIBLE SIDE EFFECTS
Diuretics (water pills) *Hydrochlorthiazide (HydroDIURIL) Dyazide, Microzide, and others* *Spironolactone (Aldactone)* *Triamterene (Dyrenium, Dyazide, and others)* *Furosemide (Lasix)* *Bumetanide (Bumex)*	Acts on the kidneys to cause excess sodium (and consequently excess water) to be eliminated in the urine. Reduction in the total body sodium and water quantity usually reduces blood pressure. Very useful in other states of water excess, such as congestive heart failure. Most often the first drug chosen to treat hypertension.	Dehydration; dry mouth; depletion of minerals such as potassium; increased blood sugar; increased uric acid. Urinary frequency.
Beta Adreneric Blockers (beta blockers)	Partially block selected effects of adrenalin (epinephrine) on the body, thus reducing blood pressure, heart rate, and workload of the heart. Combines very well with diuretics. Other uses include migraine prevention, treatment of stage fright, and treatment of certain types of tremors. Have been shown to reduce the risk of second heart attack. Useful for treating angina pectoris and certain cardiac arrythmias.	Cannot be used in asthmatics (makes wheezing worse), can cause fatigue, depression, exercise intolerance, excessively slowed heart rate, and is the most likely of the anti-hypertensives to produce erectile dysfunction.

127

Blood Pressure Drugs (continued)

NAME	EXPLANATION AND USE	POSSIBLE SIDE EFFECTS
Calcium Channel Blockers **Verapamil (Calan, Verelan, Covera HS, and others)** **Dilitazem (Cardizem, Tiazac, and others)** **Amlodipine (Norvasc)** **Nifedipine (Procardia, Adalat CC, and others)**	Block the rate of inflow of calcium ions into the smooth muscle cells, causing those muscles to relax. Blood vessel walls, composed of smooth muscle, relax, lowering blood pressure. Other uses include prevention of migraine headaches, treatment/prevention of angina pectoris, and treatment of some heartbeat arrythmias.	Constipation, fatigue, swelling, lightheadedness.
Angiotensin Converting Enzyme Inhibitors (ACE inhibitors) **Quinapril (Accupril)** **Ramipril (Altace)** **Captopril (Capoten)** **Benazepril (Lotensin)** **Fosinopril (Monopril)** **Lisinopril (Prinivil, Zestril)** **Enalapril (Vasotec)**	Interferes with production of angiotensin II, a very potent artery constrictor. With less angiotensin II available, blood pressure usually drops. Also used as part of the treatment of congestive heart failure and to protect the kidneys in diabetics. Members of this drug class are virtually interchangeable.	Cough (the main limitation of its usefulness), elevation of potassium, worsening of kidney failure. Seldom produces erectile dysfunction (a good drug choice for fifties men). Should never be used in pregnancy.
Alpha adrenergic blockers (alpha blockers) **Prazosin (Minipress)** **Terazosin (Hytrin)** **Doxazosin (Cardura)**	Blocks selected adrenalin effects, allowing smooth muscle to relax, thus dilating arteries and lowering blood pressure. Most frequent use currently is in urinary hesitancy associated with benign prostatic enlargement, where the relaxation of muscles at the bladder outlet allows better bladder emptying.	Too rapid reduction of blood pressure, especially after the initial dose, may result in fainting. Also, dizziness, fatigue, leg swelling.

Blood Pressure Drugs (continued)

NAME	EXPLANATION AND USE	POSSIBLE SIDE EFFECTS
Combined Alpha/Beta Blocker Labetalol (Normodyne, Trandate)	Combines the effects of alpha-1 and beta adrenergic blockade, thus providing a dual action in lowering blood pressure. Combines well with other antihypertensives, and may, in Gordon's opinion, be underused.	Cannot be used in asthmatics, caution in diabetics. Also, fatigue, depression, erectile dysfunction, exercise intolerance.
Angiotensin Receptor Blocker (ARB) Losartan (Cozaar) Valsartan (Diovan) Irbesartan (Avapro) and others	The newest of the commonly used antihypertensives, this class blocks the effect of angiotensin (see ACEs). Usually well tolerated, relatively high cost limit use. Uses other than for hypertension, such as in congestive heart failure and to protect the kidneys of diabetics, remain under investigation, but will probably prove out.	May increase vulnerability to viral infection, GI complaints, fatigue. Seldom causes erectile dysfunction. Should never be used in pregnancy.

Respiratory Drugs

NAME	EXPLANATION AND USE	POSSIBLE SIDE EFFECTS
Antihistamines (prescription, nonsedating) Loratidine (Claritin) Fexofenadine (Allegra) Cetirizine (Zyrtec)	Blocks the effect of histamine, a chemical produced by the body and that's important in producing inflammation, especially of the type that we associate with allergic reactions (hay fever, hives).	Can produce drowsiness in some, may thicken secretions. Also headache, nausea.

Respiratory Drugs (continued)

NAME	EXPLANATION AND USE	POSSIBLE SIDE EFFECTS
Antihistamines (sedating—mostly available over the counter) **Diphenhydramine (Benadryl) and others** **Chlorpheniramine (Deconamine, Cholor-Trimeton, Duravent, and others)** **Brompheniramine (Dimetapp, Bromfed, Rondec)** **Hydroxyzine (Atarax, Visatril)**	Although mostly available over the counter, because of their sedating properties, they are actually not as well tolerated as the prescription nonsedating antihistamines. They have been available for a long time, so their relative safety is well established.	Sedation, excessive thickening of secretions, urinary hesitancy.
Nasal Steroids **Beclomethasone (Beconase, Vancenase)** **Flunisolide (Nasarel)** **Budesonide (Rhinocort)** **Mometasone furoate (Nasonex)** **Triamcinalone (Nasacort)** **Fluticasone (Flonase)**	Reduce inflammation on contact with the nasal mucous membranes, relieving allergic nasal symptoms. Can be used seasonally or steadily, although ineffective when used on an "as needed" basis.	Nasal irritation, nosebleed, headache, cough.
Inhaled corticosteroids (for asthma) **Beclomethasone (Vanceril, Beclovent)** **Triamcinalone (Azmacort)** **Flunisolide (Aerobid)** **Fluticasone (Flovent)** **Budesonide (Pulmicort)**	Reduce inflammation on contact with the bronchial mucous membranes, thus controlling a cause of asthma. Indicated for asthma that is symptomatic on more than just isolated occasions. Does not help acute asthma attacks.	Throat irritation, cough, oral yeast infections (always rinse mouth with water after use), headache.

130

Respiratory Drugs (continued)

NAME	EXPLANATION AND USE	POSSIBLE SIDE EFFECTS
Inhaled bronchodilators (for asthma) **Albuterol (Ventolin, Proventil)** **Pirbuterol (Maxair)** **Metaproterenol (Alupent)**	Used primarily via the inhaled route, these drugs mimic adrenaline effects, providing bonchodilation quickly when needed. Relatively short acting and having no effect upon inflammation (an important cause of asthma), these drugs in their inhaled form should be used primarily for "rescue" from an acte asthma attack; other methods should be added for management of chronic asthma.	Primarily related to their adrenaline-mimicking effect, includes increased heart rate, increased blood pressure, tremor, nervousness, cough.
Salmeterol (Serevent)	A long-acting bronchodila-tor useful in the mainte-nance treatment of asth-ma. Not to be used for acute asthma attacks.	Tremor, cough, nasal and throat irritation.
Leukotriene inhibitors **Zafirlukast (Accolate)** **Montelukast (Singulair)** **Zileuton (Zyflo)**	Interfere with a step in the chemical cascade that produces inflammation, these nonsteroidal drugs are used to treat and pre-vent chronic asthma. Although not yet approved by the FDA for this use, they can be used for the treatement and prevention of allergic inflammation that's both chronic and seasonal (hay fever).	Headache, fatigue, GI complaints.

THE GOOD NEWS

- In the last fifty years, science and the public have joined forces to make tremendous strides against heart attack and stroke—decreasing both by double digits and nearly pushing stroke out of the fifties and sixties age groups. The battlefield is high blood pressure (hypertension) and high cholesterol (hypercholesterolemia), and the weapons are better diagnostics, great new drugs, and public awareness about heart attack, stroke, and the importance of diet and exercise.

- Worth double mention: New drugs to control high blood pressure and high cholesterol are incredibly effective and are usually relatively nonintrusive in day-to-day life.

- Most risk factors for heart attack and stroke—smoking, high blood pressure, high cholesterol, and obesity—are within the control of everyone. Even the risk factor of heredity isn't set in stone. You can't change the heredity cards you've been dealt, but you can choose how to play those cards. Plus, heredity only plays a 30 percent role in your overall health—the rest is up to you.

- Heart-attack death rates in fifties males have decreased by 20 percent in the last ten years.

- Because of special clot-busting drugs, if you do suffer a heart attack, there is a better chance of surviving without permanent heart muscle damage than ever before.

- With the proper use of drugs, diet, and exercise, and by not smoking, arterial damage (which leads to heart attack and stroke) can be halted. In some cases it can even be reversed.

- A simple aspirin a day can reduce your risk of heart attack and stroke. (Check with your doctor first, though, and see the aspirin sidebar in this chapter for details.)

- Moderate drinking—two or fewer drinks a day—can actually help reduce your chance of heart attack and stroke. (Do *not* start drinking if you haven't before, and see the alcohol sidebar in this chapter for details.)

132

The Cardiovascular and Respiratory Networks

- Lungs that are taken care of will last a very long lifetime without the need of aids such as extra oxygen.

- Those who do not smoke and avoid other air pollutants have very little statistical chance of contracting chronic bronchitis, emphysema, or even lung cancer. (Remembering that tiny percentage category of "shit happens.")

- If you do everything right and have healthy blood vessels, heart, and lungs, you have very little statistical chance of heart attack and stroke in your fifties or even your sixties. (Remembering once again the bugaboo of "shit happens.")

4: THE DIGESTIVE AND URINARY TRACTS

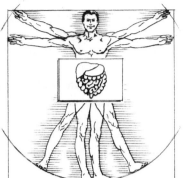

They Don't Need to Be Mysterious

BACKGROUND BASICS

The digestive and urinary tracts definitely separate the men from the boys, the doctors from the patients, the brave-hearted from the squeamish, the knowing from the unknowing. No other body parts and functions are so mysterious to the common man.

- What's your gurgling stomach *really* doing?
- Why does your lower abdomen suddenly cramp up like you're giving birth?
- And how come your mighty Mississippi has shriveled to a lowly stream?

Every guy certainly knows how digestion starts: food and drink go in. That part we definitely have down pat. And we sure know how it ends, so we'll skip this opportunity for a crass joke. But most fifties males don't know squat about what goes on between the start and finish of digestion.

An interesting phenomenon is that many male patients seem afraid to find out about their own digestive and urinary tracts, as if merely learning what's going on somehow creates, or exposes, problems they didn't know existed. Rest assured, knowing the truth about what's going on inside your body isn't going to cause any cancers to grow or polyps to form. In fact, the knowledge you gain from this chapter can help you to aid your internal systems in functioning better, as well as make you more aware of the early signs of two of the leading causes of death in men over fifty: prostate cancer and colon cancer. And early detection, as many of you do know, means stacking the survival odds in your favor.

So, if you want to trust the health of your digestive and urinary tracts to fate, skip to another chapter; if you want to take an active role in keeping them—and yourself—healthy, read on.

If you think of the musculoskeletal system as the foundation of the body, and the lungs and heart as the delivery system, the digestive and urinary tracts are basically the processing plants of the human body. They take raw material and convert it into either usable substances or waste that's eliminated. Sounds simple, but it's not. Our body's digestive and urinary tracts are like finely-tuned manufacturing plants, where conveyor belts move at lightning speed and machinery works with great precision. Most times our systems run with no one apparently at the controls, but as you've heard on late-night TV ads, operators are, indeed, standing by. In your body's case, they're in the background, taking action only when chemical changes dictate they do so.

How does all this relate to the average male in his fifties?

Unfortunately, this is the time when many first signs of trouble—both the nuisance variety and the life-threatening kind—appear.

Top Five Digestive and/or Urinary Situations Faced By Fifties Males (In Order of Frequency)

1. **Heartburn**—which is more accurately called acid reflux (backup) or GERD (gastroesophageal reflux disease).

2. **Prostate problems**—from the annoying to the life-challenging.

3. **Ulcers**—many of which are now curable after a scientific breakthrough.

4. **Kidney stones**—still one of man's most painful experiences.

5. **Gallstones**—also no picnic when it comes to pain.

Another potential digestive/urinary problem for our age group—and growing every year—is viral hepatitis. While the peak age for contracting various forms of hepatitis is in the twenties, there are certain clichéd mid-life activities men sometimes engage in that go hand-in-hand with a higher risk of contracting various forms of hepatitis:

- Deciding to have a once-in-a-lifetime sexual adventure before getting too old could spell hepatitis B or C.

- Getting a tattoo to go with that mid-life Harley Davidson could mean hep C.

- Traveling—even a relatively innocuous journey by a corporate executive faithful to his partner—could be a recipe for a number of hepatitis strains.

Hepatitis aside, digestive and urinary problems aren't usually very exotic. Plenty of fifties males are initiated into the indignities of hemorrhoids and constipation, while others find themselves struggling to understand—and control—periodic bouts of severe cramps and/or diarrhea. Then there's the infamous dribbles, which are almost as embarrassing as those spontaneous high school erections, but with no textbooks to hide the situation. And not to be forgotten is the frustration of urinary hesitancy, in which the body's desire to go isn't matched by its ability to do so.

When it's all said and done, digestive and urinary problems might make you feel like your body is turning against you. Don't worry, it's not a real rebellion, it's just a few small insurrections that usually can be handled without too much difficulty.

Before you can fully comprehend this, though, it might be a good idea to get a general overview of how the entire system functions.

How Does It All Work?— Tagging Along with a Late Night Snack

You can't sleep because that last piece of rare roast beef is whispering your name over and over. Forgetting the well-planned diet, you head for the kitchen and make a great-looking sandwich. After this satisfying snack, you tiptoe back to bed, carefully slide between the sheets, making sure not to awaken your unsuspecting partner, then drift off to a contented sleep, totally oblivious to the chain reaction you've just started in your body's digestive and urinary tracts.

For those stout-hearted fellows who want to know the details, in all their glory and gore, here's an abbreviated version of what happens to that sandwich. As you chew it (the more chews the better), it mixes with saliva, which moistens the food and begins the digestive process. When you swallow, the sandwich enters the:

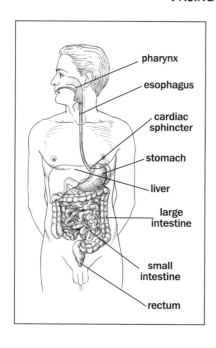

pharynx

esophagus

cardiac
sphincter

stomach

liver

large
intestine

small
intestine

rectum

Esophagus—your throat, which, through a series of well-orchestrated contractions, sends the food down through the:

Lower Esophageal Sphincter (LES)—This is a kind of trap door that keeps stomach contents and stomach acids from coming back up into the esophagus. The food then enters the:

Stomach—An expandable sack-like organ with muscle layers that churn up the sandwich with acid secretions. The process begins breaking down the food into liquid form, and some nutrients begin to be absorbed through the stomach lining into the blood, which then goes to the liver for processing. Back in the stomach, the puree of roast beef now moves through the:

Pyloric Sphincter—a muscular ring that separates the stomach from the duodenum. The sandwich then enters the:

Duodenum—the first part of the small intestine, where the sandwich is deluged with stomach acid, bile from the liver, pancreatic juices from the pancreas, and intestinal juices—all to help with the chemical breakdown of the food molecules.

At this stage, some need-to-know elements are:

Bile—a thick, bitter fluid made by the liver, stored in the gallbladder, and secreted into the duodenum to break down fats, it prepares them for further digestion down the line.

Liver—Your largest internal organ, and one of the most complex, the liver not only produces bile, but does numerous other jobs, including filtering nutrients coming in via the blood system from the stomach and intestine, and breaking them down into usable components.

Pancreas—Not only the producer of pancreatic juice, which contains digestive enzymes, it also secretes the hormones insulin and glucagon.

The now unrecognizable sandwich travels from the duodenum into the:

Small Intestine—Also known as the small bowel, this is actually the longest part of the digestive tract, measuring about twenty-four feet, and is the major site for food digestion and absorption. As the liquified sandwich moves through the tract via wave-like contractions, nutrients from the sandwich are absorbed through the wall lining and into the blood. The blood then passes through the liver for filtering. The material still remaining in the small intestine continues on into the:

Large Intestine—Also known as the large bowel or colon, this portion of the digestive tract includes the appendix, the rectum, and the anus. Here is where most of the water is extracted from the food. It's absorbed through the wall lining into the blood, which goes on to be filtered through the:

Kidneys—Two bean-shaped organs that do numerous jobs, one of which is to filter and purify blood and excrete the impurities, along with water, creating a product called urine. The urine is stored in the bladder before it's expelled from the body through the penis.

The material remaining in the large intestine is now solidifying into waste matter that is moved along by contractions that ultimately expel it from the body in a bowel movement.

Time from Start to Finish: Depending upon numerous variables, such as the kind of food ingested and individual system variances, the time from swallowing to complete digestion is approximately four to six hours.

WHERE AND HOW PROBLEMS OCCUR, TREATMENT OPTIONS, AND PREVENTIVE MEASURES

The Mouth

During the fifties decade, many men find their mouth has gone through some changes since they were young. While these changes might include everything from being less likely to fit a foot in there to feeling freer to express opinions, the following remarks will be limited to the physiological changes or problems that might be faced.

Sore Tongue and/or Loss of Taste Buds

Moderately common in men in our age group, a sore tongue is a superficial soreness of the surface that you can't quite put your finger on. Rarely, though, does it signify anything serious among fifties males. The condition is also called "geographic tongue" because the erosion of certain mucous membranes that it causes creates a kind of geographic or map-like pattern on the tongue. Minor food allergies, often to acidic foods like some fruits and vegetables, can bring on the condition. A vitamin B-12 deficiency can cause tongue soreness as well as atrophy of taste buds, meaning loss of taste. A common reversible cause of taste loss is taking too many vitamins, particularly vitamin C, which can irritate your tongue or make it hurt. Normally, your sense of taste will return once the excess vitamins have been purged from your system.

Treatment/Prevention. While your doctor can help diagnose the cause, this is where patient awareness helps. Be conscious of the kind and amount of vitamins you take, as well as the foods that are eaten just prior to the start of symptoms.

Periodontal Disease

Probably the biggest dental problem for men in their fifties is periodontal, or gum, disease. A regression of the gums, it's usually caused by low-grade infections near or around the gums, typically brought on by poor dental hygiene and heightened by long-term smoking or use of chewing tobacco. Smoking and tobacco chewing make the gums vulnerable to disease, not only because of chronic irritation, but because they constrict the blood vessels, that help to keep gums properly nourished and healthy. No matter what the cause, gum disease is the most common cause of tooth loss for fifties males.

Treatment/Prevention. Those who do contract periodontal disease might face, depending on the severity, periodontal restoration by a gum specialist—surgically transferring gum tissue from an undiseased area to a diseased area. Prevention is the key and is relatively easy, consisting of regular trips to the dentist and nightly flossing. On the other side of the coin, you don't want to overdo things—too strenuous brushing with an overly stiff toothbrush can also cause gum regression (damage). Most times, preventive flossing gets rid of the disease's bacterial causes before they can do their damage. A wonderfully simple but powerful statement to remember is: Clean teeth don't deteriorate. And if they're clean that probably means the gums are in good shape as well.

Mouth Cancers

Tumors of the mouth include those of the cheek, gum, and lips. These cancers aren't rare in our age group, but they are usually confined to tobacco users and/or heavy drinkers. The combination of excessive alcohol and tobacco—especially smokeless or chewing tobacco in this case—seems to have a synergistic effect on certain of these cancers. Because the fifties decade is when men begin to reap the whirlwind of

---

DRINK HOW MUCH?
PROPER HYDRATION

You've probably heard it before, but everyone should drink about six to eight glasses (ten ounces each) of fluid a day to keep properly hydrated. Generally speaking, water is best, because it handles hydration without extras such as calories or sugars that are usually found in juices, sports drinks, and iced tea. Coffee and alcoholic drinks don't really help, because they stimulate dehydration with their diuretic effects (translation: They make you urinate more often).

A few points about hydration you might not be aware of:

- Your body loses more than three pints (fifty ounces) of fluid a day without even trying.

- Thirst lags behind hydration—by the time you're thirsty you're probably down about four pints (sixty-four ounces).

- It's best to sip all day rather than gulp down large amounts of fluid periodically. All-day sipping is good for the system and it helps avoid excessive nighttime urinating.

- Properly hydrated, you should urinate once or twice per half a day of work.

- Constant thirst and constant urinating—without just cause—warrants a check for diabetes through a blood test and/or urinalysis.

About fifteen minutes prior to starting heavy exertion that makes you sweat, you should drink about eight to ten ounces of water, then down another eight to ten ounces every fifteen minutes or so while you're sweating. Our sweat rate can reach fifty or more ounces per hour, while our stomach is capable of delivering only thirty-five to fifty ounces of fluid per hour, meaning we can sweat faster than our bodies can provide fluid.

---

past behaviors, it's critical that those who have smoked or are still smoking be aware of such things as sore gums and even sore throats that won't go away or hang around longer than usual—they might be early warning signs of cancer.

Treatment/Prevention. Prevention includes having regular dental checkups, being aware of abnormalities in your mouth, stopping smoking, and watching your alcohol intake.

The Esophagus and Stomach

The esophagus, also known as the throat or gullet, is a muscular canal only about ten inches long. When you swallow, you set off an intricate series of wave-like contractions in the throat that help food and drink move down the canal. Normally these contractions function like a brand-new Slinky toy gliding down a set of stairs. As you get older, though, these synchronized movements can get fouled up for a variety of reasons, causing difficulty in swallowing. The relative good news is that most males of our age group will have to wait twenty or thirty years before they might face this problem.

The stomach is situated in the upper left part of the abdomen and has muscular walls, which toss food together with strong stomach acids. A stout mucous lining protects the stomach from its own acids, which continue the process of breaking down the food. This is where the food really takes a beating—and occasionally fights back. When it does, there's usually some external discomfort involved, which can be anything from gas and bloating to heartburn.

Stomach Gas, Bloating, Rumbling

What causes stomach gas, and how is it different from more serious problems, like acid reflux (backup)?

Gas is usually caused by air introduced into your stomach during the digestion process. Normally, this happens when you swallow air. Causes can include chewing gum (which generates more saliva, making you swallow more), nervousness (think of how some actors portray anxiety by excessive swallowing), or by sipping things like hot liquids. Some people swallow air habitually without even realizing it. After you've swallowed the air, it mixes with the food and acids and gives you a full sensation that can be extremely unpleasant at times.

Bloating is usually caused by overeating or overconsuming a variety of foods including fatty foods that slow the stomach's emptying. While bloating is different from swallowing air, the two conditions do create the same unpleasant full sensation.

Stomach rumbling—with the scientific name, borborygmi, sounding like the condition—is a condition that some people worry about. There's little cause for concern. It's basically the noisy passage of trapped gas and/or digesting food through the incredible kinks and loops of the digestive tract.

Treatment/Prevention. For bloating or trapped gas in the stomach, the over-the-counter products and home remedies mentioned for the following acid reflux section work well. Additionally, burping or belching, while socially unacceptable, can release some of the gas and relieve the pressure sensation. Best of all, burping and belching can be done in the privacy of your own home, which leaves your social status intact, but might reinforce your partner's belief that you haven't made it too far up the evolutionary scale. A home remedy is to drink a carbonated beverage, which adds to the trapped gas bubble and may make it easier to belch up.

Heartburn/Acid Reflux

An old adage states that all good things have a down side. Nowhere is this better illustrated than in the digestive tract. That pizza tasted *so good* as you were savoring every mouthful—why does it come back to haunt you a few hours later? And it can do so with a vengeance, waking you from a sound sleep with a surprisingly painful burning sensation in the chest, usually below the breastbone.

If, for the sake of this section, we agree that this chest pain is *not* a heart attack (which it could be, so please see chapter 3 for heart details), then the most likely culprit is heartburn or acid reflux (backup).

Typically, acid is produced by the stomach in response to the actions of chewing and swallowing, and the presence of food. The acid is part of the long and involved digestive process that breaks down food so your body can use the nutrients. The production of even a small amount of stomach acid is what gives you a hungry feeling.

When you swallow, the food goes down your throat and through the critical component, the lower esophageal sphincter (LES), which keeps the stomach's contents and acids from backing up into your throat.

If everything works perfectly, there is little chance of acid backup. Unfortunately, by the time you've reached your fifties, the possibility of physical lapses in the digestive mechanisms is substantial. In fact, it would be a surprise if *any* American male has reached his fifties without at least a few cases of heartburn.

What Causes Heartburn?

Simply put, it's food and digestive acids backing up into your throat.

That's a problem—and a serious one at times—because while the stomach is built to withstand contact with those acids, the throat is not. When the food and acid make contact with the throat's lining, they cause a burning sensation. Somebody eons ago thought the pain came from the heart, so the feeling became known as "heartburn." Later, people with a scientific orientation added more technically accurate names: acid reflux (backup) and gastroesophageal reflux disease (GERD).

No matter what the name, the pain is still the same—and normally, so is the cause. Most times the blame lies squarely with LES (the lower esophageal sphincter, i.e., the trapdoor between the esophagus and stomach), which causes acid backup by relaxing at the wrong time. Normally, LES only relaxes when you're swallowing, so food can pass from the throat to your stomach. At all other times, it's supposed to remain firmly closed, so nothing can come back into your throat from your stomach.

When the LES trapdoor is weak, limp, or chemically unstimulated to do its job correctly, acid backup will occur. Numerous elements and/or conditions can do this to LES.

Four Major Causes of Problems with LES

- **Overeating**—A full, completely expanded stomach will naturally put more pressure on the LES trapdoor, especially because it lies right where the stomach takes a relatively sharp turn. If LES is already weakened or limp, the added pressure is all that's necessary to get acid backup. This means, of course, that you might want to rethink eating that last piece of pie, which will take you from being merely full to really stuffed.

- **Overweight**—Men with large bellies have a greater chance of having heartburn, because the excess weight puts pressure on and around the LES trapdoor in ways that aren't normal. There are even people with a relatively narrow range—maybe three to five pounds—above which they have acid reflux and below which they don't. Staying at a good, healthy weight solves this problem.

- **Gravity**—If you eat a big meal and then lie down, you're likely to get acid backup even if you are skinny and young. If you're in your fifties and overweight, you're definitely in for some heartburn. Generally speaking, it's not a good idea to eat a meal and then go to bed. You should try to stay upright for around two to three hours to help digest your meal. A short, nonstrenuous walk is also a good idea, because it gets you away from the table and keeps you upright.

- **Certain Substances**—Chemically, some substances have a relaxing affect on the LES trapdoor, which can bring on acid reflux. These include nicotine; alcohol (certain kinds like red wine are said to have a greater effect than others); chocolate; coffee (not caffeine, so you don't get a break with decaf); tea to a

144

certain degree; citrus fruits and juices; tomatoes and tomato products; and peppermint, as in the after-dinner mint. In addition, rich and fatty foods (those that are known as "stick-to-your-ribs" fare) are culprits, because they sit in your stomach for a longer period of time than other foods. Keep in mind that this is not to say you can't eat these foods, just that if you're prone to acid reflux, they are the substances known to have a detrimental effect. And no matter what food you do eat, remember to chew adequately—many of us were subconsciously trained as children to eat quickly, meaning the food takes longer to digest because it isn't properly chewed when it gets to the stomach.

While most heartburn is caused by problems with the LES trapdoor, it can also be the result of a hiatal hernia (a protrusion of part of the stomach through the diaphragm) or a peptic ulcer. Both commonly occur in fifties males, but they don't always cause symptoms. If the hernia causes chronic acid backup and doesn't respond to the usual measures, it can be treated surgically.

Many people think that heartburn is generally more of a nuisance than a serious problem. Actually, chronic acid reflux can cause constant pain and difficulty in swallowing, esophageal (throat) ulcers, and muscle hypertrophy (enlargement) of the lower portion of your throat. Chronic reflux is also a contributing factor in the development of esophageal cancer.

When acid reflux occurs, the acid most often stays within the lower portion of the throat. In some cases, however, the stomach acid can—while you're sleeping—make its way to your larynx and into your mouth. If it reaches your mouth it can cause dental decay and bad breath. For some people—mainly the elderly—the acid can find its way into the lungs, creating a chronic cough, wheeze, or increased severity in preexisting asthma. Those with chronic asthma who aren't making any headway with the disease should remind their doctor about acid reflux into the lungs—it might be what's causing problems.

Treatment/Prevention. Acid backup can be controlled or even eliminated by taking the following steps:

- Don't smoke or chew tobacco

- Limit alcohol consumption

- Limit the intake of those foods that help relax the LES trapdoor

- Chew food adequately

- Eat smaller meals more frequently so your stomach never gets so full it puts pressure on LES

• Remain upright for two or three hours after a meal

• Maintain an ideal body weight

For those who still get heartburn, there are numerous effective over-the-counter remedies such as Pepcid AC, Tagamet, Mylanta, Maalox, Alka-Mints, Axid, Zantac, and Tums. Acid blockers such as Pepcid, Tagamet, Axid, and Zantac partially block the production of stomach acid, while conventional antacids such as Maalox, Mylanta, and Tums temporarily neutralize acid already present in your stomach. A newer generation of acid blockers, such as Prilosec, Prevacid, and Nexium, called proton pump inhibitors (PPIs), block acid production even more effectively than the earlier acid blockers (the "Pepcid Generation"). While all these can be very effective for short-term, sporadic heartburn, it should be noted that if you find you're using them every day or night for an extended period of time (more than two weeks at a stretch), they might be hiding a more serious condition, and you should check with your doctor.

If you find yourself without any over-the-counter remedies handy, try a teaspoon of plain old baking soda mixed with a glass of water. It neutralizes the acids like the store-bought products do. Even drinking a glass of water might help—it won't neutralize the acid, but it will dilute the acid and at least partially relieve the effects. Additionally, if you're in bed, elevate your head or get out of bed and sit up for a while.

Food Poisoning

At one time or another, most of us have had a sudden bout of severe diarrhea and/or felt sick to our stomachs and thrown up. Within a short period of time (six to twelve hours), however, we felt fine again. Chances are, we had a case of food poisoning. Most times, other than a temporarily upset digestive tract, our body is not much worse for wear. On very rare occasions, however, food poisoning can cause death. For our age group, food poisoning is not something to be too concerned about—it's more apt to harm the very young and the very old than the middle-aged—although anyone can get it at any time.

What Is Food Poisoning?

Food poisoning is a general, unscientific term for acute gastroenteritis, which can cause severe diarrhea, cramps, sometimes fever, malaise, nausea, and vomiting. The ailment is usually brought on by the ingestion of food or drink (often water or ice) that has been contaminated by any of several different bacteria (also see "giardiasis" in this chapter's malabsorption section). The route of contamination is fecal to oral (not something to contemplate for too long). The symptoms are due to either a true infection, which means the invasion of the bowel wall by bacteria, or, more commonly, the effects of a toxin produced by the bacteria. True infections are usually longer lived than the toxin-caused illnesses. Because both conditions cause diarrhea, dehydration can be a concern, so drinking plenty of uncontaminated water should be a priority.

Major Culprits of Intestinal Upheaval

- **Campylobacter**—The most common cause of intestinal bacterial infection in America, it usually attacks the large bowel. It can cause a severe illness with bloody diarrhea, fever, and dehydration, and affects more infants and children than fifties males.

- **Salmonella**—The second most common form of bacterial food poisoning in America, it also affects infants and the elderly more than the middle-aged. Usually less severe than campylobacter, salmonella is often associated with "tainted," or contaminated, eggs and meat (especially poultry).

- **E. Coli**—A toxin-producing bacteria, it is responsible for the infamous "Montezuma's Revenge" that many travelers get. When enough of the bugs are ingested to live for a while in the digestive tract, symptoms—such as nausea, vomiting, diarrhea, and, sometimes, fever and malaise—will occur. It's probably the commonest cause of bacterial food poisoning worldwide.

- **Staphylococcus**—Also a toxin-producing bacteria, it can cause food poisoning, with symptoms ranging from mild abdominal discomfort, nausea, and diarrhea to severe, life-threatening symptoms. Staphylococcal food poisoning often occurs when a food handler has a skin infection of the hands.

Treatment/Prevention. When a person contracts food poisoning, treatment usually revolves around handling the symptoms—especially the easing of diarrhea with products such as Pepto Bismol and Imodium—and rehydrating the person with plenty of fluids (most notably water). In many cases, a few days' time will usually take care of this situation, although in some cases (such as E. Coli) antibiotics may be used to keep the population of toxin-producing bacteria low enough so the amount of toxin is reduced to below the illness-producing level.

Ways of Avoiding Food Poisoning

- Clean thoroughly the cutting utensils and cutting surfaces used with uncooked meat and poultry before using them again for other foods (such as vegetables). Bleach-containing store-bought products may "sterilize" cutting surfaces. Wooden cutting boards should not be used, because bacteria can survive on them for a longer period of time than on other surfaces, and they are more difficult to clean.

- Store food at proper temperatures. The bacteria grow best in temperatures above 40 degrees Fahrenheit, so keeping food at below 40 degrees helps to retard bacteria.

- Cook eggs, meat, and poultry for a long enough time so that bacteria are killed off. Bacteria grow best in temperatures below 140 degrees, so make sure all meat and poultry are cooked beyond that temperature before being served.

- Wash all fresh foods, such as fruits and vegetables, before eating them.

- Avoid the local water from areas where proper water purification is not available. Remember, this means not even rinsing your mouth after brushing your teeth.

- Take products such as Pepto Bismol as a way of avoiding illnesses from toxin-causing bacteria. (Antibiotics are usually not recommended for prevention because too frequent use causes resistant strains of bacteria to develop, and an adverse reaction to an antibiotic that you might not have needed can spoil your trip. Antibiotics are used, however, for early treatment of bacterial gastroenteritis.)

The controversial practice of irradiating meat before it reaches the market would completely solve the problem of tainted meat. Gordon knows of no disadvantage to this.

Ulcers

Pain from ulcers has plagued mankind since our ancestors took their first mouthfuls of twigs and berries. And until a few years ago we weren't much closer to understanding them than our forebears were.

The Digestive and Urinary Tracts

What we did know was that, normally, your digestive tract is protected from the digestive acids by mucous membranes lining the interior of such organs as the stomach and duodenum (the first part of the small intestine). If for some reason those membranes break down, the acids attack the tissue beneath, causing inflammation and, in severe cases, bleeding into the digestive tract. Gastrointestinal tract ulcers are called peptic ulcers—meaning caused by acid. The most common of these are in the first part of the small intestine (duodenal ulcers) and in the stomach (gastric ulcers).

Typically, a person with an ulcer will feel a gnawing, burning kind of pain, that's often worse on an empty stomach, after consuming alcohol and spicy foods, or during stressful times. The pain can range from mild to extremely severe, depending on the ulcer's development, and can be relieved with certain kinds of food, milk, or antacids. For severe ulcers, treatment in the past included substantial surgery to remove a portion of the stomach to reduce its acid-production capacity.

What Causes Ulcers?

For generations, gastric ulcers were thought to develop from an excess production of acids or from a breakdown in the normal functioning of the protective mucous membrane. This breakdown was thought to be associated with stress and the taking of certain drugs, such as corticosteroids (prednisone) and nonsteroidal anti-inflammatories (most notably aspirin).

While all of these educated assumptions are still in place, in the early 1990s a major development in understanding ulcers radically changed the way we now approach ulcers and their treatment. It started with an ill-regarded theory—kicked around for years—that bacteria can actually cause ulcers. No one had tested it or proved it. In Australia, however, two doctors decided to do just that. Starting out, they knew that for any conclusions to be accepted by the scientific community they would have to follow Koch's Postulates regarding infectious diseases. Those postulates involve certain steps:

• Find and recover bacteria from the ulcers of someone.

• Grow that bacteria in the lab.

• Infect a healthy stomach with the bacteria. If they cause ulcers, the theory is proved.

• Recover the bacteria from the newly formed ulcers and grow them in the lab.

After accomplishing the first two steps, the Australian doctors made an incredibly gutsy move (literally and figuratively)—they swallowed the ulcer-causing bacteria. They're probably the only people in the world who ever rejoiced when they felt the first pains of an ulcer.

The bacteria they had discovered is now named *Helicobacter pylori*, or *H. pylori*. It has stimulated a new way of viewing ulcers, as well as creating a never-thought-possible cure for many people who have suffered lifetimes of chronic ulcer pain or endured stomach surgery for their ulcers.

Most surprising has been the extent of *H. pylori's* reach. The bacteria is capable of producing ulcers in various forms and in various areas of the digestive tract. A medical text, *GI Liver Secrets*, states that an astounding 60 to 90 percent of ulcers may be caused by *H. pylori*. And, because the bacteria most probably originates from contaminated food, it's estimated that people in developing countries have infection levels as high as 80 to 90 percent by twenty years of age. In developed countries such as America, less than 20 percent of people below the age of twenty-five have it. This increases about one percent per year, to 50 to 60 percent by age seventy.

Additionally, a long-term consequence of untreated *Helicobacter* infection might be stomach cancer, which means that it would be a treatable cause of the stomach cancer. An interesting aside is that the discovery of the bacteria might help explain the marked decrease in the incidence of stomach cancer and esophageal (throat) cancer over a period of fifty to seventy-five years. If the bacteria is the cause of those cancers, and the source is contaminated food, then it would stand to reason that as our food supply has become safer—with refrigeration, better food preparation, and the much maligned chemical preservatives—there would be fewer of these bacteria around, leading to fewer stomach and esophageal cancers.

In the light of *H. pylori's* discovery, current medical thinking now leaves only two major causes of peptic ulcers: *H. pylori*, and NSAIDs (nonsteroid anti-inflammatories—primarily aspirin). This is certainly borne out in Gordon's practice, where he's seen those with *H. pylori* completely cured and those with stomach sensitivity to aspirin and NSAIDs relieved of ulcer symptoms with the use of alternative pain medications. He's just not seeing as many ulcers nowadays, and those he does see can be handled in a straightforward manner.

Treatment/Prevention. Because the treatment for *H. pylori* ulcers is rather elaborate—involving three different antibiotics over a one-to-three-week period—it first must be proven that the bacteria is in your stomach. That's done by taking samples during a scope exam. It has now become routine that anyone who is scoped, no matter what the reason, is tested for the bacteria. Simpler testing—such as a breath test and blood test—is available but not as accurate.

GOOD OR BAD FOR YOU?
THE LOWDOWN ON CAFFEINE

Can't function before your first cup of coffee?

You're not alone. Millions of us feel we couldn't survive without this elixir of life, which gives us a "buzz" or "jolt" every morning. While we might love the smell and taste of a good cup of Joe, our bodies really know what the secret is: caffeine. Found in chocolate, tea, soft drinks, pain relievers, and diet pills, caffeine is a mild stimulant of the nervous system that can improve mental alertness, concentration, reaction time, memory, and reasoning.

For some unfortunate people, however, caffeine can cause sleep disruption, anxiety, irritability, nausea, lack of concentration, diarrhea, and heart palpitations, and it may affect blood pressure. Caffeine also acts as a diuretic, increasing urine output and speeding up dehydration. Additionally, sufferers of certain prostate and urinary tract ailments (such as enlargement of the prostate) should limit their intake of caffeine because it may irritate the urinary tract.

Then, of course, there is the matter of caffeine dependence. As with all addictive substances, there is a wide range of individual reactions and levels of dependency—one cup of coffee a day may be too much for one person, while ten cups might not faze someone else. Withdrawal symptoms may include headaches, nausea, and general fatigue at first.

A good general rule on coffee consumption: Cut back if you feel nervous or irritable or have trouble sleeping. If you feel fine, your caffeine intake is probably not doing you any harm—and it sure makes waking up a lot easier.

The Small Intestine

The small intestine is between the stomach and the large intestine and is the largest part of the digestive tract—measuring a whopping twenty-four feet of turning, looping tube. It's a major site of food digestion, where nutrients are pulled from the food and absorbed through the wall lining into the blood system. Along the route of the small intestine, which is also known as the small bowel, are the liver, gallbladder, and pancreas. Surprisingly, there are few problems associated with this large organ.

Malabsorption

The primary problems that may occur in the small intestine fall under the category of malabsorption, which means the abnormal absorption of nutrients. It's a lot harder to understand the causes of this condition than to notice the major initial symptom—chronic diarrhea.

Chronic diarrhea is different from what's called functional diarrhea. Functional diarrhea is something that won't wake people from sleep and force them to the bathroom. It usually goes away on its own. Most times, functional diarrhea is caused by nerves or maybe even too much coffee or spicy food. On the other hand, chronic diarrhea will wake you up and isn't lessened or relieved by what you eat. It is usually a sign of a more serious ailment and must be treated to go away.

There are a variety of illnesses—such as Crohn's disease—which are associated with diarrhea and are basically chronic inflammatory conditions. These, however, usually are less common in our age group than in much older and much younger age groups. If you haven't had any such problems by the time you've reached your fifties, you'll probably not have any problems until you're much older.

By far the most common malabsorption problem for fifties males—especially those who love the outdoors—is giardiasis.

GIARDIA LAMBLIA

An increasingly prevelant cause of chronic diarrhea is the Giardia organism that can be found in contaminated food and tainted water throughout the world. Many campers get it from creek water contaminated by animal feces, and it can taint home well water. Pet owners can also contract it from their furry fellow earth dwellers by—you guessed it—the fecal-to-oral route (remember to wash your hands after cleaning up the daily "presents" your dog leaves you in your backyard). Giardiasis can cause diarrhea, nausea, bloating, abdominal cramping and grumbling, flatulence, and intermittent periods of acute diarrhea. It's not the type of illness that will put you in bed or in the hospital—you'll be able to function—but you won't feel that great. A stool exam and/or urine test can diagnose giardiasis. Left untreated, the condition will not go away.

Treatment/Prevention. Very easy with the antibiotic Flagyl. Prevention means no longer drinking from that clear-looking (but probably bug-infested) mountain stream unless the water is purified or filtered first. It's also a good idea to have a home well tested each year.

The Liver

Weighing in at about five to ten pounds (or about 5 percent of our total weight), the liver is the largest internal organ in the body and one of the most complex. Divided into four lobes, it's supplied by two blood systems: One provides fresh oxygenated blood for the liver's own nutrition; the other carries nutrients from the stomach and intestines to the liver for filtering. Think of the liver as one big processing plant where raw material is converted into energy, building materials, or waste. Virtually all of what we eat and drink—most notably protein, carbohydrates, and fat— ends up passing through the liver to be filtered, cleaned, and processed. It's a true powerhouse of an organ.

Functions of the Liver

- Helps regulate the level of blood sugar, which is the body's fuel system, and stores a form of sugar for future use.

- Produces bile, which is stored in the gallbladder before it's sent to the small intestine to break down fats.

- Stores vitamins as well as synthesizes substances involved in blood clotting.

- Synthesizes the body's circulating proteins (antibodies and substances involved in inflammation and blood clotting).

- Detoxifies poisonous material and breaks down drugs and other ingested chemicals.

- Recycles worn-out red blood cells.

With all those duties, it's surprising that the liver is relatively problem free— except if the owner abuses it. The abuse usually comes in three forms:

1. **Consumption-related**—mainly the long-term abuse of alcohol.

2. **Behavior-related**—sharing of dirty needles or having unprotected sex, both of which can lead to contracting various forms of viral hepatitis. (See the following hepatitis section for details.)

3. **Accident-related**—unknowingly mixing infected bodily fluids, such as in a transfusion of tainted blood that leads to contracting a form of hepatitis. (It should be noted that, for the past decade or so, all donor blood has been screened for *known* forms of hepatitis.)

Before you start getting worried or paranoid, be aware that a fifties male who eats and drinks normally and avoids the above-mentioned behaviors shouldn't have much problem with his liver. There's even a vaccination you can get for two forms of hepatitis (A and B). Gordon recommends everyone get both, no matter what your lifestyle or frequency of travel.

While you're doing your part to help your liver, it's doing its part as well. The liver has tremendous recuperative powers that can sustain it and even rejuvenate it, to a certain extent, after mild abuses such as the occasional excess intake of alcohol (getting plastered). In fact, the liver is so forgiving that it often fails to give you warning signs if the occasional abuses are getting close to causing permanent damage. One day the liver will seem to be working fine, the next it will be shutting down—sometimes permanently—without much advance notice. That said, it

---

WATCH OUT FOR THIS COCKTAIL
DRUGS AND THE GRAPEFRUIT JUICE EFFECT

Most people know that mixing drugs—everything from over-the-counter remedies to prescription medications—can be potentially dangerous. That's why it's imperative that patients tell their doctors *all* the medications they're taking.

What isn't as well known, though, is that a simple half of a grapefruit, or one glass of grapefruit juice, can actually adversely affect some drugs. Only grapefruit juice has this effect because it is thought to inhibit certain enzymes in the liver and intestinal wall that have the job of decreasing the effectiveness of drugs. If these enzymes are inhibited, then whatever drug you're taking is much more potent, because more of the drug gets into your system. This can be a good thing or a bad thing. Either way, however, the grapefruit juice effect—which can last from twelve to twenty-four hours—is important to know about. Check with your doctor for greater details. Drugs that can possibly be affected by grapefruit juice include:

- Some antihistamines.

- Benzodiazepine drugs—psychoactive drugs that include tranquilizers such as Valium.

- Calcium channel-blocker drugs—used to lower high blood pressure.

- Statin drugs—used to lower high cholesterol.

- Some antibiotics—most notably erythromycin, which uses some of the same enzymes grapefruit juice is thought to inhibit. Because of this similarity, any drug that has a warning of possible adverse interaction with erythromycin probably means that the drug will interact with grapefruit juice as well.

should be mentioned that early, very mild damage can be detected with blood tests long before major damage has occurred. But prevention is definitely the key to keeping the liver healthy and functioning well.

Hepatitis

Generally speaking, hepatitis is an inflammation of the liver that creates symptoms such as jaundice (yellowing of the skin and the whites of the eyes), loss of appetite, abdominal discomfort, and dark urine. It may be caused by a viral infection, infestation with parasites, alcohol, drugs, toxins, transfusions of incompatible blood, or a complication of another disease. It may be mild and brief or prolonged and severe, even life-threatening.

Viral hepatitis is the most common form and has additional symptoms that include headache, fever, pain in the region of the liver (upper right part of the abdominal cavity), and loose, clay-colored stools. The virus can be passed in various ways, depending on which one of the five currently identifiable forms of viral hepatitis it is: A, B, C, D, or E.

Because D and E are unusual, the ones to be concerned with are A, B, and C. While a person who has one can also contract the others, it's important to note that A and B are fully preventable with immunization shots. Once again, Gordon recommends that everyone, no matter what age, sex, or lifestyle choices should get immunized.

HEPATITIS A

This is what physicians used to call infectious hepatitis, and it's spread through the fecal-to-oral route. Epidemics have been known to occur via contaminated water or food. While many think contracting hep A is a possibility only when traveling through countries with poor sanitation, that's not true. All it really takes is one infected restaurant worker anywhere in the world who handles food with unclean hands after going to the bathroom. Contaminated raw shellfish can also be a source of the hep A virus.

Treatment/Prevention. Most people who contract hep A have an acute attack, then recover completely, although some (rarely) have such severe cases that their liver is rapidly destroyed, and they either get a transplant or die. During the acute phase of hep A, treatment is for the symptoms only, because there is no antiviral drug that's effective. The best treatment for hep A is to not get it at all. Ten years ago, hep A wasn't preventable; today it is. Two shots, spaced six months apart, will immunize you for life.

HEPATITIS B

Because liver cancer is sometimes a delayed complication of chronic hep B, hep B is the most common preventable cause of cancer worldwide. Hepatitis B is a serious problem in the Far East, where it has reached nearly epidemic proportions, but is less common in the United States.

Hepatitis B is most commonly contracted through shared needles, shared razor blades, close living (mothers can pass it through breast feeding), and unprotected sex. You can catch it from semen and blood, but probably not from saliva. More prevalent in the gay community and the drug culture than in the average U.S. population, it can also be transmitted via accidents that can infect anyone (most notably health-care workers). At one time, hep B could be contracted by blood transfusions, but a test to detect it has been available for about thirty years, so the blood supply is protected from hep B.

Like hep A, hep B can be severe early on, usually more intense than hep A, but probably 90 percent of people get over it completely. Ten percent become carriers or develop chronic hepatitis B.

Treatment/Prevention. For the acute phase of hep B, because there is no antiviral drug that works, treatment is basically symptomatic and supportive, meaning the symptoms are treated individually. Like hep A, hep B is completely preventable through a series of shots (three for hep B) spaced over six months. It has now become a universal—albeit controversial—immunization for children. Most fifty-year-old men have not been immunized but should be.

Many of you might be thinking: "I'm not going to have sex with a stranger. I'm not going to shoot up on the corner with somebody. Why should I worry?"

The problem is that accidents do happen. What if you're traveling in a third-world country and you get into a car accident? You might end up in a primitive hospital where someone uses a dirty needle to inject you with a pain killer, or you might get a transfusion of tainted blood.

Do you want to pay for one such accident for the rest of your life? Especially when there's a way to protect yourself completely?

HEPATITIS C

Hep C has become a major issue both worldwide and in the United States. It's spread in the same ways as hep B—shared needles, unprotected sex, and transfusions. It couldn't be detected until 1993; now there's a test to detect it. Because hep C was taken out of the blood supply in 1993, people who were transfused after that are safe. Unfortunately, this also means that there's potentially a big reservoir of people who were transfused prior to that who might have the disease.

The frightening aspect of hep C is that it doesn't cause a noticeable illness in its acute phase. More often than not, it never goes away; it's a chronic illness that stays around for a long, long time. Anyone can be walking around with hep C and not know it. The only way the disease can be detected is through blood tests. It's estimated that as many as 90 percent of those infected become carriers, while only 10 percent get over hep C completely.

The worst part—yep, it gets worse—is that over a long period of time severe damage does occur to the liver, which will eventually lead to liver failure. This means that, potentially, years from now, a large group of people will experience liver failure and will need transplants.

Treatment/Prevention. Before the year 2000, hep C was basically untreatable. In early 2000, however, a treatment was developed. Using a combination of interferon (a protein produced by our immune systems to fight viruses) and ribavarin (an anti-viral drug), some hep C patients have gone from a high viral "load" (meaning lots of virus in their systems) to undetectable levels of virus—basically a "cure." The downside is that this is a very difficult, expensive, lengthy course of treatment, not unlike chemotherapy for cancer patients. On the upside, it is the first promising bit of news on the hep C front in some time.

As far as prevention goes, currently there is no immunization for hep C.

Alcohol can accelerate liver damage in both hep B and hep C, and should therefore be avoided completely by those with the diseases.

Alcoholic Liver Disease

Alcoholic liver disease can be a concern for certain males in our age group. If you've been drinking fairly heavily for thirty years, this is the decade when liver problems due to drinking can start showing up. But that depends greatly on the intake and the individual. The youngest patient Gordon ever had who died from liver failure brought on by alcoholic liver disease was twenty-seven, but he really worked overtime—drinking massive amounts—to kill his liver.

As for warning signs of alcoholic liver disease, heavy drinkers don't have a reliable "marker" like smokers do. Smokers know that after twenty pack years their odds of smoking-related diseases start rising dramatically (see chapter 8 for details and an explanation of pack years). For those who are heavy drinkers, though, there is no such marker, because the liver is very resilient and capable of healing itself for quite some time. This ability to handle sustained abuse is certainly a good thing, but it also has a downside—there's little warning before the organ suddenly begins to fail.

Because we don't know the limits of the liver, it's best not to push the outside of the envelope. Heavy drinkers should either try to reduce their consumption or quit altogether.

What Constitutes a Heavy Drinker?

Anywhere from two to six drinks a day puts you in the heavy drinker category. (A drink is either an ounce and a half of hard liquor, five ounces of wine, or ten to twelve ounces of beer.) Moderate drinkers are those who have two or fewer drinks a day. Beyond six drinks a day you get into the classification of alcoholic. While the term alcoholic can mean different things to different people, a reasonable working definition is someone whose consumption of alcohol is in some way adversely affecting his life—whether it's affecting his relationship with his family, his career, or his health.

Because the liver is so resilient until it fails, outward behaviors are often our only gauges of the internal situation. These can include a person's decreased productivity, decreased appetite, lack of interest in exercising or taking care of himself, domestic strife, and bad personal judgment (the most notable example being drinking and driving).

At the very least, all these behaviors would suggest that an honest evaluation of your alcohol consumption should be completed; at the most, they constitute reasons for giving up drinking altogether.

Studies have shown that mortality rates for moderate drinkers are actually lower than for teetotalers, mostly because of a reduction in heart disease (alcohol improves good cholesterol). This isn't to say that teetotalers should start drinking—approximately 10 percent of those who do start drinking will have a hard time controlling the quantity. Because physicians can't tell which of their patients will fall into that 10 percent group, they're reluctant to advise those who don't drink to start drinking for their health. They do, however, reassure patients who are moderate drinkers that they are not harming themselves and are probably doing themselves some good. It should also be pointed out, however, that studies have shown that, with more than two drinks a day, the mortality rate is actually higher for drinkers than for teetotalers.

No matter where you fall in the alcohol hierarchy, it's critical that you tell your doctor the truth about your consumption levels. This is one of the three areas in which many male patients lie to their doctors (the others being sex and smoking). Most times, you won't get away with it. Doctors can inevitably tell from certain blood tests, and by the way you look—the glassy, watery eyes of the heavy drinker, a florid appearing face, thin limbs, and a thick abdomen.

Treatment/Prevention. Other than abstinence, there is no treatment for alcoholic liver disease. And once the liver fails completely, the body can't live without a liver transplant. Advanced signs of the condition include difficulty fighting off infections, bleeding problems because your liver doesn't manufacture clotting factors like it used to, swelling feet, and fluid collection in the belly.

For those who want to moderate or stop their drinking, there are numerous programs to help—most notably Alcoholics Anonymous. A great first step toward any kind of control would be to speak with your doctor or therapist.

The Gallbladder

The gallbladder is a pear-shaped organ that's a scant three inches long and located on the lower surface of the liver. It's little more than a storage vessel for bile, which is produced by the liver. Eating a meal rich in fats stimulates bile to be discharged from the gallbladder into the upper part of the digestive tract (the duodenum) where the bile breaks down the fats, preparing them for further digestion. While the gallbladder is definitely small—both in size and function—it nonetheless can make itself painfully known through the dreaded attack of gallstones.

Gallstones

As our bodies age, changes in the content of our bile can cause stonelike masses to form in the gallbladder that are aptly named "gallstones." While we're not exactly sure why or how they form, it appears that diets rich in fatty foods are partly to blame. Usually not much bigger than a pea, the overwhelming majority of gallstones just sit quietly, causing no pain, and only occasionally creating a little inflammation by rubbing against the walls of the gallbladder.

Surprisingly, the smaller the gallstone the greater the possibility of trouble. That's because a small one can work its way into the duct that drains the gallbladder and cause what's known as a gallbladder attack. The pain is intense and is centered in the right upper quadrant of the abdomen, though it may also radiate to the shoulder or back. Along with the pain there's usually nausea, vomiting, and, sometimes, fever. If the stone moves to the duct between the gallbladder and the duodenum, it can back up bile into the liver and eventually into the blood stream, which can cause a person to become jaundiced (yellow-skinned). Biliary infections can complicate gallstone disease and the addition of fever to the above symptoms raises that possibility. An infected gallbladder or bile tract is a medical emergency.

The decade of the forties is when gallstones first begin forming, and normally they are more prevalent in women. Doctors have an expression—fair, fat, fertile, and forty—to describe the most common traits of sufferers. This doesn't mean, however, that men are out of the woods. In fact, if they're ever going to suffer this ailment, males in their fifties are probably at the peak time to do so.

Treatment/Prevention. Because a gallstone attack is usually so severe, it will land you in an emergency room. There is a drug that can dissolve the stones, but once you stop taking the drug the stones come back, and there's some evidence that suggests the drug raises cholesterol.

Surgery is far and away the most common treatment and probably the best option. A variety of surgical techniques can be used, but the most satisfactory is a laparoscopic technique that uses a tubelike device through a small incision to remove the entire gallbladder. Typically, those who have this surgery don't form gallstones again—probably because there's no reservoir (the gallbladder) left where the stones can form. This surgery is considered relatively routine, and recovery time is usually short (one to two weeks, with usually only one night in the hospital).

As to living without a gallbladder: You're better off living without one than living with a diseased one, because that will just bring back the stones and all

---

WHERE DOES IT GO?
GI TRACT EXAMS

- **An Upper GI Series**—A workhorse used for seventy-five years, it gives a reverse X-ray image to spot if the throat (esophagus) is ulcerated, narrowed, or irritated, or if the stomach has ulcers. It's less precise than newer techniques and can't treat what's found.

- **Esophagogastroduodenoscopy (EGD)**—A fiber-optic scope exam of the esophagus, stomach, and first part of the small bowel that provides incredibly accurate images. It can also take tissue samples and treat ailments like bleeding ulcers and a narrowed throat. Performed as an outpatient day procedure under "conscious sedation."

- **Flexible Sigmoidoscopy**—The same as the EGD, but for the lower one-third of the lower bowel. The scope is inserted through the rectum and used to spot potentially precancerous polyps (abnormal growths), cancers, and diverticuli (outpouchings in the bowel lining). Usually performed by primary-care physicians as an office procedure. With no nerve ends in the lower bowel, no anesthesia is required. Strongly recommend-ed for every male starting at fifty, and should be repeated every three to five years.

- **Colonoscopy**—A longer version of the sigmoidoscope, a colonoscope can travel further up the colon. It's a day procedure in a hospital or clinic under conscious sedation. The gastroenterologist will immediately remove any polyps and can do other treatments also. Usually done only after a sigmoidoscopy has found polyps, or for other unexplained signs and symptoms, such as blood in the stools.

their attendant complications. A possible consequence of not having a gallbladder is some degree of intolerance to fatty food, which usually causes bouts of diarrhea, but that's a symptom often associated with gallstone disease anyway. Diarrhea can occasionally occur after a gallbladder's been removed, but it typically goes away after a while. At the rare times when it doesn't vanish, it can be treated easily.

Prevention of gallstones includes reduction of fat in the diet, the drinking of coffee (some evidence suggests it reduces the incidence of gallstones), and the usual measure of choosing one's parents wisely (gallstones seem to have an hereditary link).

The Pancreas

At nearly twice the size (six inches) of the gallbladder, the pancreas provides two important services: It secretes pancreatic juice, which contains enzymes used in the digestive tract, and it produces the hormones insulin (which regulates the breakdown of sugar) and glucagon (which counters the effects of excessive insulin).

Pancreatitis

Relatively speaking, males in our age group have little to worry about when it comes to the pancreas. The exception is the closet drinker, binge drinker, or alcoholic, whose drinking can bring on pancreatitis, an inflammation of the organ usually marked by nausea, vomiting, and intense abdominal pain that often spreads to the back. It is easily detected by simple blood tests. Pancreatitis can also be caused by gallstones, certain drugs, high levels of cholesterol and triglycerides, and certain infections. Sixty to eighty percent of cases are due to alcohol or gallstones, approximately equally divided between the two.

Treatment/Prevention. Depending on the severity and cause of the pancreatitis, treatment may include hospitalization, intensive medical care, and the taking of pain-relieving drugs. Acute pancreatitis is invariably severe enough to require hospitalization and carries an impressively high mortality rate. Emergency surgery is sometimes required to treat the complications of pancreatitis.

Prevention includes taking charge of your fat intake to prevent gallstones, maintaining good cholesterol levels, and controlling alcohol consumption.

Diabetes

Already afflicting more than sixteen million Americans (with 2,200 new cases diagnosed every day and approximately 500 deaths a day), diabetes is now considered by some physicians to be approaching epidemic proportions in America. There are two primary forms of the disease: type 1 (previously called juvenile-onset diabetes) and type 2 (known as adult onset diabetes, maturity-onset diabetes, and/or noninsulin dependent diabetes).

Insulin and Diabetes

Both types of diabetes are related to insulin. Insulin is a hormone produced by the pancreas that allows sugar (glucose) to enter cells so it can be used for fuel. If sugar can't enter the cells, the cells must use an alternative source of fuel, namely fat. When fat is burned for energy without sugar, an overproduction of acid may occur.

That, in itself, is a life-threatening situation, but to compound matters, the sugar that doesn't get into the cells begins to accumulate in the blood and urine, dangerously thickening both liquids. Trying to rectify the situation, the body demands water (creating constant thirst) and continually tries to rid the system of the sugar via the urine (creating frequent urination). This happens in both forms of diabetes and, unfortunately, does real harm to the body.

The most insidious part of adult onset (Type 2) diabetes is that often symptoms don't show up until damage—sometimes severe and permanent—has been done to numerous systems and organs. The overload of sugar in the blood can cause havoc with the blood vessels, both the large ones that supply the heart and extremities (most notably the legs) and the tiny blood vessels in places such as the eyes, hands, and feet. This can lead to everything from heart disease and eye damage (including blindness) to foot ulcers, nerve damage, and kidney problems. What can be especially traumatic for men is that diabetes can create erection problems, due to blood vessel damage, in 50 to 60 percent of cases, according to the American Diabetes Foundation Association. If left unchecked, both forms of diabetes can cause death.

While Type 1 and Type 2 diabetes can have similar consequences, they do come from two different problems.

The Difference Between Type 1 and Type 2 Diabetes

Type 1 diabetes is a condition in which the pancreas stops producing insulin. Without insulin a person will die, so insulin must be injected regularly into a Type 1 diabetic. Because Type 1 normally develops in young people, a man in our age group who hasn't yet developed Type 1 probably won't, while a fifties man who contracted Type 1 when he was younger will have become an expert manager of the condition long before reaching fifty.

The Digestive and Urinary Tracts

Type 2 diabetes is another matter altogether, afflicting mostly people in their forties or fifties and with the peak incidence of diagnosis taking place in the fifties. It strikes men and women approximately equally. In Type 2 the body's cells have developed an insulin resistance, so that they do not allow sugar in—even with insulin sitting outside telling them to let the sugar in. This causes some of the same dangerous situations as Type 1. The insulin resistance results in an overproduction of insulin (the body's attempt to compensate) and eventual failure of insulin production.

Contributing Factors to Developing Type 2 Diabetes

- **Genetic Predisposition.** If someone in your family has had diabetes, your chances of getting it increase. Often this is a difficult component to pin down because of inaccurate, unknown, or incomplete family histories.

- **Increasing Age.** Type 2 becomes more prevalent as we become older, usually striking in the forties and fifties. This, however, has now begun to change as the medical community records more and more Type 2 cases developing in overweight teenagers.

- **Being Overweight.** It can be as little as ten to thirty pounds overweight, although most cases are linked with obesity (at least 20 percent overweight). The Centers for Disease Control and Prevention in Atlanta announced in 2001 that there is dramatic evidence showing that Type 2 diabetes is so much on the rise in all age groups (jumping 33 percent nationally to 6.5 percent from 1990 to 1998) that it is becoming epidemic and seems to correspond to the drastic rise in obesity in America (from 12 percent of the population in 1991 to 20 percent in 1999).

- **High Levels of Cholesterol.** While not all people with high cholesterol have diabetes, nearly all Type 2 diabetics have high cholesterol—due in large part to the overweight factor.

With Type 2 diabetes there are no symptoms until the disease is relatively far advanced. This means the blood sugar level will be extremely high—300 to 400 mg per deciliter—compared to the upper limit of normal fasting blood sugar of 110. Additionally, if sugar is found in the urine, then it's often the case that the person's blood sugar level is already in the 200s. This is why having periodic blood and urine tests that check for sugar levels is critical to catching diabetes before it does any permanent damage.

163

Possible Type 2 Diabetes Symptoms

- Fatigue

- Water-weight loss

- Constant thirst

- Frequent urination

- Increased skin and yeast infections

It should be stressed that diabetes has dire consequences (approximately 500 deaths a day in America), which can be prevented by early detection and aggressive treatment.

Treatment/Prevention. There is no cure for diabetes, but treatments are available. With Type 1 diabetes the treatment is straightforward—supply insulin to the body. If this is done correctly, diabetes can be kept under control with minimal damage to the body.

For most Type 2 diabetics, the treatment is nearly as uncomplicated as with Type 1—although it's harder to implement. In the majority of Type 2 cases, exercise and attaining a healthy weight through proper eating habits will usually control the diabetes. Exercise does magical things to the body's ability to use insulin properly. And with a proper diet—and the subsequent weight loss that should follow—sugar levels may reach safe and healthy ranges. In some cases, the body actually returns to properly utilizing insulin.

Unfortunately, many Type 2 diabetics—like many other overweight people—find it difficult to follow an effective diet and exercise program. This is where a relationship with a physician willing to help develop and sustain such programs can be crucial to successfully controlling diabetes. Additionally, if the diet and exercise fail, the doctor now has a small arsenal of drugs available.

How Diabetes Drugs Work

Bombard the system with insulin. As mentioned earlier, in Type 2 diabetes the problem isn't usually a lack of insulin; it's the body's inability to utilize existing insulin. But until recently, there was no way to directly deal with this body malfunction. The only treatment doctors had was to overload the body with insulin as a way of forcing the system to function properly. It worked with limited benefit.

Make the pancreas produce more insulin. This is done through sulfonylurea drugs. It is a little better than periodically injecting the body with insulin, but not much.

Reduce the rate at which the liver makes sugar. This is done with a biguanide class of drug (most notably Glucophage). These drugs also seem to lower the cell's insulin resistance. These drugs are a step-up from simply pumping insulin into the system.

Attack the cell's insulin resistance. The thiazolidinedione class of drugs (notably Avandia and Actos) has revolutionized treatment of Type 2 diabetes by going to the cause of disease—the cells' resistance to insulin. The drugs can be used alone or in combination with other drugs. An added benefit is that these drugs have some positive effects on cholesterol levels as well.

As for the prevention of diabetes, it can't be done yet—although scientists are looking into identifying the predisposing genes. You can, however, drastically reduce your risks of getting Type 2 diabetes by maintaining a healthy weight through a well-balanced diet and a good exercise program (see chapter 8 for details). It also wouldn't hurt to find out as much as possible about your family history in relation to diabetes. If you know you have a genetic predisposition, you'll also know to be periodically monitored and tested to catch it at its earliest if it shows up.

The Large Intestine

Often referred to as the colon or large bowel, the large intestine gets its name not from its length (the small intestine easily wins that contest at 24 feet) but from its girth (one to two inches in diameter), which is substantially larger than the small intestine. Just like its big name, the large intestine can also have a large number of problems, many of which specifically visit men in our age group.

Digestively speaking, the large bowel has a relatively easy job, extracting water and electrolytes such as calcium, salt, and potassium from the sludge (fecal matter) sent to it by the small intestine. As that process is happening, the waste begins to solidify and is moved along by contractions in the lining wall, ultimately being eliminated from the body as a bowel movement or stool.

Problems associated with the large intestine run the gamut from annoying (diarrhea, constipation, and hemorrhoids) to more severe (diverticulosis) to down-right life-threatening (colon cancer, which is the third leading cause of cancer death in men). The fifties decade is where many of these problems first start showing themselves. It is also when early detection can have the most impact.

For some of these ailments—especially colon cancer—a scope exam is the best way of early detection. When a person is "scoped," a fiber-optic endoscope (tubelike device) is inserted into the colon by way of the rectum, so that a doctor can inspect the lining of the colon for polyps (growth or nodules), tumors, or other abnormal lesions. While doing this, a doctor can take a sample of anything that looks suspicious, as well as perform certain treatments, such as cauterizing (sealing up with heat) any bleeding sites—all through the use of the scope.

There are two basic scoping exams: One is called a flexible sigmoidoscopy, which is done to inspect the lower portion of the large intestine. This exam requires a scope of about two feet in length and can usually be performed by your family physician in an office visit. The other exam, called a colonoscopy, is a complete examination of the entire colon. It requires a scope about five or six feet long and is handled as an outpatient procedure done in a more hospital-like setting.

Every man who turns fifty should have a flexible sigmoidoscopy, with repeat performances every five years thereafter (sooner if symptoms warrant). He should also have a stool analyzed for blood every year.

Flatulence

No, it's not abnormal. We fifties males get a lot of grief from our partners, but there really isn't any proof that we pass more gas than they do. There's also no proof that people who complain about having gas all the time produce more gas than people who don't complain about it. They just may feel it more.

Treatment/Prevention. One thing science does know about this topic is that there are certain gas-producing foods. They include the cruciferous (cross-shaped) vegetables that are relatively rich in antioxidant vitamins and fiber and have been touted as part of a good anticancer diet. These are Brussels sprouts, cauliflower, beans, cabbage, and broccoli. Additionally, gas producers include wheat products like bread and pasta, as well as apples. Because of all these items, it's generally understood that vegetarians have more gas (a bad thing) as well as more bowel movements (a good thing) than meat eaters.

What Causes Gas and How To Prevent It

The culprit in all this is complex carbohydrates. They can't always be easily digested in the small intestine, so they move on into the large intestine where they become fermented. This, of course, causes a bloating feeling and produces gas.

For people who are extraordinarily sensitive to gas-producing vegetables and who want to eat them or can't avoid them, there's an enzyme product called Beano that actually breaks down the complex carbohydrates into simpler sugars that can be digested more readily. This occurs before the offending substance reaches the colon, so there's nothing to ferment. Beano is sold over the counter and comes in liquid or tablet form. You take it with a meal, and it seems to work quite well.

Another cause of gas is lactose intolerance, meaning your digestive tract can't properly digest the sugar (lactose) that's in milk. A fair number of people are lactose intolerant, and it becomes more common with age. Most children are not, but as people get older they tolerate milk less and less well. This intolerance is highest of all in people whose genetic background is from the tropical areas of the world—so blacks and Mediterranean peoples tend to have a higher incidence than people whose origin is in the northern hemisphere, particularly the far north.

Many times you can make the diagnosis of milk-sugar intolerance by yourself, but some people may need the help of a doctor to distinguish the condition from something more significant. Simply avoiding milk and milk products works. For those who won't or can't do that, there's lactase (the enzyme that helps digest the lactose in milk), which you can put in milk to solve the problem. There are even products that already have it added. Milk that has lactase in it will taste a little sweeter than regular milk.

No matter what produces gas in you, undoubtedly there will come a time when you feel the need to let it rip, but you'll be in a situation that doesn't tolerate such behavior. At times like that, you might wonder, "Is it harmful to my system to hold in gas?"

Not really. If you've eaten something fartogenic and you're producing a fair amount of gas, but you have to hold it in for a couple of hours, you're definitely going to feel pretty uncomfortable, crampy even. That's the main danger. But don't worry, it won't back up and cause a fart embolism in your brain.

Hemorrhoids

The scourge of fifties males everywhere, hemorrhoids are the swelling of one or more of the hemorrhoidal veins, which are a network of veins around the anus and the rectum. Like veins everywhere, they're thin-walled and relatively passive structures. This means they can, under certain circumstances, become engorged with blood, expanding out like a balloon overfilled with water. Swelling is compounded when those blood-engorged veins can't empty.

What Causes Hemorrhoids?

- **Straining at the stool (pushing too hard to aid a bowel movement)** increases the pressure that prevents those veins from emptying.

- **Sitting for long periods of time on American-style toilets** acts basically like a tourniquet, cutting off blood flow between your bum and the rest of the body.

- **Sitting in a stationary position for a long time** restricts blood flow (this includes everything from protracted sales meetings and long airplane flights to long-haul truck driving and heavy-equipment operating).

Ultimately, the dilated blood vessels become inflamed and the tissue around them swells, so you end up with a protruding vein. As most of you already know, this not only can be very painful but also sometimes makes it difficult to pass a stool. Additionally, the protruding vein can bleed and get irritated or cause itching when your buttocks rub against each other as you walk or run.

There are two kinds of hemorrhoids: external and internal. The dividing mark is the so-called "dentate line" (just inside the anal sphincter). Internal hemorrhoids don't really hurt, because the bowel wall has no pain receptors, while external hemorroids can hurt worse than sitting on a spike.

Treatment/Prevention. Soaking in warm water (sitz baths) helps, as do products like Preparation H, which act to shrink the protruding veins. Suppositories can help internal hemorrhoids.

Some external hemorrhoids can become clotted, causing what's called thrombosed hemorrhoids. They can be so excruciatingly painful that any doctor who performs the in-office tiny incision to remove the clot makes a friend for life—the relief from pain is nearly instantaneous and overwhelming to the sufferer.

Other types of surgery can also come into play for severe hemorrhoids. Because of great advances in the last ten to fifteen years, there is seldom any need for the formal and relatively major operation of a hemorrhoidectomy. Now there are numerous smaller procedures that can be done to individual hemorrhoids—everything from injecting them with a solution that shrinks them to rubber-banding them off above the anal sphincter.

Hemorrhoid Prevention Strategies

- Increasing the intake of water and roughage

• Exercising more

• Not straining at the stool

• Not sitting for prolonged periods of time anywhere

Irritable Bowel Syndrome

This is a rather long, ominous name for a very common condition of the large intestine. Known also as "functional bowel syndrome" or "spastic colon," it's characterized by recurrent abdominal cramps and alternating bouts of diarrhea and constipation. Having no known organic cause, IBS can be associated with emotional stress and poor living habits, such as not enough water and roughage in the diet and not enough exercise. It can also be a result of poor bowel habits (not going when the urge hits). The condition is usually more prevalent in earlier age groups than the fifties. If a fifties male comes in complaining of IBS-like symptoms, the physician should consider IBS, but he or she also needs to consider that it might be something more severe, such as diverticulitis or colon cancer.

Treatment/Prevention. The treatment is similar to what's prescribed for preventing colon cancer and diverticulitis: Eat plenty of roughage, drink lots of water, exercise, and use a bulk additive. It helps if you take an active role in the condition—pay attention to what your digestive tract likes and doesn't like; some people are intolerant of some foods, such as lactose (milk sugar). Eating meals regularly (not skipping meals) can be helpful, because your GI tract wants your "eating life" to be predictable.

Blood in the Stool/Urine

Never, ever ignore blood in the stool or urine. Think of it this way: If you're bleeding—and we *know* you're not menstruating—then it has to come from *somewhere*. Blood can indicate a wide variety of ailments, so you should have it checked out immediately. In fact, it is such an important warning sign that it's automatically tested for in routine urinalyses and stool examinations.

What can blood in the stool or urine indicate?

In men younger than fifty, there are numerous relatively minor reasons why there might be blood in urine or stools.

Blood in the Urine Might Mean

- A spot of irritation in the lining of the urethra (the urine tube), the prostate, or the bladder

- Kidney stones

- Urinary tract infections (UTIs)

- That you've been exercising—this can occasionally cause benign microscopic blood in urine (but not in stools)

Blood in the Stool Might Mean

- A small fissure or "tear" of the anus (often caused by passing a hard stool)

- Lower bowel inflammation

- A small hemorrhoid that's popped or become irritated

With men fifty and older, however, there is a much higher degree of probability that the presence of blood indicates something serious, such as cancer or a bleeding ulcer. Particular types of cancer include bladder cancer, kidney cancer, and colon cancer (prostate cancer doesn't normally cause blood in the urine). Because blood in the urine or stool can sometimes be the *only* early warning sign when it comes to cancer, it's absolutely critical that you inform your doctor if you see anything suspicious.

Bleeding ulcers can also cause blood in the stools, which will make the stools black and tar-like rather than red. While we now know that many ulcers are caused by bacteria (see the ulcer section in this chapter), we also know that bleeding ulcers can be caused by use of OTC anti-inflammatories, which inhibit a substance that protects the stomach from its own acids. This problem can be particularly prevalent in fifties males—many of whom take an abundance of pain relievers to soothe bodies that are being pushed as if they were still thirty years old.

Bleeding in the Urinary Tract

If visible bleeding takes place in the urinary tract, most times it's completely painless—even when it's the passing of a blood clot. Visually, the blood can be quite obvious, making your stream red, maroon, or coffee-colored. It can also be in microscopic amounts that are invisible to the unaided eye. If you pass a blood clot and happen to be looking when it happens, you'll see an actual small mass of reddish material, but if you miss the passing, there's a strong likelihood you won't see anything abnormal afterward. That does *not* mean your problem has gone away. In fact, clots can be the first signs of bladder cancer.

Generally speaking, it's more common not to see blood than it is to see it—that's why doctors do urinalyses as often as they do. It always helps, though, for you to keep a watchful eye on your own situation. Normally, your urine should be a light yellow. If it's bright yellow, that could be caused by the intake of certain vitamins (such as C), or it could be an indication you're underhydrated. Almost clear urine can mean that you're overhydrated. An interesting note is that, in some people, eating beets can make your urine red for a short time.

Bleeding in the Digestive Tract

As for blood in your stool, that too can be either noticeable or invisible. If it's visible, its particular appearance will indicate the general area of concern: When a stool is nearly black or tar-colored the bleeding is probably going on somewhere between your throat and duodenum (the start of your small intestine); when a stool is maroon or bright red, the bleeding is between the duodenum and your anus. Bright red typically means it's coming from somewhere close to the anus—often a hemorrhoid or polyp. Many times there is no pain associated with bleeding in the stool, although that's not always the case.

Other reasons for the presence of blood in stools include ulcerative colitis or Crohn's disease and bleeding from a diverticulum (see below).

Treatment/Prevention. Once it's been established that bleeding is taking place somewhere in the gastrointestinal tract, one of the best ways to pinpoint the problem is through a scope exam via a tubelike device. The technology has reached such a level that many times the situation can be corrected the moment it's found. Bleeding ulcers are a good example: The scoping doctor finds the ulcer, injects adrenaline into the base of the ulcer to constrict bleeding, then cauterizes it (heats it), which seals it—all through the scope.

Diverticulitis

As mentioned earlier, the large intestine uses contractions to move along the nearly digested food through its tract. For a variety of reasons—including hereditary predisposition, a diet poor in roughage, and chronic constipation—there are times when the bowel contracts on an empty space or a mass of hard stool. When this happens, it leads to back pressure. If there are weaknesses in the colon's wall lining—specifically where arteries come in—then that back pressure, over time, can create outpouchings. It's like when you squeeze a balloon and suddenly one spot bulges out. That bulge, when it happens in the large intestine, is called a "diverticulum," and the condition of having them is called "diverticulosis."

Diverticulosis is a common condition by the half-century mark—probably half the people in America have a few diverticuli. They're fairly common among fifties males. Most times they don't cause problems. If, however, one or more of them gets inflamed, it's called diverticulitis. Symptoms include cramp-like abdominal pain, fever, and diarrhea or constipation. The most severe cases—which can be life-threatening—occur when a diverticulum ruptures and infection of fecal matter takes place outside the colon's walls. This is accompanied by fever and persistent, rather severe pain that's usually localized to the left lower quadrant of the abdomen.

Treatment/Prevention. Many times, inflamed diverticuli can be treated with "bowel rest" (no eating—nutrients are supplied through a tube into a vein) and antibiotics. Prevention of diverticulosis is similar to prevention of colon cancer: Eat lots of roughage, drink plenty of water, exercise, and use a bulk additive.

Ruptured diverticuli usually call for surgery to remove the affected part of the colon and to clean up the infection caused by release of the fecal matter. If there's enough leakage from the ruptured diverticulum, a temporary colostomy might be required. That's where fecal matter is eliminated from the body through a hole in your side so the bowel's infected area can heal properly. Once healing has taken place, your bowel can be surgically put back together again.

Colon Cancer

See chapter 7 for details.

The Kidneys

Only about four-and-a-half inches long, two-and-a-half inches wide, and one inch thick, the two bean-shaped organs that make up the kidneys have important jobs to do. Primarily, they filter wastes from the blood and eliminate them, along with water, in urine. The cleansing process is handled by an incredible one million filtering units. Besides cleansing the blood, the kidneys also regulate the water, electrolyte, and pH balance of the body. You can live without one kidney, but life cannot be sustained, unaided, without at least one functioning kidney.

Problems that can occur include inflammation, infection, the formation of kidney stones, and kidney cancer. None of these ailments affect men in our age group any more than any other segment of the population, but all are possible and can be serious. We also know that nonsteroidal anti-inflammatories (NSAIDs) can

YOUR SOON-TO-BE-CLOSE FRIEND
THE BULK ADDITIVE

Did you ever think you'd worry about your bowel movements? We didn't either. If you have bowel problems—constipation, diarrhea, or both—and your doctor has found nothing wrong, try bulk additives. Many think they're only for relieving constipation. That's just wrong.

Bulk additives are composed mainly of fiber (usually indigestible fiber) that promotes stool cohesiveness. They work in both extremes—softening a hard stool (constipation) or firming up a soft or runny stool (diarrhea). The best-known bulk additive is Metamucil. Known as the best friend of the seventies set, it can also work wonders for our age group—anyone, really. It not only restores normal bowel movements, but, arguably, reduces the risk of:

- **Diverticulosis.** It makes stools more uniform in amount and consistency, which helps avoid those isolated areas where the bowel wall contracts on an empty space or on a hard stool (conditions right for the bulging out of diverticulum).

- **Hemorrhoids.** Well-formed stools lead to less straining at the stool, which lessens your chances of hemorrhoids forming.

- **Colon cancer (possibly).** Uniform stool shape and size speeds transit time, meaning less time for potentially carcinogenic agents to be in contact with the bowel wall.

What in bulk additives makes all this happen? Psyllium husks. Grown nearly exclusively in India, psyllium's uniqueness is that it's very water soluble—much more so than wheat bran or oat bran. While it's true that some people experience bloating or gas when taking psyllium, it still works well in solving many cases of bowel problems that have no known causes.

have adverse kidney effects, so long-term users should periodically have blood tests to check kidney functions.

Kidney Stones

A common affliction that's not especially age-related, kidney stones do happen more in men than in women. The cause, in most cases, is thought to be overproduction of a substance called oxalate, a byproduct of metabolism. Excessive oxalate may be hereditary, or it may be brought on by diet.

If you have the most common type of kidney stone, calcium oxalate, your doctor may recommend a low oxalate diet (a rather complex diet). Increasing the amount of calcium in the diet may help, and staying well hydrated (plenty of water in the system) is very important. A kidney stone "belt" (where stone formation is quite prevalent) covers the southeastern U.S. and might be linked to the same area's incredibly high intake of iced tea. It's possible that large quantities of tea—especially cold, not hot—might predispose people to kidney stones. It's also possible that other dietary factors may be responsible for this southeast peculiarity. Because of the hot climate in the Southeastern United States, dehydration may also play a role.

Getting a Kidney Stone

No matter how stones form, one thing is certain—and is verified by every person who's ever had one—passing a stone is one of the most painful experiences known to man or woman. For men, the pain is located on one flank or the other and will radiate down toward the testicles and into them. The pain is extreme, to the point where you won't be able to function.

The pain is generated when the stone, which forms in the collecting system of the kidney, tries to pass through the ureter—a muscular tube that carries urine from the kidney down to the bladder. The ureter is about a foot long and is relatively narrow and rather rigid. Stones can be as small as a grain of sand and still get stuck in this tube. Once a stone gets into the bladder, there's no pain, and it usually passes through the penis when you urinate without any problems. But the foot-long ureter journey the stone needs to travel can take anywhere from a few hours to a few days. In the case of larger stones, it truly can be an impossible journey.

Plain X rays, ultrasound, or X rays enhanced by a radio-opaque contrast injected into the veins can "see" the stone and determine if it will be able to pass without help. CT scanning has begun to replace the other imaging tests for detecting kidney stones (it's quicker, more accurate, and there's less risk of allergic reactions to the intravenous contrast media used with the radio-opaque injection). The tests can also tell if you have other stones waiting in the wings to make their painful presence known. Normally, only one stone passes at a time, but if you've had one stone, there's a good chance your kidneys can form others in the future—not a very comforting thought.

Keep in mind, though, that kidney stones do *not* mean the kidneys are malfunctioning.

Presumably, it's the chemical content of the urine and the inability of the body under certain circumstances to keep all the minerals in solution that's the problem.

Treatment/Prevention. When a kidney stone gets stuck trying to sneak out of a kidney, the pain will likely be the only thing you'll be aware of, although blood in the urine can also occur. It will probably hurt so intensely that you'll immediately head for an emergency room. They'll usually treat you with pain medication, have you drink a lot of water, and determine which test is best for you. They'll also keep you from getting into bed because general movement actually helps—although the pain might tell you otherwise. Once the stone's size has been discovered, and it's been determined whether the stone's a lone warrior or a scout for a whole division, then a procedure is chosen.

For a single small stone, letting it pass with time is usually the best course of action. For those stones that are permanently stuck or those taking an inordinate amount of time to pass, surgery may be called for. In many cases, the stone is retrieved via a scope that enters through the penis and goes through the bladder into the ureter. Ultrasound from outside your body (called lithotripsy) can be used to break up a stone that is stuck in the kidney, but then you still have to pass the shards, which can still be painful.

If you're part of the let-it-pass group, once it hits the bladder the pain will instantly go away. Within a few times of urinating it will make its final—and non-painful—journey out of your body. If at all possible, collect the stone for analysis to rule out certain rare, but serious, conditions. A tip on retrieval: Urinate into a clean container, strain the urine through a tea towel or paint strainer, and don't look for that five-inch boulder you think it should be—it'll probably be no bigger than a piece of gravel.

No one who's passed a stone would ever wish the ailment on his worst enemy—the point being that it's best to try and avoid them in the first place. The best prevention is probably drinking more liquids—typically water.

Kidney Cancer

We don't know how or why this relatively rare cancer develops. Most importantly, early detection is a key to survival, and one of the few early warning signs is blood in the urine. Another is a vague pain in the mid-back area.

Treatment/Prevention. Not much good news to report here. If diagnosed early enough, surgery may be curative. Irradiation (X ray) and chemotherapy are relatively ineffective for this cancer.

The Bladder

Think of the bladder as an elastic holding tank with muscular walls that can squeeze it empty when you urinate. That's how it's supposed to work. By the time you've reached your fifties, though, the bladder is feeling about the same as some of your muscles—a little tired of constant abuse and being pushed to too many limits.

Think about it: How many times were the beer and conversation flowing so well that you just *couldn't* leave to hit the head? How many times was it a critical play that couldn't be missed for a stand at a urinal? Or how about that presentation at work that wouldn't allow a quick run to the john? When you count them all up, you've been putting a cork in it for a lot of years.

Well, buddy, sorry to say, but it's the start of payback time.

In the fifties decade, the bladder is like a balloon that's seen too many helium fill-ups: It starts losing some of its zing. The sphincters (trapdoors) that control

POKED AND PRODDED
IMPORTANT DIGESTIVE/URINARY DIAGNOSTIC TESTS

Prostate exams:

• PSA (Prostate Specific Antigen) Test—Starting at age fifty, every male should have this simple, inexpensive blood test annually. A result outside normal ranges (zero to four) or a drastic increase from last year's result does not necessarily mean prostate cancer, it just indicates the need for further tests.

• **Digital Exam**—This old annual standby, where your primary-care physician feels your prostate with his finger for any abnormalities (primarily enlargement), is an important part of diagnosing problems.

• **Ultrasound**—This is the gold standard of prostate testing and is often combined with a biopsy. Most times done in a urologist's office, an ultrasound does not require anesthesia.

• **Urinalysis**—One of the easiest, most common tests, the urinalysis provides a tremendous amount of information: It detects blood in the urine, which can indicate various diseases, including cancer; it helps spot the warning signs of ailments such as diabetes, urinary infection, and kidney disease; and it can reveal the presence of crystals, which are the building blocks for kidney stones.

• **Stool analysis for blood**—Like the urinalysis, this is recommended annually for every male over fifty. Presence of blood in the stools can indicate anything from bowel cancer to hemorrhoids.

the release of urine from the bladder aren't exactly snapping open like they used to. And the muscular wall linings aren't as strong as they used to be. While most of these problems don't fully show themselves until a decade or two later, they do give owners a few hints of what's to come. (For urinary flow problems, see the next section on the prostate.)

Bladder Cancer

See chapter 7 for details.

The Prostate

When you were twenty, if some old guy had come up and told you that a walnut-sized gland was the root of your sexual pleasure, and that someday it would give

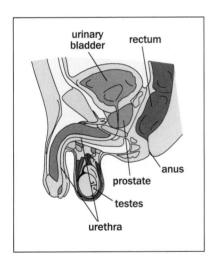

you all kinds of pain, trouble, and maybe even break your heart, you'd have laughed in his face. Today—thirty to forty years later—you're tempted to go find some teenage boys and straighten them out.

By now many of you are intimately acquainted with the prostate. For those lucky few who have yet to experience any troubles in this area, here's the scoop. The prostate is only a few inches in diameter and wraps around the neck of the urethra (the tube that carries urine from the bladder out through the penis). Its main function is to provide the fluid through which our big-headed sperm friends swim.

Reasons Why the Prostate Causes Problems

- **Location.** Hiding near the middle of the pelvic region, it's hard to get at and treat.

- **Size and Composition.** Being small doesn't help treatment. Added to that is an interior maze of intricate pools and reservoirs, where infectious bacteria can never be touched. Because of these two factors, treating prostate infections can be extremely challenging.

- **Swelling.** Over time it swells, both naturally and from inflammation. This can cause the prostate to strangle the urethra, restricting the free flow of urine.

- **Avascular.** Not a lot of blood flows to the prostate reservoirs, so treatment using the blood stream (antibiotics) can be difficult and prolonged.

- **Nerve Complications.** Not only does the prostate wrap around the urethra, it also wraps around many of the hair-sized nerves that aid in creating erections. If the prostate has to be removed, it's a real challenge not to touch these nerves which, if damaged or cut means that . . . well, you get the picture.

Trouble Starting Your Stream

Remember when you were a kid and you were standing in front of a line of urinals, and you had trouble getting started? As we get older, that situation can recur with more and more frequency. It can be embarrassing, frustrating, and at times somewhat painful. It may be okay once the stream's started, but getting it going may be hard. It may also be hard to get rid of the last dribbles. In fact, you may get rid of them in the embarrassing dribbles-down-the-pant-leg syndrome—a merit badge of age that you really don't want to earn.

Causes of difficulty in getting the stream started can be physiologically based and/or psychologically based.

When it comes to the physical causes, many fifties males know that swelling of the prostate (see the following sections on BPH and prostatitis) can cause the problem by blocking the urethra. Fewer may know that it can be a failure of the bladder outlet sphincter (trapdoor) that lies at the neck of the urethra. Fewer still realize it can be caused by taking antihistamines or decongestants, which work on the smooth muscle of the bladder outlet, restricting the relaxation necessary for the free flow of the urine. Other, less commonly used drugs, can also cause problems.

Psychologically-based reasons are, by their very nature, harder to pin down. The hesitancy we faced as a child might have become a greater worry. To a certain extent the physical can lead to the mental: You can have a physically-based problem that leads you to be so concerned that it actually causes the problem. That's called a self-fulfilling prophecy—where your obsessing over the problem ends up causing it.

Treatment/Prevention. Both sides of the condition can be treated, but you should consult your doctor in either case. See the following BPH and prostatitis section for further details regarding treatment for the physically based problem. One thing you should not do is consciously push while urinating—you might be inadvertently contracting muscles that actually constrict the bladder sphincter, making the problem worse.

Incontinence and the Infamous Dribbles

Thankfully, incontinence, or the inability to control urination, is a relatively rare event in men. Women are approximately five times more susceptible to the condition than men. It's important to remember, though, that male incontinence can happen at any age and is not necessarily a natural part of growing older. It is *not* a disease, but rather a symptom or side effect of some other medical condition.

The mechanics of the situation involve the urethral sphincter muscles. The big job of these muscles is to keep urine in the bladder. They do so by remaining tightly closed until called upon to open—either for the passage of sperm or urine. If these muscles relax at the wrong time, urine will leak out.

Causes of Male Incontinence

- Parkinson's disease, diabetes, and Alzheimer's disease

- Prostate problems such as an enlarged prostate (BPH) may contribute to incontinence

- Prostate cancer surgery (but it's rarely permanent)

- Urinary tract infections, or UTIs

- Constipation, in rare cases

- Spinal cord injuries

- Some medicines, especially alpha adrenergic blockers (see the drug chart at the end of this chapter), which have the tendency to relax the sphincter muscles, which can cause the problem

- Emotional issues, such as stress

While incontinence can involve the leakage of large or small amounts of urine, generally speaking, the condition informally known as "the dribbles"—the leaking of a few drops of urine that usually ends up as a temporary stain on the front of your trousers immediately after urinating—is *not* a sign of incontinence.

By the time we reach our fifties, most males will have experienced the occasional case of the dribbles. It is not abnormal or anything to be too concerned about. More of an embarrassment (especially when emerging from a very public rest room) than a real medical condition, the dribbles are usually no more than a result of the sphincter muscles not snapping shut as quickly and efficiently as they once did. In this case, age does play a contributing role—the older we get, the less muscle control we might experience throughout our bodies.

Treatment/Prevention. Men with incontinence should take heart. Many of its causes can now be treated and cured—with antibiotics for UTIs, for example—so it's important to consult a doctor. Conditions that can't be treated can be managed well with any number of constantly improving absorbent products that can be worn in relative comfort without being detected.

For men suffering the embarrassment of the dribbles, a change of habit—giving yourself more time to shake off the last drops of urine—might do the trick.

ARE THERE PERSONAL TRAINERS FOR THESE?
KEGEL EXERCISES

In the 1950s, gynecologist Arnold Kegel developed an exercise to help women overcome the incontinence (the inability to control urination) that can develop after childbirth.

In typical male fashion, we men simply appropriated the concept for our own use. Kegels exercise the pubococcygeal (PC) muscles, which run from your pubic bone to your tail bone. They control the flow of urine and sperm through the urethra (the tube inside the penis).

To get a sense of the PC muscles, try stopping the flow of urine in midstream. That's them. Do that same stopping action to exercise the PC muscles from various positions (standing, sitting) when you're not urinating, and make sure your buttock, thigh, and stomach muscles are completely relaxed when doing so.

There are two exercises: One is to contract the PC muscles quickly and release them quickly; the other is to contract and hold the muscles for five to ten seconds before releasing them. Do both exercises until they're nearly automatic. Results should be seen in a few months. Reportedly, they can help men:

• Cure the infamous dribbles that occur just after urinating.

• Aid in handling or even curing incontinence.

Others might consider wearing an absorbent underwear pad. While an absorbent pad is, admittedly, a bit of overkill, it certainly would take care of any and all potential dribble stains.

Benign Prostatic Hypertrophy (BPH)

This long-winded term is what doctors use to describe the gradual increase in size of the prostate, which is probably inevitable and a normal part of aging. As the prostate enlarges, it steadily strangles the urethra, restricting the flow of urine from the bladder to the penis. Many times this starts to happen to men in their fifties, and by the sixties, probably 20 to 30 percent of men have BPH.

Symptoms include difficulty starting your urinary stream, which might start as a trickle and never get up to the roaring river you used to have when you were young. Another symptom is getting up numerous times during the night to go to the bathroom. Frequent night urination is usually due to not being able to completely empty the bladder at one time—if you're only draining off 20 or 30 percent each time you go, it doesn't take much to top off the bladder again.

Some men worry that having BPH predisposes them to prostate cancer. There is no scientific evidence linking the two, although both ailments tend to occur in the same age group.

Treatment/Prevention. Traditionally, the standard treatment for BPH was surgery. While this could include removing the prostate completely, it usually meant going in through the opening of the penis and paring away the inside of the gland to increase the bore of the channel. Called TUR (transurethral resection), or TURP (transurethral resection of the prostate), it's still done today but less often, because of various effective medications that are much less intrusive. What has replaced surgery is drug therapy (for more details see this chapter's drug chart).

Drugs Used for BPH

• **Alpha-adrenergic blockers.** They relax smooth muscle, so they work on the bladder outlet sphincter (trapdoor) to relax it, which allows urine to pass more freely. (These alpha blockers also have had some effectiveness in treating high blood pressure.) Don't worry, these drugs that work on the smooth muscle do so in such a mild way that they will not make you lose control when you urinate.

• **Flomax (tamsulosin).** A newer drug brought out in the late 1990s, it's also an alpha-adrenergic blocker. It seems to work more on the sphincter and less on the blood pressure than the other alpha-adrenergic blockers do.

• **Proscar (finasteride).** This drug blocks the effects of male hormone on the prostatic tissue and is reputed to shrink the size of an enlarged prostate gland over time. Under a different name, Propecia, it's prescribed to treat male pattern baldness. Gordon has not found it to be a miracle drug for either use.

Prostatitis

An inflammation or irritation of the prostate, prostatitis (also referred to as chronic prostatitis), is often caused by an infection of the gland and is frequently hard to define. It's probably more than one illness, but each of them fits into the same category, because they all have the same symptoms: pain in the lower abdomen or groin, frequency of urination or retention of urine, and, in severe cases, fever and chills. Generally speaking, infection in prostatitis may or may not be present—often it is in the acute phase—but the symptoms may linger long after the infection has been successfully treated. This means the symptoms tend to last for months. Relatively common in fifties males, prostatitis can start in much younger men and plague them for a long time.

One form, called bacterial prostatitis is caused by—you guessed it!— bacteria, which can come from various sources. These include a microscopic breach in the lower bowel that allows bacteria from feces to infect the prostate. The most common method of infection is from a urinary tract infection or STD (sexually transmitted disease). Rarer is a urinary tract infection or a problem somewhere else in the body (such as a sinus infection) with bacterial spread through the blood stream.

There seem to be some activities that predispose people to prostate infection. Straining at the stool can foster the lower bowel breach. This means that chronic constipation should be treated so there's less chance of rectal pushing during extended toilet visits. Sitting for long periods of time—especially sitting with any kind of vibrations (such as truck drivers and heavy machine operators experience) also seems to lead to prostatitis.

Treatment/Prevention. While this is many times a hard and frustrating ailment to treat, antibiotics are the treatment of choice, usually for longer periods of time than other illnesses (six or eight weeks sometimes). Additionally, treatment of chronic prostatitis includes staying away from certain items that tend to cause urinary tract irritations: coffee, tea, alcohol, and tobacco.

Prevention includes making sure you're properly hydrated, staying away from prolonged sitting (by getting up often and stretching), avoiding the urinary irritants listed above, and voiding your seminal fluid (having an ejaculation) a few

times a week. In some chronic cases in which antibiotics haven't been totally successful, the treatment switches to the use of anti-inflammatories for pain, small
amounts of zinc supplements (200 mg a day), vitamin C (250-500 mg a day),
plenty of water (see this chapter's hydration sidebar for details), and alpha-block-
ers, which can be helpful by relaxing the smooth muscles of the prostate and bladder outlet, without causing incontinence.

GOING WITH THE FLOW
URINARY SELF-HELP TIPS

Something's definitely wrong down below: You're urinating more than usual,
or you can't start the stream (although the desire to urinate is driving you
crazy), or you can't empty completely when you do go. Whatever the
specifics, you know something isn't working right.

First: Go talk to your doctor. It could be anything from a bladder infection
to a sexually transmitted disease; from chronic prostatitis to serious kidney
problems. Second: Try some of the following urinary self-help tips. They
won't harm you and they just might help:

- **Drink cranberry or blueberry juice (or take a supplement).** Chemicals
  within them prevent bacteria from "clumping," which is necessary for scattered bacteria in the bladder to invade the bladder wall and cause an actual infection.

- **Take a zinc supplement.** For years, urologists have recommended zinc
  (200 mg a day) for chronic prostatitis. The reasoning is a little nebulous,
  but the positive results are there.

- **Take vitamin C.** 250 to 500 mg a day seem to help, but we're not
  exactly sure why.

- **Try the herbal supplement, saw palmetto.** It may have some benefit for symptoms of benign prostatic hypertrophy (enlargement of the
  prostate), but the scientific evidence is still somewhat sketchy. Follow
  what's recommended on the bottle.

- **Restrict your intake of coffee.** Caffeine may cause local irritation.

Bladder/kidney infections are not trivial. These infections always require a
medical evaluation for proper treatment. Every problem can be managed, if
not cured.

Prostate Cancer

See chapter 7 for details.

The Penis and Testes

While we all know that our penis and testicles are officially part of the digestive and urinary tracts—and we're glad of that—we also know that they play a much greater role in our sexual lives. With that thought in mind, see chapter 5 for an examination of these very special male organs.

Testicular Cancer

See chapter 7 for details.

REAL LIFE TALES

Number One: A Reluctant Poster Child for Scientific Advancements in Ulcer Treatments

Simon is fifty-seven years old, a pharmacist, and about fifty pounds overweight. Much of his weight problem can be traced back to an ankle, broken in his early twenties, which never regained its original mobility. This stiff, painful ankle has not only made it difficult for Simon to exercise but has also caused him to rely on over-the-counter pain medicines, such as aspirin and ibuprofen. The onset of arthritis years ago certainly hasn't helped Simon's overall health.

Lastly—and the reason why this story is in the digestive and urinary chapter—Simon has suffered since the 1960s from ulcer disease. He has constantly been plagued by ulcers that have caused stomach upset, pain, and, in a few cases, internal bleeding. His entire adult life has been adversely affected by this ailment. Compounding the ulcer problem is the fact that the pain medicines for his ankle and arthritis are NSAIDs (nonselective nonsteroidal anti-inflammatory drugs), which cause stomach upset and ulcers, because they inhibit a compound that protects the stomach's lining. While Simon has never had surgery to correct the ulcers, he has been scoped with a tube inserted through the throat and into the stomach numerous times so that the doctor can assess the situation and seal off any ulcers that are bleeding.

In the 1960s, when Simon first came to a doctor for his ulcers, treatment was limited to three somewhat dubious options: conventional antacids; the periodic intake of milk and high fat foods, called the Sippy Diet; or surgery. While on the

Sippy Diet, Simon began to gain the weight that he's never been able to shed.

In the 1970s, Simon experienced the first real benefit from a scientific break-through—Tagamet was developed to inhibit stomach acid secretions. For twenty years, Simon basically lived on Tagamet, and his quality of life improved significantly, although he still suffered from flare ups of ulcers.

Then, only a few years ago, ulcer theory was turned on its ear with the Australian discovery that many ulcers are caused by a bacterium, *H. pylori*, rather than by stomach acid and/or stress. Simon was tested and found to be positive for the bacteria. After undergoing the rather major triple antibiotic therapy required, Simon was finally free of ulcers for the first time in thirty years.

The story doesn't end there, however. Because of Simon's reliance on NSAIDs for his ankle and arthritis, after three or four years without ulcers, he developed another one—this time caused not by bacteria but by the NSAIDs.

Just when Simon was resigning himself to a life never completely free of stomach upset and ulcers, along came another scientific breakthrough: Celebrex, a painkiller that works without inhibiting the compound that protects the stomach's lining. Pain relief no longer had to be married to stomach upset and possible ulcer formation. (See this chapter's drug chart for details.)

Looking back over forty years, Simon has climbed a kind of scientific evolutionary ladder, benefitting at each rung by what has been discovered. Today, while still overweight, Simon is now ulcer free, relatively pain free, and working toward shedding his unwanted pounds.

Number Two: Dealing with the Problem Child of Men's Health—The Prostate

Pat is fifty-two, in good physical shape, and works out every day. He's at a good weight, has never smoked, and drinks alcohol only moderately. He's a retail store owner who spends a fair amount of the day sitting, many times on a hard stool.

Gradually, over the course of a few weeks, he begins to notice some urinary problems that aren't too dramatic, but are certainly annoying. He has difficulty completely emptying his bladder, or a few minutes after urinating he gets the sensation that he needs to go again, but nothing happens when he goes back to the bathroom. At night he awakens two, sometimes three, times to heed nature's call. All together, a frustrating experience that Pat wants to live without.

After a few weeks of gradually worsening symptoms, Pat goes to see his doctor. Past history reveals that Pat has had a few acute episodes of prostatitis (infection of the prostate) in which similar symptoms were much more pronounced. Each of these incidents seemed to be successfully treated with antibiotics, because there were long intervals with no symptoms. But over the years a pattern is beginning to form: onset of symptoms, drug treatment, no symptoms, then gradual reintroduction of symptoms.

Pat's exams show nothing: He has no fever, which would have been one sign of acute prostatitis. The urinalysis and the prostate cancer PSA (prostate specific antigen) test come back normal. The digital exam reveals that Pat's prostate is a little soft and swollen but nothing to be concerned about, because the other tests are negative. Sexually, Pat is functioning normally. A trip to a urologist confirms nothing is seriously wrong.

Once again Pat is put on antibiotics, this time for a lengthy six weeks because the prostate is involved (hard to reach, hard to treat), and because he's had the symptoms for a relatively long period of time. Pat experiences relief from the symptoms within a few days of starting the drug. It's nothing overly dramatic, just a gradual fading of the symptoms.

Unfortunately, within three weeks of finishing the antibiotics, Pat is having the same problems again.

This time, other potential remedies are tried—anti-inflammatories (ibuprofen, 200 to 400 mg three times a day), 200 mg daily of zinc, 250 to 500 mg a day of vitamin C, and the prescribed alpha blocker called Flomax, which relaxes urinary outflow (translation: It helps him to completely empty his bladder when he goes to the bathroom).

A year down the road, Pat is relatively well off. He's not on antibiotics, but he remains on Flomax. He's now paying close attention to certain items: hydration (how much water he drinks in a day) to aid in better urinary flow; substances that might irritate the urinary tract, such as coffee, tea, and alcohol; and sitting for long periods of time without a break.

Pat's coming to grips with a health problem that will probably never be completely out of his life—chronic, nonbacterial prostatitis. More a product of age and circumstances than anything else, Pat's urinary problems are definitely manageable but, realistically, never completely curable. Besides managing his problem through awareness and drugs, Pat is also better off because he knows he doesn't have cancer, he knows he doesn't have something contagious, and he knows there's no provable infection.

Not exactly the resolution Pat would have dreamed of, but probably the best he can get when it comes to the problem child of men's health—the prostate.

Number Three: Do You Really Want VIP Medical Treatment?

Cliff is fifty years old, works as a computer analyst, and has a brother who's a physician (Gordon Ehlers). Not wanting to go through the regular medical channels, with all the questions, lab tests, and paperwork, Cliff calls his brother to report chest pains when he jogs. His brother, justifiably worried, and wanting to get right to the problem, skips the routine office visit, where certain established protocols (such as taking a complete history, asking a barrage of questions, and ordering standard lab tests) would have been done.

Instead, the doctor—who knows Cliff has never smoked, isn't overweight, and has good cholesterol and a good family history—invites Cliff for a run. Three quarters of a mile into an easy jog, Cliff says he just can't make it; the pain in his chest is too much.

To the doctor, this seems to spell angina, a condition where the heart muscle is deprived of adequate oxygen because of a blocked or partially blocked coronary artery (see chapter 3 for details). The doctor immediately gets Cliff to take a tread-mill test, which elicits the same painful response. The test seems to confirm the brother's initial diagnosis.

Treadmill test in hand, Cliff goes to see a cardiologist friend of his brother's who reviews the tests and says Cliff needs a cardiac catheterization (insertion into a leg artery of a tube that goes up to the heart). This, along with some dye injected into the arteries, will reveal where the presumed coronary problem is located.

Scheduled for this relatively serious procedure, Cliff gets a standard pre-operative blood workup done. That's when the cardiologist calls the brother and pops a surprising question: "Did you know Cliff is anemic?"

The brother gets Cliff on the phone. "How are you feeling?" he asks.

Cliff admits to being tired all the time. He says he thought it was stress and his lack of exercise, so he had been pushing himself to exercise more, but that had brought on the chest pains.

"Have you been bleeding in your stool or urine?" the brother queries.

"Ah . . . yeah," Cliff replies.

"How often?"

"Every time I go."

"Why didn't you tell me?"

"I figured it was only hemorrhoids. . . . I was embarrassed to say anything."

Turns out Cliff had a pretty severe case of hemorrhoids, which was causing his anemia. Because anemia is the deficiency of oxygen-carrying material in the blood, this meant that every time Cliff exercised, his blood couldn't get enough oxygen to his heart to keep up—hence, the chest pains and the test results show-ing heart muscle deprived of oxygen. After relatively minor hemorrhoid surgery, Cliff returned to his normal, healthy self.

If Cliff had received the standard, non-VIP medical treatment, his condition would have been caught long before surgery was scheduled. In this case, the cau-tionary tale speaks not only to the patient, but to the doctor as well—not to men-tion anyone else who hopes for, or expects, special treatment from relatives or friends in the medical community.

KNOWING WHAT YOU PUT IN YOUR MOUTH— A DRUG CHART

Stomach Drugs

NAME	EXPLANATION AND USE	POSSIBLE SIDE EFFECTS
H2 Blocker Drugs (Available by prescription and, in lower doses, OTC) **Cimetidine (Tagamet)** **Ranitidine (Zantac)** **Famotidine (Pepcid)** **Nizatidine (Axid)**	Blocks production of a portion of the stomach acid. Used to treat heartburn (GERD), ulcers, gastritis, and esophagitis.	Headache, agitation, disorientation, and impotence.
Proton Pump Inhibitor Drugs (Prescription only) **Omeprazole (Prilosec)** **Lansoprazole (Prevacid)** **Pantoprazole (Protonix)** **Rabeprazole (Aciphex)** **Esomeprazole (Nexium)**	Expensive and only available in oral form. Inhibit stomach-acid production much more effectively than the H2 blockers. Used to treat ulcers, esophagitis, gastritis, and as part of the treatment of *H. pylori*. Can be used to protect against NSAID-induced GI irritation.	Diarrhea, bloating, headache.
Prostaglandin Analogues (Prescription only) **Misoprostol (Cytotec)**	Used to offset the ulcer-producing effects of the NSAIDS. Available as a combination with a NSAID (diclofenac), in a drug called Arthrotec.	Headache, diarrhea, and bloating. Should never be prescribed for a pregnant patient.
Prokinetic Drugs (Prescription only) **Reglan (Metoclopramide)**	Prevents gastroesophageal reflux by promoting stomach emptying and tightening of the lower esophageal sphincter (LES).	Headache, diarrhea, bloating, restlessness, drowsiness, and Parkinson's disease-like symptoms.

The Digestive and Urinary Tracts

NAME	EXPLANATION AND USE	POSSIBLE SIDE EFFECTS
Antacids **(All OTC)** **Maalox, Mylanta, Tums, Rolaids, and many others.**	Neutralize stomach acid on contact, relieving heartburn and acid-type symptoms. Duration of effect limited by how long the antacid stays in the stomach.	Diarrhea and absorption difficulties with certain drugs.
Pepto-Bismol **(Bismuth Subsalicylate)**	Works as a mild antacid, relieves stomach upset, and diarrhea. Mild anti-bacterial effect useful (with other drugs) in treating *H. pylori,* and in prevention of traveler's diarrhea.	Causes dark tongue and dark stools; may interfere with absorption of certain drugs.

Urinary Tract Drugs

NAME	EXPLANATION AND USE	POSSIBLE SIDE EFFECTS
Alpha-Adrenergic **Blockers** **Terazosin (Hytrin)** **Doxazosin (Cardura)**	Used to relax bladder outlet smooth muscle, enhancing urinary outflow in prostatic enlargement.	May lower blood pressure, causing fatigue and lightheadedness.
Tamsulosin (Flomax)		Fewer side effects than Hytrin or Cardura.
Prostate-Related Drug **Finasteride (Proscar)**	Used to reduce the size of an enlarged prostate by blocking tissue conversion of inactive testosterone to active testosterone at the prostate level. Used under a different name (Propecia) to treat male pattern baldness.	Impotence, decreased libido.

THE GOOD NEWS

- You do not have to accept many digestive and urinary tract problems as a product of age. It is true that a tremendous number of ailments related to these two systems can begin to surface in the fifties decade, but knowing how your digestive and urinary tracts function—and why they malfunction—will lead to better maintenance of both. Well-maintained digestive and urinary tracts will give you very little trouble.

- Over-the-counter drugs are becoming more and more effective in tackling bouts of mild intestinal upsets.

- Heartburn, or acid reflux (backup), is preventable and/or curable.

- A new class of pain-relieving anti-inflammatory drugs (brand names Celebrex and Vioxx; see the drug chart in the musculoskeletal chapter for details) has been developed that does not upset the stomach as much or promote ulcer formation.

- Because of a scientific breakthrough in ulcer theory, many ulcers are now curable.

- The liver has incredible recuperative, rejuvenative powers, so that mild abuses, such as the occasional excessive intake of alcohol, can be negated.

- Controlled, moderate drinking (two or less drinks a day) has a beneficial effect on your health (although if you don't drink now, you shouldn't start—10 percent of the population has trouble controlling their drinking, and you don't know if you fall into that 10 percent).

- Vaccinations can now protect you from contracting the very serious diseases of hepatitis A and B.

- While colon cancer is still the third leading cause of cancer death in men, the introduction of relatively easy exams, such as the sigmoidoscopy (which can be performed during a regular doctor visit) and colonoscopy (which is done in a day-surgery procedure), have begun to have a real impact on the mortality rates—the death rate is up to 60 percent lower in screened versus unscreened populations.

The Digestive and Urinary Tracts

• If caught in time, most digestive and urinary tract cancers are definitely survivable (early detection and/or prevention are the key factors here).

• Good bulk additives, such as Metamucil, work to alleviate not only constipation but diarrhea as well—smoothing out the ups and downs of any digestive tract, no matter what the age.

• The majority of urinary tract problems, such as hesitancy, restricted flow, and/or not being able to completely empty the bladder, are all very treatable.

• Today, the treatment options for prostate cancer do not automatically spell impotency, and even if that is a result, impotency can, many times, be cured as well.

5: SEXUAL ISSUES, ENERGY, AND MALE MENOPAUSE

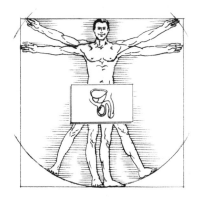

Making A Smooth Transition Into Senior Status

BACKGROUND BASICS

Who to believe?

Biologists tell us the sexual drive—the drive to reproduce—is one of life's most basic, primeval motivators. Social scientists tell us sex is an "elective" activity that can and should be constrained, restrained, and sometimes even stifled depending upon the particular situation.

The answer, of course, is they're both right. No two ways about it, your sex drive is a tremendously complex and integral part of who you are. Many have probably heard the remarkable stat (who thought this one up?) that a teenage boy has a sexual thought flash through his head every ten seconds—ah, the good old days.

By the time that kid reaches fifty, though, the old synapses just aren't snapping like they used to. While no one's studied how often fifties men think about sex, we all know personally that every ten seconds just ain't happening anymore. The change is probably a survival skill—there would be a lot more coronaries if we fifties males were having sexual thoughts every ten seconds. It also signals that most of us have learned there's more to life than just having sex.

No matter how our sex drive has changed, though, it's still important to us men. But it is something that should be integrated into our lives, not boxed up or looked at as a separate entity. It is neither all important nor unimportant. And our sex drive doesn't just influence our sexual life. Critical elements of our sex drive—most notably testosterone—play huge roles in our overall health, energy, and attitude that go way beyond sex.

The Equipment—Taking Stock

You gotta admit, this part of our body is pretty incredible. Where else can you find "equipment" that can bring so much personal joy and pleasure, and never wears out? Sure, it can temporarily run down, but given adequate rest, it's usually ready to get back in the game.

Truth be told, while most of us have been enamored with our sex organs ever since we experienced our first orgasm, most of us don't know much about how they actually function. Only when some, or all, of the system breaks down do we suddenly want to know how our sexual organs work, what's currently wrong, and how the problem can be fixed—pronto!

What's What with Our Equipment

The penis. The "big kahuna" of genitalia is made up mainly of soft, spongy tissue covered in loose skin that can shrink in times of flight-or-fight, or expand and grow rigid during an erection. Parts of the penis include the:

Urethra. An eight-inch tube that leads from the bladder through the penis to the exterior. At appropriate times, it carries either sperm or urine.

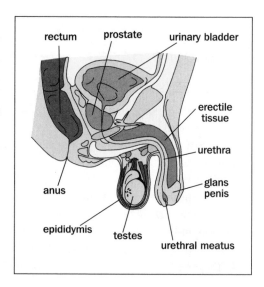

Meatus. The penis opening at the end of the urethra—yep, it actually has a name.

Glans. The bulbous tip, or head, of the penis, responsible for much of the penile sensation.

Foreskin. A thin, stretchable fold of skin that covers the glans when the penis is soft and rolls back when the glans expands during an erection. The foreskin can be removed for religious, social, or medical reasons—usually when a boy is only a few days old—in a surgical procedure called circumcision.

The scrotum. The sac that hangs at the base of the penis. It's divided into two compartments, each of which holds a testis, or testicle. Normally, the left testicle and its compartment are a little larger and hang lower than the right.

The testes. Most men have two testes, or testicles. They produce sperm cells and the male sex hormone called testosterone.

The epididymis. A long and coiled tube attached to each testicle, inside of which sperm are stored and mature. Each epididymis leads to a:

Vas deferens. A tube that winds into the pelvic area and carries the sperm into two short ejaculatory ducts that pass through the prostate.

The seminal vesicles. These two small sacs sit at the junction between the vas deferens and the prostate. They store seminal fluid, a nourishing solution that helps the sperm "swim" when they are ejaculated.

Semen. The thick, whitish secretion that comes out of the urethra during ejaculation. Semen is comprised of sperm from the testes and fluids from the prostate and seminal vesicles. These are mixed at the base of the urethra, just below the prostate.

Corpora cavernosa. Two cavernous chambers located on either side of the urethra, which, when filled (engorged) with blood, cause an erection to occur.

SCIENCE COMES
TO THE LOCKER ROOM
PENIS MEASUREMENT DETAILS

We all know that size *should not* matter—especially to you, and hopefully not to your partner—but our society seems to have a "bigger is better"complex. For the curious, here are some details. For those who do believe size equates to performance and "manliness," there are whole new worlds of perspective out there worth exploring.

- Visual evidence in X-rated movies aside, the largest erection that has been scientifically measured came in at twelve inches long (not as big as you thought, huh?). The smallest, with testicles and normal functioning, was only half-an-inch long.

- The average size of an erect penis is 5.1 inches long and 1.6 inches in diameter.

- Penis size is not reflected in overall body size or in any parts—including thumbs, fingers, toes, ear lobes, feet, or noses. (Where *do* these sexual myths come from?)

- Erect penis size is not reflected in flaccid (soft) penis size—a penis that is long when soft can sometimes gain only a couple of inches, while a penis that's small when flaccid can sometimes gain as much as three to four inches.

- The size of erection, the hardness, and the degree of angle (which varies widely) will diminish slightly with age, but functioning is not affected.

Lastly, women have consistently stated in surveys that size does not matter, and that it's much more important to have a caring partner with a good sense of humor who's willing to talk and share his feelings than someone who's hung like a horse. Believe them.

Sexual Issues, Energy, and Male Menopause

Sexual Changes—
An Overview of What the Fifties Bring

While the general physical changes of life are outlined elsewhere in this book, the sexual changes our age group will be facing are outlined here. The good news is that, normally, the changes are relatively few and inconsequential:

• Slight decrease in the angle and in the rigidity, or hardness, of erections.

• Slight increase in the speed at which an erection wilts after orgasm.

• Slight increase in the time needed to become erect after an orgasm.

• Slight decrease in the number of orgasms normally experienced in one night.

• Shift in stimulation—fantasizing alone will not always create an erection in a fifties male; manual stimulation may now be necessary.

Don't worry, these are changes that most of us wouldn't even notice without attention being focused on them. Anyone with an already normal, healthy sex life can rest assured that these changes will do nothing to affect that. In fact, many fifties men actually report that while they do have fewer orgasms than when they were younger, each one seems to be more intense and pleasurable. Maybe greater appreciation brings greater joy?

Male Menopause—Myth or Reality?

Do fifties men experience male menopause?

Strictly speaking, no. Since we don't have a menstrual cycle, we can't go through a cessation of menstruation.

But the answer is a qualified yes if the question is refocused and rephrased: Do fifties men go through a significant change in their lives—both physically and psychologically—that is similar to what women go through when they hit menopause?

A good starting point for determining if there is male menopause—and what that might entail—is to look at what society now considers female menopause to be.

Strictly speaking, the word "menopause" simply means the end of menstruation, when a woman's body no longer produces a monthly flow of blood (commonly known as a "period") from the uterus. This usually happens between the ages of forty-five and fifty-five. Today, however, menopause has also come to refer to an entire stage of a woman's life, a stage that is reflected in numerous physical and psychological changes:

- Hormonal changes, most notably a drastic decrease of estrogen (which is responsible for menstruation and female features such as breasts).

- Cessation of ovulation, or the periodic release of an egg from the ovaries.

- Hot flashes, heart palpitations, and dryness of vaginal membranes that normally come with the hormonal changes.

- Emotional upheavals, which may be the result of hormonal imbalances.

Physical Aspects of Male Menopause

Many believe that the broadening of the meaning of menopause to include a wide range of elements has left the door open for men to appropriate the term for their own particular stage in life. Adding legitimacy to the claim is the similarity of the physical and psychological changes that the sexes share during this period between forty-five and fifty-five.

Taking first the basic hormonal changes, estrogen has a direct male equivalent in testosterone, the male sex hormone. Both are produced by both sexes—women produce a little testosterone along with large quantities of estrogen, while men produce a small amount of estrogen with copious amounts of testosterone.

Testosterone in males is produced mostly by the testicles along with a little by the adrenal gland. Responsible for the development of our sex organs, facial hair, and deep voices, testosterone also maintains our sex drive. Additionally, many believe testosterone is the key ingredient in setting the degree, or level, of our general "maleness"—that intangible quality comprised of such characteristics as assertiveness, aggressiveness, and linear thinking (not, as some might think, our fashion sense, ability to change a flat tire, or hesitancy to talk about our emotions).

The level of testosterone in the male body peaks during puberty, creating a kind of controlled internal havoc that many of us can still recall with a mixture of humor and embarrassment. Remember that crazed, frantic feeling that permeated every waking hour? *Testosterone.* Remember that great feeling of release when mixing it up in sports? *Testosterone.* Remember those sexual fantasies about your shapely seventh-grade math teacher? Yep. *Testosterone.*

After the peak puberty years, testosterone levels off and stays that way until around fifty. Then it starts a slow, steady decline. The decrease is usually slight—

Sexual Issues, Energy, and Male Menopause

about 1 percent per year—but by the time you've reached seventy-five, your testosterone levels can be nearly one-third of what they were when you were seventeen. And 48 percent of healthy men age fifty to seventy have testosterone levels below the lowest levels in younger men.

Usually, the decline is nothing to worry about. Up to 80 percent of males stay within normal levels for their entire lives (unlike women, 100 percent of whom do experience a drastic drop in estrogen that triggers menopause). Because the testosterone decline in men is so gradual, there are often no symptoms. With that said, however, there are some men who do experience symptoms.

Possible Symptoms of Lowered Testosterone

• Loss of sexual desire and fewer erections, or inability to achieve erections

• Insomnia and/or fatigue

• General feeling of anxiety, fear, and/or not thinking clearly

• Loss of muscle and bone mass

• Weight gain

For fifties men worried about their testosterone level, it can be measured, and there is replacement therapy (similar to estrogen replacement therapy for women), but often the chances are good that the problems lie elsewhere, such as kidney or liver disease, or even in their minds.

Psychological Aspects of Male Menopause

Moving from the hormonal to the psychological aspects of male menopause is like going from the relative foundation of a sandy beach to the fluidity of a quicksand pit. As with female menopause, the changes that occur in fifties men often include elements of a mid-life crisis. This lends credibility to the thought that male menopause is a legitimate stage in a man's life. The only truly refutable point is that the word "menopause" doesn't strictly fit males. With this thought in mind, some experts have begun to coin the word "andropause" (*andro*, Greek for male or masculine) as a suitable substitute. Good idea, but it just doesn't have the same "ring" to it.

WHERE AND HOW PROBLEMS OCCUR, TREATMENT OPTIONS, AND PREVENTIVE MEASURES

Understanding You, Your Partner, and What's Going On

For those men in our age group who have never thought about what they're like as lovers—and let's hope that's a very small group—this section might be worth reading.

For those of us who have thought about the topic . . . we are, of course, fine lovers. We understand the differences between the sexes. We're patient. We take our time. We think of our partner's enjoyment first. We can't wait to "snuggle" afterward.

Yeah, right, and Bill Clinton never inhaled.

So, maybe we *all* might want to skim this section.

(It should be noted that we certainly do not put ourselves forward as "doctors of love." We have, however, spent a great deal of time reading, researching, and, in Gordon's case, listening to patients—both men and women—on this critical subject. The following is a compilation of the best information, suggestions, advice, and tips we've come across.)

One of the overriding themes that comes from studying the topics of sex and the sexes is that there is an incredible diversity in sexual reactions, not only between the sexes but among them. Because of the complex physiological and psychological nature of sex, each individual's sexual response is nearly as personalized as his or her fingerprints.

With that said, however, there is still plenty of room to make some broad generalizations about the sexes and sexual response. (Apologies to those who don't fall within these parameters.) The most obvious place to start identifying the differences between men and women is in the three critical stages of lovemaking.

Sexual Response—Arousal

Men: Initially, our minds can expand with surprising agility to link an incredibly diverse (and seemingly nonsexual) number of "things" to sexual arousal. Basically, we can get aroused at just about anything. And nearly all mental images or visuals (such as pornographic material) can cause initial stimulation. Once arousal has begun, however, we seem to focus on the sense of touch, and we circle our erogenous wagons around one very well-defined and prominent area. Face it, there aren't too many male erogenous zones beside the penis—although our senses of smell, taste, and hearing can add a lot for many men, as can the stimulation of the anal area and the prostate (as massaged through the bowel wall).

Sexual Issues, Energy, and Male Menopause

Women: Initially, a woman's arousal can be triggered by an incredibly focused experience—such as seeing a partner's forearm, nape of the neck, or smile in a different way. Or seeing the partner tenderly playing with children, or performing an act of kindness. Even a particular scent or a great sense of humor can get the ball rolling. Then, as arousal begins, women seem to expand their tactile arousal to include nearly every part of their body. Properly done, a kiss or touch on the back of a knee, an upper arm, or the small of the back can be as arousing to a woman as one placed on a more obvious erogenous area (breast, mouth, vagina).

Sexual Response—Orgasm

Men: If we think about it—and this is one place where we're usually not in the thinking mode—besides some random toe curling, the focus of the male orgasm sensation is centered within the penis.

Women: While orgasm for a woman certainly starts with clitoral sensation or vaginal contractions, the sensations created in a good, earth-shaking kind of orgasm seem to embrace every cell and hair follicle of her being.

Sexual Response—Post Orgasm

Men: It's a cliché but mainly true that after orgasm most men up through their twenties are simply thinking about doing it again. We men in our fifties tend toward sleep because we've entered the "refractory period," a time when we cannot respond to sexual stimulation, and our bodies start to replenish sperm and seminal fluid. As we all know, this refractory period can be as short as a few minutes in our younger brethren to as long as a few hours in our older compatriots. Some of us find that the time between an orgasm and the first stirrings of another arousal are the moments of greatest clarity and clearest thinking.

Women: It's also a cliché, and usually true, that after sex most women would like to be held, caressed, murmured to—in part as confirmation that the sex that just took place was more than just sex.

This is *not* to say that the sexes can't cross the lines and share in each other's processes. Quite the contrary. Those who understand and appreciate the differences between the sexes can, many times, actually end up getting a taste for how the other half experiences the sexual process.

When it comes to how sex is viewed, the differences between the sexes are legendary. There's an old joke about a married couple talking to a therapist. The woman complains, "Doctor, he wants it all the time; we have sex once a week." The man complains, "Doctor, she never wants it; we have sex once a week."

How to reconcile those different perspectives?

Communication is the key. Honest and open discussion with your partner about both of your needs, wants, and desires is critical to bridging the gap between our ways of thinking. If you're having trouble even talking about the topic, try asking your partner questions that reflect what you would really like to talk about. And then listen—truly listen—to what your partner is saying. A way to test whether or not you really heard what was said is to immediately repeat in your own words what your partner just said. You might be surprised by the differences revealed from such an exercise.

If you are still having trouble talking with your partner about sensitive issues, consider seeing a therapist, either separately or jointly. There is a wide variety of licensed practitioners offering a stunning array of therapies—everything from religious guidance and traditional psychoanalytical counseling to hypnotherapy and sexual surrogate training. Your regular doctor can help you find the best therapist to fit your particular situation.

Masturbation

One of the great things about reaching your fifties is that you can confidently put to rest certain myths that might have been drilled into you as a child. You now know with great assurance that masturbating will not grow hair on your palms—although that bit about going blind gained some credibility in the forties when your arms weren't long enough for reading anymore.

While most men do masturbate at least occasionally, it is one of the few activities we all share in but don't talk about—not even to our partners or regular doctor. There is an unspoken stigma or embarrassment about masturbation that comes from vague, and unjustified, feelings of guilt. Many of you might appreciate that, scientifically speaking, occasional or periodic masturbation is quite the opposite. It's normal, healthy (as long as it doesn't become a compulsion), maintains sperm quantity and quality, and sustains a healthy prostate by preventing congestive prostatitis (a condition where prostatic fluid builds up to cause inflammation and congestion).

On the downside, there's one major point to keep in mind: Masturbation is, by its very nature, a focused, narcissistic, goal-oriented activity that can lead some to forget that sex with a partner should be slower, more focused on the other person, and less goal-oriented.

Being A Better Partner

What is "good" sex? How often should you be having sex? Can you heighten the sexual experience for you and your partner?

Sexual Issues, Energy, and Male Menopause

Interesting—and tough—questions to answer. They're tough because we are all so individual in our sexual interests, preferences, and responses. The most important gauge is how you and your partner feel about your sex life. If you both feel it is healthy, active, and satisfying, then you have no problem—regardless of the type or frequency of sexual activity.

The first major attempt to quantify and qualify the American sexual experience was the Kinsey report. Released to the public in 1948, it was seen as radical, controversial, and somewhat titillating. This certainly couldn't be said about the language used—the definition of orgasm, "an explosive discharge of neuromuscular tension," didn't do much even for men's usually overactive imaginations.

The report did challenge some well-established myths—for example, that women weren't that interested in sex—and forced people to re-examine the concept of what was "normal" sexual behavior. At the time, the overwhelming majority of Americans only practiced vaginal intercourse. More than fifty years later, though, sexual practices have changed, expanding from traditional vaginal sex to include the now commonplace mutual masturbation and oral sex—fellatio (sucking the penis or otherwise stimulating it with the mouth) and cunnilingus (stimulating the vagina and clitoris with the mouth). The practice of anal sex (penile penetration of the anus) has risen as well (as many as 8 to 10 percent of Americans practice it regularly now), but in a much smaller proportion of the population than the practice of oral sex.

As to sexual frequency, various studies have shown a wide range, depending on numerous factors.

Weekly Frequency of Intercourse in Couples

- 18-24 years old, a little more than three times a week

- 25-34 years old, nearly three times a week

- 35-44 years, two times

- 45 years and over, one time

Another study reported that about one-third of Americans have sex at least twice a week, another one-third have sex a few times a month, and the rest have sex a few times a year.

It's obvious that there is no hard and fast rule here. You're the only one who knows whether or not you're getting enough sex. Just remember that the grass isn't always greener on the other side. If you're a married man longing for those sexually active days when you were single, keep this in mind: Married couples or those living together actually have more sex on average than single people.

How can you improve your sex life? The following are some ideas. It's important to note, however, that you should never approach a relationship with the thought of manipulating your partner into more sex. Your actions, of course, should always be generated from a genuine feeling of love and respect.

Suggestions for a Better Sex Life

Remember the mental. The mind is the key to real sexual excitement. Don't neglect your partner's mind—spend as much time seducing and exciting it as you do your partner's body.

Reverse roles. Every chance you get, try and put yourself in your partner's shoes psychologically. When you understand your partner (both sexually and non-sexually), you go a long way toward understanding how he or she will respond sexually. In the physical realm of sexual activities, consider doing to your partner what you've dreamed or hoped your partner would do to you.

Talk. Tell your partner about your feelings and thoughts when it comes to sex.

Listen. Ask your partner—then make sure to listen—about his or her feelings and thoughts regarding sex.

Relearn. A new partner will not necessarily respond to the same techniques and stimuli that a previous partner enjoyed. Experimenting to learn what turns your new partner on can be just as exciting for you as it can be for her or him.

Anticipate. You can enjoy and appreciate sexual anticipation, and even work toward using it as part of long-range, all-day foreplay.

Massage. Take the time to massage various parts of your partner's body—everything from hands or feet to face and back. Make sure that not all massages culminate in sex—show your partner that you can give pleasure without always having to receive a sexual reward.

Enjoy. Sex should be filled with large quantities of sheer joy and fun. Try using sex "toys," mutual masturbation, or even humor to stimulate variation and prolong arousal time.

New positions. If you normally have sex in the same way, try new positions or sexual techniques.

Sexual Issues, Energy, and Male Menopause

New places and times. If you always have sex in the bedroom in the morning, try the kitchen or laundry room in the afternoon. Spring for a night in a hotel, even if it's just down the street. You might be surprised at how a change of scenery can do wonders for a sagging libido in you and/or your partner.

Be creative. Think beyond the norm, outside the box, over the top. As long as it won't hurt anyone, make anyone uncomfortable, make anyone do something they don't want to do, why not consider it?

For those looking for shortcuts—a.k.a. aphrodisiacs—to stimulate a partner, there really aren't any. The Food and Drug Administration has stated that aphrodisiacs don't exist (and we can all trust the government, can't we?), and in 1990 it banned any product claiming to enhance sexual performance or libido.

"Houston, We Have Lift Off!"
What Exactly Is An Erection?

Why can't you just will an erection to life? Because an erection is controlled by the parasympathetic nervous system—the same outfit that handles pupil movement in your eyes. Without sexual stimulation—mental and/or physical—nothing's going to happen down below.

That's not to say things can't move at lightning speed. As most of us still remember from our misspent youth, we can actually get an erection in as little as five to ten seconds.

Technically, an erection is when blood gushes into two spongy, cave-like areas of the penis, which immediately fill up with blood and expand. At the same time, the soft tissues and veins of the penis constrict slightly to keep the blood from leaking out of the spongy areas as the valves of the vein leading out of the penis stay shut. These steps aid in maintaining an erection. Once ejaculation (release of sperm) occurs, the blood returns to what it was doing before, or goes off to a well-deserved nap. Interesting note: You can have an orgasm (albeit a "dry" one) without a prostate, but you normally can't have an orgasm without an erection.

Starting in the late forties/early fifties, the frequency of erections does decrease, the hardness of the erection does diminish, and the speed at which an erection wilts after sex does increase—but none significantly enough to preclude a healthy sex life. It's also completely normal for men in their fifties to find fantasizing by itself doesn't produce an erection every time anymore. Actual physical touch of some kind will probably be needed. So don't worry if you're a little slower off the mark now—take it as a sign that you're supposed to savor each experience.

When it comes right down to it, the best aphrodisiac is good health—don't smoke, drink only moderately, eat right, exercise, learn to handle stress, and learn to relax. When you maintain good overall health, you'll generally have good, healthy sexual functioning as well.

When the Game Goes Bad

Just as your sexual organs can bring you great pleasure, they can also bring you great pain—both literally and figuratively.

Loss of Sexual Desire

It's hard to believe that a typical teenaged boy's sex-crazed mind could someday become a mind with no real interest in sex. Unfortunately, this loss of sexual desire, or libido, can happen—and at nearly every age of life—although it's most likely to strike men over sixty than younger ones.

Admittedly, as part of the natural aging process, there is usually a decrease in sexual appetite or interest and a slight diminishing in physical responsiveness, but there is no scientific reason why even a healthy 100-year-old male can't enjoy sexual thoughts, urges, and orgasms.

There is no need to panic if you suddenly realize your sexual drive isn't as strong as it was thirty years ago. If you still find yourself getting sexually aroused, generating and maintaining an erection, and enjoying orgasms on a regular or consistent basis, then you're probably fine—no need to worry if you're having only a few sexual thoughts a day, versus hundreds.

If, however, you never seem to think about sex anymore, if visuals that once were exciting aren't, or if your partner's assistance doesn't even help, then there probably is a problem. There might be a problem even if you can still become aroused or interested in sex occasionally, but not consistently. Accompanying symptoms may include fear, anxiety, or panic about having sex, as well as a loss of energy and a general decrease in your enthusiasm toward life.

While the loss of libido can be somewhat nebulous, it is all too real for those who suffer from it, and it can be especially difficult for the sufferer's partner. The ailment can be caused by physiological factors, psychological factors, or a combination of both, and can be similar to those that cause erectile dysfunction (see the following ED section).

Sexual Issues, Energy, and Male Menopause

Physical Causes of Diminished Libido

• Fatigue

• Reaction to certain medications, alcohol, and illegal drugs, such as marijuana

• Illness or disease, most commonly diabetes and blood vessel disease

• Decreased levels of the male sex hormone testosterone

Psychologically based causes are, by their very nature, harder to pin down, but they have just as much impact as the physical causes. They can include preoccupation, depression, or relationship and/or job problems that create stress and tension.

Treatment/Prevention. Whatever the cause, most, if not all, decreased sexual desire can be treated successfully. The best starting point is to be examined by a doctor. If the causes are physical, there are numerous and varied ways of correcting the problem (supplementing the testosterone, changing an offending medication, treating an illness). If the underlying causes are psychological, treatment can include anything from drug therapy to psychoanalysis.

Premature Ejaculation

One of the benefits of getting older is that you get past certain points in which a particular ailment, illness, or disease is prevalent. This is the case with men in our age group and premature ejaculation, the most common sexual problem. It's just not usual for fifties males to experience such a problem—it's normally associated more with our younger brothers in their teens or twenties. Premature ejaculation can take place at any stage during love making, and there is no set time table that indicates the ejaculation is premature. Pure and simple, if you ejaculate before you want to, that's premature ejaculation. The cause is normally performance anxiety or too much excitement about the coming sexual event.

If you think you might be suffering from this ailment, ask yourself: Is it *really* a problem? It's been reported that the average American couple spends only about five to ten minutes on sex—start to finish. While that's a rather depressing statistic—we all need to slow down and enjoy it a bit more—if you and your partner are happy having sex within that time frame, and you ejaculate during that time frame, then you do *not* have a premature ejaculation problem. It's only a problem if you don't want to ejaculate and you do.

Treatment/Prevention. Here is where home remedies usually work wonders. If you have an understanding partner who wants to help, the two of you can work toward giving yourself more self-control. Work on getting aroused, then cooling down, getting aroused, then cooling down, with the goal of lengthening the time spent with an erection and no ejaculation. When you get the feeling that you're about to ejaculate, stop what you're doing until it subsides (the old standbys: Think about baseball or the Queen Mum), or you, or your partner, can softly squeeze either the base or tip of the penis until the feeling goes away.

Other methods include: masturbating before intercourse, because the second erection will usually last longer than the first; or using a condom, which decreases your sensitivity (not to mention reducing the risk of sexually transmitted diseases). Medications, such as certain antidepressants (known as SSRIs) can also be used to delay ejaculation.

Erectile Dysfunction (ED)

When Bob Dole—war hero, U.S. Senator from Kansas, and Republican presidential candidate—went on TV to talk about erectile dysfunction (the inability to have or sustain an erection), some thought he was discrediting his position. The vast majority of people, though, saw it otherwise—as a courageous act from a courageous man.

Political correctness aside for a moment, most men innately understand that nothing physical goes so much to the heart of being a man as an erection. The endless jokes that tie an erection to being a man only underscore just how important this relationship really is. Rightly or wrongly, there is something about the ability to "get it up" that makes us who we are as men.

This has significance in numerous aspects of our lives. For one thing, if something does go wrong with the physical process, it can have wide-reaching—and devastating—ramifications for the sufferer.

The good news is twofold: First, ED is relatively rare—a 1980s study of predominately white, well-educated, happily married American couples showed that only about 7 percent of men experienced ED; and second, nearly all cases of ED, no matter how severe or what the cause, can now be improved, if not cured.

Scientifically, the process of generating and maintaining an erection has two critical components: the parasympathetic nervous system and the blood vessels. Without these two, nothing would ever happen—and our lives would definitely be a lot less joyous.

The parasympathetic nervous system is a purely automatic operation that also handles the dilating and constricting of your eyes's pupils. This means that—contrary to what you may think or feel—an erection is not entirely under voluntary control. We—and our partners—can certainly try to spur on the parasympathetic nervous system with such things as sexual fantasies, sexually explicit visuals, extensive touching, and other exhilarating activities, but if the parasympathetic isn't "in the mood," our efforts are all wasted.

Even if the parasympathetic is in the right frame of mind to do its job, if the blood vessels aren't healthy enough to bring the blood to the penis and aid in "containing" the blood in the penis until ejaculation takes place, you've got a problem.

Four Ways Your Sexual System Can Break Down

Psychological factors. Job stress, pressure to perform, relationship tension can all be factors in failure to get or sustain an erection.

Vascular problems. If the penis's artery or veins are damaged or blocked, then ED can occur.

Nerve damage. Accidents and certain diseases like diabetes can cause nerve damage that will affect the erection process.

Hormones. If your testosterone level is significantly decreased, you won't have the sexual desire necessary to generate an erection.

It's also important to understand that ED comes in varying degrees. Most of us have probably at one time or another experienced a temporary breakdown of the system. The majority of these cases usually point to the cause, and to the fact that the ED is only temporary.

Causes of Temporary Erectile Dysfunction

Too much alcohol. Drinking can raise the level of excitement and lower inhibitions, but too much can mean the main actor won't be taking center stage that night.

Too little sleep. Fatigue can affect the ability to get or sustain an erection.

Too much guilt. Those tempted to stray outside of a committed relationship may find that their conscience might well get the better of their desires, wrecking the party.

More Serious Causes of Erectile Dysfunction

Surgery. In operations where the prostate is removed, there is a chance that certain nerves necessary for creating an erection will be damaged or severed.

Smoking. Long-term smokers will have some degree of blood vessel blockage or damage that might lead to erection problems.

Diseases. Diabetes can have an affect on the peripheral nervous system, while high blood pressure and heart disease can affect blood vessels, creating ED.

Illnesses. Flu and similar ailments can cause temporary ED.

Drugs. Certain drugs—legal and illegal—can cause ED problems.

As noted before, erections also change with age, but those changes should not be viewed as the beginning or early warning signs of erectile dysfunction.

By far the biggest problem with ED is that the causes of the problem don't stay confined to their own spaces. A diabetic or a person who's undergone prostate surgery can have a physically based ED that is made worse by his dwelling on the problem. A psychologically caused ED can turn into a vicious cycle that is hard to break—an occasional performance problem can be obsessed upon so much that it causes performance anxiety, which, in turn, creates another failed attempt.

One study showed that 64 percent of men with ED waited a year before seeing a doctor. If ED occurs suddenly, it probably is psychologically based. If the problem develops slowly, it is usually physiologically based. If the problem comes and goes occasionally, it's probably stress or fatigue. If it's a chronic problem, lasting six weeks or longer, you need to see your family doctor or internist (specialist in internal medicine).

Treatment/Prevention. Nearly every case of ED, regardless of the cause, can be helped in some way, if not completely cured. It's all a matter of first identifying the underlying reason. This means that the ED sufferer must first get over the feelings of embarrassment and/or shame that are usually associated with the problem and talk openly to his doctor.

The physician will first approach the problem from the physical side, looking for any signs of illness, as well as checking the patient's blood pressure, liver functions, size and shape of the testicles, and testosterone level. The doctor will also ask a series of questions to help determine the cause or causes. This is the time when the patient must be completely honest so the doctor can make an accurate diagnosis. It is also important—regardless of whether or not the doctor asks—to mention other problems that might not appear to be associated. (Example: If the patient also feels pain in his legs when walking up hill, the pain can indicate vascular damage that may be the culprit behind the ED.)

Sexual Issues, Energy, and Male Menopause

Treatment for ED can vary and involve two or three approaches at once, depending on the cause. If the ED is psychologically based, traditional one-on-one discussion therapy and/or marriage counseling has helped many men and their partners. Additionally, reputable sex therapy clinics have proven to be of great value in restoring some men to normal sexual functioning.

Treatment for Physically Based ED Depends on the Problem

Low testosterone level. Hormone replacement therapy, similar in concept to estrogen replacement therapy for women, is usually a quick and relatively easy way of correcting the problem, although getting the optimum dosage can take some adjustment time.

Vascular damage or blockage. Depending upon the degree of damage or blockage, either drugs to attack the blockage or surgery to remove the blockage or repair the damaged blood vessels will often improve the condition, if not cure it.

Nerve damage. Whether it results from an accident, a disease such as diabetes, or surgery (prostate removal), nerve damage that leads to ED can be overcome. Historically, that has meant use of penile implants, most notably one that keeps the penis semirigid all the time, and one that can be pumped up (both have their pros and cons); or an injection of an erection-causing drug directly into the penis (not an easy thing for a guy to do, nor very spontaneous for that matter). Today, many men suffering from this type of ED are now using the highly successful drug Viagra, considered by many to be a true "miracle" drug (see the following section for details).

Another option to overcoming ED that has not yet been fully scientifically tested is Yohimbine. It's an extract from the bark of an African tree that is supposed to, over time, aid in the creation of erections. It has to be taken regularly, typically three times a day. This should be approached with some caution, however, because there have been reports of painfully hard erections that last too long.

Viagra, Miracle Drug

There's probably not one American man in his fifties who hasn't heard of Viagra, the first oral medication for overcoming erectile dysfunction. Viagra is such an important drug that it warrants its own section among this book's ED treatment and prevention options.

When Viagra first hit the market in early 1998, the demand was overwhelming.

In the first three months alone, close to three million prescriptions were written across the country. In Gordon's practice, for the first six months there wasn't a day that went by that he didn't write a Viagra prescription. Viagra also seems to have become our decade's drug of choice—80 percent of all Viagra prescriptions being written are for men fifty or older.

From all reports—nationally, locally, and within Gordon's own patient base—the results have been nothing less than astounding. Officially, the success rate is an astounding 70 percent. Many men who have struggled for years, sometimes decades, with the mental and/or physical problems of erectile dysfunction have now found a way to return to normal sexual functioning.

How Viagra Works

Simply put, the drug increases the nitric oxide in the circulatory system. Nitric oxide is a chemical that affects the cells lining the arteries, redirecting (shunting) the flow of blood to the body part that needs it most. When you're exercising, for example, your muscles need more oxygen, so blood is sent to the muscles. When you've just eaten, blood goes to the digestive tract to aid digestion. When you want an erection, nitric oxide redirects the blood to your penis and—voilà! You've got an erection.

Does this mean that Viagra causes erections?

Not exactly. That soft caress or favorite fantasy is still a necessary trigger, but when it comes down to the mechanics of an erection, the nitric oxide does a lot of the real work corralling the blood and sending it into the right chute.

The usual dosage for Viagra starts at one 50 mg pill, but that can be modified up or down, depending on effectiveness. Manufacturer's directions say to take it about one hour before sexual activity, but that, too, can be adjusted to fit individual reaction times. The effect of Viagra usually lasts from four to six hours or until orgasm. Gordon's patients often find that the effects may last longer than originally expected—often eight to twelve hours—with a second or even a third erection/ejaculation possible.

Side effects are not common, but they do include low blood pressure, flushed skin, headaches, nausea, and visual problems such as tinted vision. The Food and Drug Administration and the manufacturer both have warned that Viagra is potentially dangerous when combined with nitroglycerin used for heart conditions. If you take any nitrates in any form, you should *not* take Viagra. For all other ED sufferers, however, it seems to be perfectly safe and is just the miracle drug they've been waiting for.

A note to those sexually healthy thrill seekers dying to ask: "Will it enhance an erection or orgasm in someone who doesn't suffer from ED?" Viagra is not a recreational sexual drug, nor should it be used as one. Viagra might give the normal fifties man's erection a little bit of a boost, but it definitely is *not* an aphrodisiac that improves or enhances sensations, feelings, or orgasms. And no, it won't give you the teenaged ability to go at it all night.

In late 2000 it was reported that a new drug, Vardenafil, has been developed that is nine times more potent than Viagra, can help create an erection in twenty minutes, has a 75 percent success rate in early trials, and has fewer side effects. If all goes well, it should be on the market in 2002.

Sexually Transmitted Diseases (STD)

Currently there are approximately twenty to thirty STDs (depending on how they're defined), many of which have little in common other than sexual contact as the method, or pathway, of infection. The various microorganisms that can cause STDs spread from one person to another when the infected person's blood, semen, or vaginal secretions come into contact with another person's blood or other bodily fluids. This means that the most common route of STD infection is through sexual contact, particularly when it involves one of the body's orifices— mouth, rectum, meatus (penis opening), or vagina.

As many of us have heard, since the advent of AIDS in the 1980s, many STDs have shown a decrease in new cases—attributable, no doubt, to better awareness, education, medical care, and probably a fear factor that has driven many to practice safer sex practices (see the safer sex sidebar in this chapter for details). Unfortunately, some STDs are starting to show increases again, indicating the need for constant vigilance.

Possible Signs of an STD

- An unusual discharge from the penis or vagina

- An itching or soreness of the anus, penis, or vagina

- Any kind of sore, ulcer, or rash on or around the genitals, mouth, or anus

- Increased frequency of urination

- Pain or a burning feeling when urinating

- Swollen glands in the groin

Often these symptoms are caused by ailments other than sexually transmitted diseases, but if you experience any of them, you should be checked out. And don't be lulled into nonaction because the symptom goes away. Some of the STDs have a latent stage where damage is being done but symptoms have disappeared. Just as critically, if you do have an STD, and your symptoms have vanished, you're probably still able to infect others, so going for a doctor's exam is not only in your best interests, but in those of your partner(s) as well.

If you do find yourself with an STD, don't panic: All of them are treatable, the majority are curable, and you are definitely not alone—it's estimated that one in four people will catch an STD at least once in their life time. Most importantly, though, you should act responsibly and inform every partner who is (or was) at risk—regardless of how that information might affect you or any relationships you're currently in. Additionally, if you have contracted an incurable STD (such as genital herpes or AIDS), or you have an as-yet-untreated STD, you should act responsibly by informing all potential partners before having sex and always following safer sex practices (see the safer sex sidebar in this chapter).

This is one time when being in your fifties is a good thing—more than 85 percent of STDs occur in people aged fifteen to twenty-nine. Let's hope part of the reason we aren't getting STDs as much as younger men is because we're wising up a little.

Following are the most common STDs. Keep in mind that all of them can be prevented by adhering to safer sex practices.

CHLAMYDIA

A bacterial infection acquired primarily through vaginal or anal intercourse, it can also be spread to other parts of the body through touching. (The bacteria that causes chlamydia can also cause NGU, an infection of the urethra; see the following section for details.) In its various forms, chlamydia is the most common cause of reported venereal infection in America, infecting between four and eight million people every year. Most women with chlamydia do not exhibit symptoms, while up to 50 percent of men do not either. Those men who do may experience a stinging sensation at the end of the penis, a watery discharge from the penis, swollen testicles, increased urination, and painful urination—usually within three weeks of being infected. Those at high risk for chlamydia include people who have become sexually active at an early age and anyone who is promiscuous.

Untreated chlamydia can lead to fever, headaches, pain in the groin, a general feeling of malaise, sterility, urinary tract infections, and permanent damage because of complications affecting the lungs, liver, or heart.

Because chlamydia can be easily confused with gonorrhea, a culture or DNA probe and urinalysis is necessary for diagnosis. Sometimes, however, testing is skipped, as it can be faster and easier to simply treat the man's symptoms. If they go away, then all partners are tested and/or treated as well—although testing is usually done (and is recommended).

Treatment/Prevention. Antibiotics are the normal course of treatment.

NONGONOCOCCAL URETHRITIS (NGU)

An infection of the urethra, NGU is usually caused by the same bacterium that's responsible for chlamydia and is often spread by anal, oral, or vaginal intercourse. However, not all NGU symptoms are sexually caused. Some cases of urethral irritation can be due to allergic reactions to soap, spermicides, or vaginal fluids.

No matter what the cause, the symptoms are the same: discharge from the penis, a burning or itching around the penis opening, and a burning while urinating. In a few months' time, these symptoms might go away, but NGU is still there and can ultimately cause arthritis, infections of the prostate gland, and permanent damage to reproductive organs in both men and women.

Because NGU symptoms are the same as those of gonorrhea, tests can be done on the discharge to determine which it is.

Treatment/Prevention. Antibiotics are effective in curing NGU.

HERPES

Strictly speaking, this is not classified as an STD, but it is typically passed on by, or associated with, sexual activity. A viral infection spread by contact with an infected area, herpes may or may not show visible signs of infection. The two most notable forms of herpes are HSV-1, or oral herpes, which causes fever blisters and cold sores in the mouth and on the lips, and HSV-2, or genital herpes. Both HSV-1 and HSV-2 can be spread from the mouth to the genitals and vice versa, usually through oral sex, but also through kissing.

Genital herpes, which infects about half-a-million Americans annually, usually begins about a week after exposure, with tingling and itching around the genitals, followed by genital sores on the penis, the anus, or buttocks about four to fourteen days after exposure to the virus. Fever and headaches might be present. The sores, which ooze a highly contagious fluid, heal within about ten days. After the initial attack, some suffers never have another outbreak, while many others do. Subsequent outbreaks usually produce milder symptoms than the initial attack.

To prove conclusively that a person currently has oral or genital herpes, a "culture" of a lesion (sore) is done. (The doctor rubs a swab on the sore, the swab is given to a lab, and whatever is found on the swab is grown, or cultured. If what grows is one of the herpes viruses, then the person knows they have the infection.) This test is important, because the long-term implications for the individual of having herpes are significant. Blood testing for herpes is not as useful as a culture, because a blood test can show only that a person has had herpes in the past. It cannot tell if a person currently has the infection.

Treatment/Prevention. Herpes is incurable. The virus stays in your body indefinitely. It can hibernate forever or may cause future outbreaks, especially during times of fatigue and stress. Outbreaks can be treated with various antiviral drugs that suppress virus reproduction and shorten the length of outbreaks. Recurrences can be suppressed with daily doses of an antiherpetic drug.

GONORRHEA

Many of us know this one as "the clap." It's a bacterial infection of the urethra, rectum, mouth, or throat, passed on by vaginal, anal, or, less commonly, oral sex. Nearly a million cases a year are reported in America. It's not uncommon for one person to be infected several times in one year. Gonorrhea cannot be picked up or transferred via inanimate objects.

Symptoms appear within seven days after infection. These include a feeling of discomfort inside the penis, pain during urination, and a yellow discharge from the penis. Initially, up to 90 percent of infected women may not have symptoms. When symptoms do show up in women, they can range from increased urination, discomfort when urinating, a yellow discharge, and an unpleasant smell, to a severe pelvic infection. Left untreated, however, gonorrhea can cause infertility and infections of the joints, heart valves, and brain. Gonorrhea is usually diagnosed through lab testing of a discharge or a smear of an affected area.

Treatment/Prevention. Antibiotics do the trick. Your doctor might treat you for chlamydia as well, because many people with gonorrhea also have a chlamydia infection. Gonorrhea is one STD that has been showing significant resistance to antibiotics.

HIV AND AIDS

HIV (human immunodeficiency virus) is the virus that in its last stage of development causes AIDS (acquired immune deficiency syndrome). The virus resides in blood, saliva, semen, and vaginal secretions, and attacks the body's immune system. It can be spread when an infected person's bodily fluids come in contact with an uninfected person's bodily fluids through such means as anal, oral, or vaginal intercourse, blood transfusions, or the use of contaminated needles. It can even be transferred from mother to baby. In heterosexual relations, HIV is more easily spread from man to woman than from woman to man.

IS IT REALLY WORTH IT?
PRACTICING SAFER SEX

In this age of incurable HIV and AIDS, where sex can, quite literally, equal death, experts say there is no "safe" sex (other than masturbation), only "safer" sex. While the following points might be difficult to contemplate in the heat of passion, they should be considered:

- **Selection.** Is that mysterious stranger worth it? How about that tantalizing coworker? Do all passions need to be satisfied? Only you can make such judgments.

- **Preparation.** If you're not in a strictly monogamous relationship, *always* use a lubricated latex condom. Latex is more effective than lambskin in protecting you from the HIV virus, and lubrication helps prevent condom tearing. Use water-based lubricants, as oil-based ones can damage condoms and vaginal tissue. Added protection: the greased double hull—two condoms used simultaneously with spermicide to help kill the HIV virus.

- **Implementation.** Receptive anal sex is the single riskiest sex act for transferring HIV. Oral sex can also be highly risky, so use a condom over the genitals and "look before you leap" (for sores, warts, or other abnormalities), although this won't catch everything. Wash all affected areas before, between and after anal, oral, and vaginal sex. Urinate immediately after sex.

- **Alternatives.** If not in a strictly monogamous relationship, consider abstinence or "outercourse"—non-penetration activities such as masturbation (solo and mutual)—and the use of sex toys (not shared).

What Happens after HIV Infection

The stats tell a grim story: More than 50 percent of HIV-positive people will develop AIDS within ten years of infection, and approximately 80 percent of all those who develop full-blown AIDS will die within two years. Worldwide, by the end of 2000, an estimated thirty-six million people are living with AIDS and an incredible 21.8 million have died. In America, there have been 438,000 AIDS-related deaths. Ninety percent of HIV-infected people live in developing countries that have little, if any, access to drug therapy. In industrialized nations—and specifically in America—the spread of HIV has been drastically reduced from its initial onset in the 1980s.

Usually, no symptoms appear in the initial stage of HIV infection, which can last from one to ten years, although some people develop a flu-like illness that can produce fever, night sweats, fatigue, muscle aches, headaches, swollen lymph nodes, sore throat, and diarrhea. This will clear up in about three weeks. While many HIV-infected men experience little disease progression for years and feel fine, they still can infect others. Viral replication occurs at a remarkable rate during this "latent" stage.

When HIV enters its final stage of full-blown AIDS, the immune system breaks down completely, opening the way for numerous infections and certain cancers.

Blood tests can detect the antibodies the body produces to fight HIV. It usually takes about one to three months from the moment of infection for the antibodies to appear, although it may take as long as six months. Those in high risk groups should consider periodic testing.

High risk groups include bisexual and homosexual males, intravenous drug users and their sexual partners, prostitutes, and hemophiliacs who may have received transfusions of infected blood (prior to 1985). Anal sex and multiple sex partners definitely increase the spread of the virus. Once the virus has taken hold, HIV can be passed on to heterosexual people who do not appear to fall into any high-risk group. A sad truth is that anyone who has sex with anyone who has had a previous partner is at risk of contracting HIV, although heterosexuals in a strictly monogamous relationship have little to fear. HIV cannot be contracted from toilet seats, handshaking, or even kissing.

Treatment/Prevention. While currently HIV and AIDS are incurable, treatment is getting better and more effective at slowing the growth rate of the virus and treating some of the symptoms. Researchers are also getting closer and closer to finding a vaccine for HIV. In the meantime, however, prevention is critical and once again revolves around safer sex practices. The only absolute protection from HIV is celibacy. An important note is that if you do test positive, it means you have developed antibodies to HIV—it does not mean you have AIDS. It is extremely important that those in high-risk groups be tested regularly. Early diagnosis allows antiviral treatment to be started early in the course of the disease, slowing the progress of the disease and reducing the risk of transmission to others.

GENITAL WARTS

Not exclusively an STD, genital warts are spread through sexual contact and are benign growths on or around the genitals and/or anus. Caused by a virus called human papillomavirus (HPV), genital warts, or venereal warts, can come in clusters and are normally painless. In some cases, they grow big enough to block the opening of the urethra.

Treatment/Prevention. The HPV virus has no cure, but genital warts can be removed via laser, freezing, or medication. Even without treatment, however, genital warts usually disappear in time. The HPV virus has implications in the development of cervical cancer in women; whether as cause and effect or as a "marker" for higher risk individuals is not yet known.

HEPATITIS B

This is a virus acquired through exposure to infected blood, semen, vaginal secretions, usually via sexual contact. Nonsexual transmission can occur with exposure to blood via shared needles or razors. More than 1.5 million Americans have hep B, and one-third of carriers have no symptoms but can be highly contagious. Symptoms can include fever, headaches, muscle aches, fatigue, loss of appetite, vomiting, and diarrhea. Advanced symptoms include dark urine, clay-colored stools, abdominal pain, and yellowing of the skin and whites of the eyes. (See chapter 4 for hepatitis details.) Hepatitis B can be detected through a blood test.

Treatment/Prevention. While the hep B virus may remain in your body for life, most infections clear up on their own in eight weeks. About 10 percent do become chronic and may lead to cirrhosis (liver disease) and liver cancer. Acute or severe infections are treated with bed rest and plenty of fluids. Prevention is easy: a vaccination series, which is strongly recommended for everyone (as is the vaccination series for its cousin, hepatitis A).

SYPHILIS

Caused by a bacterium that likes the warm, moist linings of genital passages, the syphilis bacterium dies quickly once outside the body. It cannot be spread via objects such as toilet seats, towels, or cups. Syphilis is a serious STD that can cause permanent damage to vital organs and even death. The normal method of infection is by vaginal, anal, or oral sex, kissing, or skin contact with open sores. About 100,000 new cases are documented each year. An incubation period, with no sign of symptoms, can last from nine to ninety days.

Four Stages to Syphilis

• **The primary stage** is when the first symptoms appear. A shallow, painless ulcer that oozes a clear fluid (not blood) and heals within a month without treatment will show up at the site of initial infection. During this time, the person feels fine.

- **The secondary stage** occurs when the bacteria have spread throughout the body, and the person begins to feel generally unwell. Symptoms can include a rash on the palms, the soles of the feet, or sometimes on the mouth; a sore throat; and swollen glands. Wart-like growths may appear on the genitals. All these symptoms will eventually disappear without treatment.

- **The latent stage** can last from months to decades and is marked by no symptoms. After a year or two in this stage, most people stop being infectious, although syphilis can still be detected by blood tests.

WHO ARE YOU GOING TO ASK?
GETTING ANSWERS TO SEXUAL QUESTIONS

Okay, you have a sexual problem, concern, or question. Who are you going to ask? Your partner? A friend? A family member? How about your doctor?

The June 1999 issue of the *Journal of the American Medical Association* reported on a U.S. survey of 500 adults, twenty-five years of age or older. A hefty 71 percent felt their doctor would dismiss any concerns about sexual problems they might bring up. Nevertheless, 85 percent said they would talk to a doctor if they had sexual problems, even if they might not get treatment.

Such cynical perceptions of the medical profession belie the years of preparation a medical doctor goes through before hanging up a shingle. Physicians are trained professionals. No matter how young or inexperienced they look, they have tremendous knowledge and resources available. And they want to help. A few points to keep in mind:

- **Analyze the problem.** Before the doctor visit, try to objectively look at the problem, think about possible causes, and try to identify ancillary problems.

- **Be honest.** Put aside shame and embarrassment; a doctor can't diagnose accurately without correct and complete information. The stakes are too high to lie.

- **Be concise and complete.** Respecting a doctor's limited time, keep the explanation brief, while making sure to include everything you think might be relevant.

Keep in mind, help is available. All sexual problems can be improved, if not always cured. The doctor's arsenal of options includes psychiatric, pharmacological, and hormonal forms of treatment. And doctors are there to listen and help.

• **The tertiary stage** usually occurs in about one-third of those not yet treated. Here, the disease does permanent damage to the bones and joints, the heart, brain, eyes, and nervous system. Treatment is usually still possible even in this late stage.

Syphilis can be hard to detect because symptoms can be mild or indistinct. Blood tests for antibodies or testing of sores for bacteria doesn't always work, so repeat testing can be important.

Treatment/Prevention. Penicillin is the usual, and quite effective, treatment for the disease. The penicillin is given in doses that are dictated by what stage the disease is in. While treatment does bring about cure, it will not reverse the damage syphilis has done before treatment.

REAL LIFE TALES

Number One: Dodging One Sexual Bullet Sometimes Puts You in the Path of Another

Richard is a successful lawyer who's fifty-two years old. He's been married for twenty-five years and loves his wife.

He makes a trip to Chicago and spends a few weeks there involved in a case. During that time, he works closely with others lawyers, ultimately becoming attracted to one female attorney in particular. It's a mutual attraction and soon Richard is in bed, enjoying the delights of someone new. While there are numerous sexual rendezvous during the trip, Richard and his partner know this is not a long-lasting relationship, merely an enjoyable break from somewhat dull, but generally satisfying, marriages.

When Richard gets home, he resumes sexual relations with his wife. In short order, however, she develops vaginitis, an inflammation of the vagina that can have a variety of possible causes. Before the test results come back, Richard is overwhelmed with guilt and confesses to his wife about the Chicago affair.

Richard's wife is, to say the least, upset and angry—justifiably so. Lucky for Richard, she agrees to marriage counseling. That's where he finds out that it isn't just the unfaithfulness that upsets her; it's also the how-could-you-expose-me-to-microorganisms-from-another-person issue.

Now, after concluding the marriage counseling, they have decided to stay together. Richard considers the whole episode to be grievously unfortunate and very traumatic (so much so that he was on antidepressants for a while). He wouldn't wish the experience on anyone. But, ironically, he also believes that he came out of the situation with a stronger sense of what his marriage is all about.

And what about the vaginitis?

Test results showed it to be a garden variety that was easily cured. Richard probably did bring something home, but most likely it was simply a different strain of a common vaginal bacteria that upset his wife's own bacterial balance of nature, causing an infection.

Richard and his wife were tested for every kind of sexually transmitted disease and got a clean bill of health. In this case, Richard definitely dodged the huge STD bullet, but while doing so, he had also stepped into the path of the equally dangerous infidelity bullet.

Number Two: Letting Two Good Years of Sex Slip By

Todd is fifty-eight and a geologist. Generally his health is okay, he's relatively fit, just a few pounds overweight, and is trying to keep it all under control.

During a routine office visit, Todd is told he has high blood pressure. Because high blood pressure is a "silent killer" that usually causes no symptoms but wreaks havoc on blood vessels, it should be treated as soon as it's found. Todd's blood pressure is not yet in the dangerous range, but it's high enough that it demands action.

Todd is immediately given medicine to bring it down. No complaints on Todd's part, but during the next few years his blood pressure fluctuates, and it never seems to get completely under control. The doctor is somewhat frustrated, and Todd isn't saying much.

Finally, after some in-depth questioning from the doctor, Todd admits he is finding it difficult to get and maintain erections while on the blood pressure medicine (a common side effect of some blood pressure drugs). Because of this important fact, Todd is doing a little self-medicating—periodically skipping his daily dose so he can have satisfactory erections.

Today, blood pressure drugs come in such a vast array that with a change in prescription, Todd has his blood pressure under control *and* has the ability to get and maintain erections.

Both the doctor and Todd were remiss in this case: the doctor for not asking the right questions, and Todd for not sharing all the pertinent facts with his doctor and for self-medicating (never a good idea without talking to the doctor first).

Number Three: Why Fight Loss of Your Sex Drive? It's Just Aging, Isn't It?

Mario is a painter. At fifty-nine years old, he's a relatively big man, bordering on fat, who takes medicine for high blood pressure and a little arthritis. For the past few years he's been feeling a little tired and a little depressed at times. He doesn't believe he's thinking as clearly as he used to. It's also been two years since he and his wife have had sex, but his lost libido doesn't bother him much, and his wife has never been too interested anyway. In Mario's book, these are all symptoms of getting old that he needs to learn to live with. Why fight it? he thinks, it's just aging.

During a routine office visit, however, he does tell the doctor about tenderness around his breasts. The doctor finds there is some actual breast tissue developing (as opposed to mere fat that imitates the look of breasts). With extensive questioning, Mario reveals all the physical and mental changes that have been going on during the last three years.

The blood pressure drug Mario takes is not known for the side effect of breast enlargement, and he doesn't take any of the herbal remedies or over-the-counter antacids that are known for that (if taken long enough in large enough quantities). So the doctor tests Mario's hormone levels—his testosterone might be down, or a feminizing hormone may be up.

Turns out Mario's testosterone is very low. While most men never experience a significant drop in their testosterone level, Mario is a real-life case of male menopause.

Within a short time of starting testosterone replacement therapy, Mario is back to a normal he hasn't known in years (more energy, better stamina)—and it feels great. His sex drive is back, which is a good thing, of course, but now he'll face a partner who's not that interested in sex. Some stories don't have a completely satisfying ending.

KNOWING WHAT YOU PUT IN YOUR MOUTH—
A DRUG CHART

Erectile Dysfunction Drugs

NAME	EXPLANATION AND USE	POSSIBLE SIDE EFFECTS
Sildenafil (Viagra)	Allows selective dilation of blood vessels of the erectile tissues of the penis, allowing engorgement with blood to concur, thus promoting an erection. Enhanced release of nitric oxide by the endothelial (blood vessel lining) cells is the mechanism of action.	Minor headache, bluish tint to vision, lowered blood pressure is possible. Must not be used by anyone taking nitroglycerin in any form. Generally, remarkably well tolerated by takers.
Alprostadil (Muse)	Dilates blood vessels less selectively than Viagra, so must be used locally (rather than in oral form). Muse is a suppository inserted in the urethra after urination, just before needed. Not surprisingly, Viagra has proven to be useful in more men than either Muse or Caverject (see below).	Urethral irritation, penile pain, dizziness, and, rarely, a painful and prolonged erection.
Alprostadil (Caverject)	The same drug as Muse, but delivered by self-administered needle injection directly into the penis. Trial and error is sometimes required to find the optimum dose.	Local pain and scarring are possible; increased risk of infection or bleeding at the injection site, prolonged painful erection.

Sexual Issues, Energy, and Male Menopause

THE GOOD NEWS

- If treated right, our sexual equipment should never "wear out," no matter how old we get.

- While it's true that the number, size, and hardness of our erections do diminish slightly with age, these changes are hardly noticeable and do not adversely affect our sexual functioning.

- Whatever the cause, sexual problems such as erectile dysfunction and more than average loss of sexual desire can usually be treated successfully.

- If you find yourself with a sexually transmitted disease, don't panic. All of them are treatable, and the majority are curable. Just remember to act responsibly toward your past, current, and future sexual partners.

- Eighty percent of all males stay within normal levels of testosterone for their entire lives.

6: MENTAL STATE AND CHANGING PATTERNS

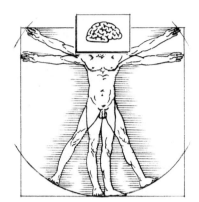

From Stress and Depression to Hair Loss and Headaches

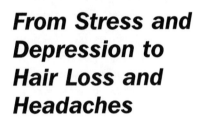

An obvious truth is that in your fifties you're a different person than you were in your twenties. It's obvious because we can see the physical changes every time we look in the mirror: Where did the hair go? Where *did* the wrinkles come from? Whose turkey neck is that? These physical changes reflect what's happening at the cellular level—supposedly, within every ten years every cell in your body dies, is removed, replaced, or changed in some way, making you a truly different person every ten years or so.

Within the psychological realm, shifts in perspective or outlook probably match, if not surpass, the physical changes that have taken place over the years, although they might be harder to identify and define. It's natural, though, for our thinking to shift as our bodies—and the world around us—change. Many of these changes will be specific to you, as your general outlook on life (positive or negative) dictates how you view and react to the physical changes that take place in your fifties.

There are, however, some age-specific psychological changes that can be applied generally—in the broadest sense—to men in our age group. Like the long-distance runner who has gotten far enough from the starting gate to settle into his rhythm to run *his* race, many men in their fifties seem to have gained some positive psychological perspectives.

Possible Insights Gained by the Time You Reach Your Fifties

A Sense of Relief—"I've made it this far." Most of us have reached the fifties without being struck by cancer, an oncoming train, or some life-threatening or life-changing disease. Realization of this can bring on an internal, almost subconscious sense of relief regarding physical well-being. (Those with a propensity toward hypochondria should try using this positive review of the past to gain a more positive view of current physical health.)

A Sense of Calm—"I know who I am." When it comes to the twisting and confusing pathways known as career and relationships (family, friends, lovers), many of us will have somehow stumbled onto relatively safe and secure pathways. Traditionally, the fifties is an age decade of career zeniths, completion of child rearing, and recommitment to established love relationships—all normally a result of better understanding of who you are and what you want out of life. Ironically, this self-awareness can lead either to greater appreciation of the status quo or a rejection of it to go and find what is really desired. Both directions can bring a sense of calm self-assurance.

A General Clarity of View—"I know where I'm going." The relief and calm that many men in our age group feel can lead to a general sense of being able to see ahead, know where you're going, and chart the potential obstacles. This sense of purpose and direction comes from the accumulated insights gained from analyzing past experiences.

A Sense of Perspective—"I know life's not all about sex." As we enter our fifties, one of the normal changes is that we don't think about sex as much as we used to. And our equipment doesn't act and react as fast as it did. This might actually be a good thing. It might mean we can finally start turning our considerable brain power toward seeing other perspectives and sides of life: Cuddling is pretty nice; emotional intimacy feels good. Having someone who really listens (at least occasionally) is sometimes even better than having sex. And a face that has no lines or wrinkles isn't half as interesting as one that does. A wise man once said, "Boys, once you stop thinking about [sex] all the time, life'll get much simpler." All of which leads to the thought that there truly is life beyond sex (not be confused with life *without* sex—a very different animal).

228

Mental State and Changing Patterns

Admittedly, these four perspectives don't all fall into place for every male in our age group—and even if they do, there are still many other questions and concerns that make life uncertain. But gaining any of these four can you give renewed strength to better deal with mental issues such as stress, depression, and/or changing-pattern issues such as hair loss and sleep disruption.

WHERE AND HOW PROBLEMS OCCUR, TREATMENT OPTIONS, AND PREVENTIVE MEASURES

Mental State

Fatigue and Energy

It's true that as you enter our age group many of your body parts begin to make you stand up and take notice, but your tight muscles, sore joints, and declining eyesight are, in most cases, still more of a nuisance than they are life-changing. More importantly, though, your overall energy level and basic attitude toward life should not be drastically different as you travel toward your sixties. In fact, there are many men who report a kind of "second wind" in their fifties that reenergizes them both physically and mentally.

On the other side of the coin, if you are feeling tired or run-down there can be many reasons why.

Common Causes of Fatigue

• **Lack of sleep**

• **Not enough exercise**

• **Poor eating**

• **Normal daily tension**

The kind of fatigue these symptoms reflect can be brought on by extremes: too little or, less often, too much sleep; too little or, less often, too much exercise; and too much or, less often, too little eating. Generally speaking, this is where self-help can work wonders. If the fatigue is a result of one or more of those four highlighted situations, a little self-analysis can identify where your problem lies. Once that's accomplished, it's only a matter of making the necessary changes.

If you make the appropriate changes and don't notice a return to your normal levels of energy and attitude within a week or two, it might be time to see a doctor and look into other causes.

Other Causes of Fatigue

• **Lack of fitness**

• **Stress, beyond normal daily tensions**

• **Depression**

• **Presence of illness, including most diseases**

In fact, fatigue can be a symptom of nearly every disease or serious ailment, so it should not be treated lightly. By far the number one cause of fatigue is lack of fitness, with lack of sleep coming in second. However, fatigue should never be passed off as just part of growing old—fatigue is *not* a natural result of aging.

Treatment/Prevention. If you've identified lack of sleep as the cause of your fatigue, you're not alone—approximately one-third of all adults suffer from regular insomnia. That's probably because our overall amount of sleep has been decreasing over the past two decades due to our highly stressed and overworked society. While sleep requirements are highly individual, most people need six to nine hours a night (see the sleep section in this chapter for details).

If you have identified lack of exercise or poor nutrition as the cause of your fatigue, see chapter 8 for exercise and diet suggestions. If the cause is stress, see the following section. If you think your fatigue is a symptom of a disease, see your doctor.

How can you tell if fatigue is disease-related?

If it lasts for more than a week, doesn't respond to changes you've made, interferes with your life in any way, or is accompanied by specific physical symptoms, then it could mean something serious is going on in your body. A trip to the doctor is advised.

Obviously, it's best to avoid fatigue altogether. This, of course, is easier said than done. However, there are numerous courses of action you can take to keep yourself energized, upbeat, and fatigue-free.

Preventing Fatigue

Work within your own rhythms. Some people are morning people, others function better at night. By the time you've reached our age group you should definitely know the conditions under which you function best. Work on developing an environment that brings out your best. Schedule difficult tasks during your peak times.

Start with a good breakfast. Your mother was right, breakfast is important. Fruit, cereal, and skim milk will give you a lot more get-up-and-go than a Danish and coffee. (See chapter 8 for dietary details.)

Take periodic breaks. Working for long stretches without a break is actually counterproductive. Don't try to plow on through. You'll achieve more if you stop occasionally to rest and rejuvenate yourself—stretching exercises are great for this.

Follow your bliss. Paraphrasing philosopher Joseph Campbell: If you pursue your "bliss"(whatever you're passionate about), doors will open where you never thought they were, and you'll be energized in the process. If work (even small elements within work) doesn't do it for you, find a hobby that stimulates your passion.

Don't smoke, and limit your drinking. While both might seem momentarily energizing, they do more harm than good. Alcohol is a depressant, so if you're already fatigued, it's certainly not going to help your condition. It might make it worse.

Get plenty of sleep. A critical ingredient to a healthy, energized life-style. (See the section on sleep in this chapter for details.)

Stress

We all know it, have felt it, we've all had to deal with it in our own way. Stress is that nearly tangible feeling of frustration, anger, tension, or anxiety that a particular experience creates in us. The experience can come from practically anywhere and involve nearly anything.

Some Causes of Stress

• Internal doubts, fears, phobias

• Job-related concerns

• Partner difficulties

• Family tensions

• Financial problems

Even if we eat well, exercise, and get enough sleep, we can still feel the effects of stress, and some people are not as good at handling stress as others are. As we get older, stress takes a cumulative toll. As it wears us down, affecting us more and more, we begin to lose our ability to deal with it—creating a downward spiral that can cause real havoc, both mentally and physically.

What Exactly Is Stress?

Basically, it's the body's and mind's response to a perceived threat. Back in the caveman days, the threats were relatively straightforward—animal attack, club-carrying guy attack, or the occasional crazed cavewoman. Today, in our highly complicated and structured society, our minds have come to regard as threats anything perceived as endangering our physical or mental well-being—everything from doubting our ability to do a particular job to the death of a loved one.

The mind reacts to these "dangers" by implementing certain physical processes that prepare the body for action, whether it be to stand and fight, or turn and run—the old "fight or flight" scenario we've all heard about. These physical processes include the increased production of adrenaline and cortisol, stress hormones that raise the heart rate, respiration, blood pressure, and sugar levels.

As we all know, such physiological changes don't go unnoticed—it's like putting a naval vessel on "full alert," where every member of the crew becomes highly focused on an incoming crisis or attack. And by the time a "stand down" order is given, the crew—not to mention the body—is pretty well exhausted, regardless of whether the attack actually happened or not.

Side Effects of Slight Stress

• Sleeplessness

• Fatigue

• Indigestion and heartburn

• Irritable bowel syndrome

• Headaches

Mental State and Changing Patterns

• Muscle tightness and backaches

High levels of stress or stress endured for an extended period of time may produce more permanent changes in blood vessel health, resulting in such problems as high blood pressure, angina, and heart disease. It can also affect the overall immune system, so that there is a greater susceptibility to viral and bacterial infections and possibly cancer (not yet positively linked, but common sense leads us to feel the "rightness" of the connection).

Linking Stress to Overall Health

For decades science has been studying the link between stress and health. In the mid-1960s American heart specialists identified "type A"and "type B" personalities. A-types are those prone to coronary problems, because they are aggressive, ambitious, restless, and obsessively concerned about time and deadlines—meaning major stress is a daily part of their lives. B-types are more relaxed, not obsessive about time and schedules, generally less aggressive, and have learned to handle stress (or are not affected by it). Not surprisingly, it's been reported that A-types are twice as likely to suffer a severe heart attack as B-types. (In some ways, however, this may be too simplistic an approach—hostility, anger, and feelings of helplessness may actually be more important than personality types.)

Taking a different look at stress, two American psychiatrists, Thomas H. Holmes and Richard Rahe, devised a Social Readjustment Ratings Scale, which ranks forty-three stressful events in terms of their affects on the body. On a scale of one to 100, the death of a spouse rates 100, divorce is seventy-three, while a minor incident with the law an eleven. In many ways, these ratings would naturally change as we age; as we get older there is normally a greater ability to handle and deal with many stressful situations.

But all of this stress does translate into some pretty heavy medical problems. According to the National Institute of Mental Health, and other surveys, 70 to 80 percent of all visits to the doctor are for stress-related and stress-induced ailments. Reportedly, 50 percent of all illnesses in America are caused, in part, by stress.

Are You Suffering from Stress?

• Do you eat when you're not hungry?

• Do you have difficulty falling asleep?

• Do you feel fatigued most of the day?

• Do you have trouble concentrating or focusing your thoughts on a task?

• Do you suffer from recurring headaches?

• Do you lose your temper easily, have no patience, or get irritated quickly?

• Have you lost any of your sex drive?

If you answered yes to any of those questions, you could be suffering from stress and should see a doctor. (Not surprisingly, these signs can indicate depression—see the following section for details). If you're a male in our age group, there's a good chance you did answer yes to a few of those questions. While stress is not age-specific, it nonetheless can become a major issue for many men in their fifties. As mentioned earlier, coronary disease (which is age-specific to fifties men and older) often is related to prolonged exposure to high levels of stress.

Not as scientific—but just as real to many—is the anecdotal evidence that some men in our age group discover that their individual coping methods (haphazardly developed over the years) don't work anymore. A classic example is the "suffer in silence" method of "dealing" with stress—initiated because "real" men supposedly don't voice stress-related concerns or express emotions. This kind of John Wayne approach would certainly make the Duke happy, but it has put a lot of fifties men in coronary-care units, not to mention psychiatrist's offices.

For most people, a certain level of stress is okay. Most of us know that a little pressure, a little tension, a little stress can motivate us on a day-to-day basis. In fact, low-level stress can be like a couple of jolts of strong coffee—the heart gets pumping and the brain shifts into high gear. As long as the stress can be positively channeled, and no underlying negative side effects are occurring, there is no reason for concern.

However, it can be surprisingly easy for low-level stress to feel suddenly unmanageable, for the stress to become suddenly high level, or for past stress management techniques to become ineffective. When this happens, reassessment of what you're doing and development of better stress management is critical to maintaining mental and physical health.

Treatment/Prevention. Good stress management is highly individual—what works for one won't necessarily work for another. It can be self-created or developed with the help of health care professionals. When determining what might work best for you, keep in mind basic components like those that help with fatigue—eating right, getting enough sleep, avoiding tobacco, and drinking only moderately.

Mental State and Changing Patterns

Fundamental Principles to Relieve Stress

Exercising. Whether it's a workout at the gym, a run in the park, a pickup game of basketball, or even just stretching in a hotel room, physical exertion is one of the best natural ways to relieve stress.

Seeing the positive side of things. That glass-half-full concept turns out to be good for your mental and physical health. It's been shown that people who have a positive, proactive perspective on life live longer and are generally healthier than those who are constantly pessimistic. Admittedly, if you've never had a positive attitude, developing one could take a lot of hard work and effort, but the rewards will definitely be worth it.

Expressing emotions calmly and rationally. Without this release valve, stress can build up like water pressure in a steam engine.

Releasing anger in constructive ways. Count to ten before exploding. Take a few deep breaths and then exhale long and slowly—feel the tension flow out of your body. Anger, in and of itself, is not bad, it's how you handle it that counts. Bottling it up will only mean it will take its toll somewhere down the road.

Laughing. A hearty belly laugh is truly great medicine. And being able to see the humor in life is a way to avoid the negative consequences of stress. A good sense of humor also can defuse a stressful situation involving others.

Getting out. Those under stress tend to isolate themselves from the rest of the world—the "I can't deal with my friends right now" type of attitude. But getting out, relating to others, and seeing that life is going on as usual can help reduce stress.

Getting Away. When was your last vacation? Getting away from your problems for a few days can often restore a much needed sense of perspective.

Assessing yourself. Have you been avoiding your problems? Have you been refusing to talk about how you're feeling?

Assessing the stress. What are its root causes? Are the causes ones you can control and change, or are they out of your control (and, therefore, not to be worried about)? Are your problems too overwhelming to face alone?

Asking for help—from a friend, a family member, and/or a professional—when necessary. Asking for help is not a sign of "weakness," it is a sign of a mature adult realizing another perspective can be the key to unlocking the answers. Problems shared are problems nearly solved.

If you do find the stress you're under is too much to handle on your own, there are numerous options, from traditional to alternative.

Stress-Relieving Options

- Therapies—everything from traditional psychoanalysis to alternative methods, such hypnotherapy—have helped many realize that stress can be flushed from the system with the right change in attitude.

- Prescription drugs, such as antidepressants—prescribed and monitored by a doctor—have been successfully used to lower stress levels.

- Herbal remedies such as St. John's wort seem to help people relax and/or manage their stress (although science has not proven a definite link). Ask your doctor before trying herbals for stress.

- Massage, yoga, deep relaxation, and meditation can help both the mind and body relax.

When it comes to stress and how to manage it, ask yourself: Are you choosing stress without even realizing it? Sometimes, because of life-long habits or behaviors, we actually put ourselves into more stressful situations than necessary or needlessly worry about problems we have no real control over.

Good stress management includes healthy doses of personal assessment and analysis. Life is made up of an infinite number of choices. We have the ability to make different choices to create a better life for ourselves—and those around us. To truly reduce stress in your life, these changes need to be on both a large scale and a minute scale—everything from our overall outlook on life, to whether or not that rush-hour traffic jam will affect your entire day. Keep reminding yourself that each choice, no matter how seemingly insignificant, does truly make a difference in your life.

Depression

While many males in our age group find they have a renewed sense of purpose and excitement in life, there are others who feel the exact opposite. To them, reaching

Mental State and Changing Patterns

the sixth decade means that the best of life is behind them, and there's not much to look forward to other than degeneration. A small percentage of these men don't just have a negative outlook on life, they may be suffering from the very real and very serious ailment: depression.

What is Depression?

As we've all heard—and as some of us have experienced—depression can be a crippling mental disorder. It is a state of mind that is marked by a sense of sadness, discouragement, worthlessness, loneliness, despair, and/or hopelessness. Thoughts of suicide or death can be prevalent, as can sleeplessness, agitation, crying for no apparent reason, and general apathy. These feelings can create a lack of purpose, meaning, and direction, which in turn causes decreased activity and an inability to function. Depression can be particularly insidious because the sufferer doesn't feel able to do anything or initiate lifestyle or perspective changes that might help the condition. As such, depression is known as a "whole-body" illness, affecting thoughts, moods, and the body. Physical complaints such as sleep and appetite changes, and decreased energy, attention, and concentration may precede obvious mood changes.

Approximately seventeen million Americans suffer from some form of depression. Women are twice as likely to experience major depression as men. Some believe the statistical difference is due to the fact that many men won't seek help for depression—it's not the "manly" thing to do. Nevertheless, according to one study, approximately 10 percent of all males will suffer from major depression at some point in their lives. And men are three times as likely as women to choose suicide as a way of ending their depression, according to the *Journal of Clinical Psychiatry*.

What Causes Depression?

Because depression involves the brain (the most complex organ in all of nature) the causes of depression can be elusive. The biological model of depression, prevalent since the development of effective drug treatments of depression, holds that most depression is caused by a depletion of a neurotransmitter, a chemical that aids in the transmission of nerve impulses from one cell to another in the brain. The usual neurotransmitter shortage is with the chemicals serotonin and/or norepinephrine. These shortages seem to stimulate an infinite range of emotional disorders—everything from social anxiety disorder, on one end, to suicidal depression on the other. The newer antidepressant drugs (see the drug chart in this chapter) help to restore these chemical balances, and, particularly combined with some form of talk therapy, have a high rate of improvement.

Many things can cause the depletion of neurotransmitters, including a genetic predisposition; hormone disorders (menopause and male menopause); adverse life events, such as the loss of a loved one or financial adversity; and feelings of personal worthlessness or guilt (for real or imagined transgressions). Regardless of the cause, the combination of drug treatment and psychotherapy is quite helpful.

Depression's Various Forms

Situational Depression. Just as it sounds, this is a temporary state caused by a specific incident or event, such as death of a loved one, divorce, or job termination. Treatment is necessary only when the condition goes on for more than two weeks and/or begins to interfere with the person's life.

Dysthymia. When someone has more depressed days than not, and each day is more or less depression-filled (for more than two years), he is suffering from the chronic state of dysthymia. He is still functional, but he's less than "normal" and the condition can lead to major depression. A combination of therapy and antidepressants is the usual course of treatment.

Seasonal Affective Disorder (SAD). A condition where the sufferer becomes depressed during the autumn and winter because of the lack of natural light. Treatment with intensely bright light using a special apparatus can be helpful. Care should be taken regarding what light is used so that skin cancer doesn't become a possibility.

Manic Depression. Also referred to as bipolar disorder, this is where a person experiences periodic mood swings from mania (overly expressive elation or irritability, talkativeness, and hyperactivity) to depression and a decreased need for sleep. Treatment usually involves a combination of psychotherapy and mood stabilizing drugs. Prescription antidepressants may also be used, but usually not without a mood stabilizer.

Psychosis. This is a major mental disorder where the person becomes detached from reality and has impaired perceptions of life. Often hospitalization is called for, along with psychotherapy and prescription antipsychotics.

It's important to note that getting "the blues" or "feeling down" is actually a natural and normal part of life and is *not* considered to be clinical depression. While we should take these occasional bouts of mild depression seriously, we shouldn't be overly concerned about them. It's only when we can't shake the blues, and a

Mental State and Changing Patterns

sense of sadness or hopelessness permeates our entire life for more than two weeks that it becomes a problem that needs serious, professional help.

How can you tell the difference between being temporarily bummed and being seriously depressed?

See Your Physician for Possible Depression If:

• Self-help measures don't positively change the situation within a few weeks.

• You are unable to sleep properly for more than two weeks.

• You have lost interest in most activities, events, friends, lovers, or family.

• You have a general feeling of sadness throughout a day.

• You gain or lose weight without consciously trying.

• You have suicidal thoughts, or think about death a lot.

• You feel agitated, irritated, or anxious most of the time.

While some of these symptoms can be related to other ailments and normal life, they can all be associated with depression. If you are experiencing several of these symptoms, you should talk to your doctor. And remember, seeking help for depression is not something to be ashamed about. Depression is very treatable—approximately 85 percent of people with major depression significantly improve and return to productive lives, according to the American Psychiatric Association.

As a final note, it should be stressed that as science finds out more and more about the way the brain works, it becomes clearer that depression is very much a result of chemical imbalances within the brain. Most of these imbalances are now very treatable via drugs that restore the brain to proper functioning.

With that said, however, it is also acknowledged that chemical imbalances are not all of the depression equation (e.g., do emotional states stimulate chemical imbalances, or do chemical imbalances stimulate emotional states?), which is why the best course of treatment for depression is usually a combination of drugs and some form of talk therapy.

Treatment/Prevention. There are many and varied treatments for depression, depending upon factors such as the cause and degree of the depression and the patient's medical and personal history. Because of the strong link between brain chemical imbalances and depression, it's strongly advised that anyone who feels seriously depressed should first see a medical doctor to determine if there is a chemical imbalance before pursuing other courses of treatment.

In mild cases of depression, many people have found self-help books and/or various forms of psychotherapy effective. For more serious depression, usually psychotherapy, with or without prescription antidepressants (see this chapter's drug chart for details), will do the trick and return the sufferer to a more normal state of mind. Antidepressants usually reduce the symptoms so that the patient can deal with the underlying problems.

It is critical to note that those on antidepressants should carefully follow all doctor's orders regarding how and when the drug should be taken. Because antidepressants often work by stimulating certain brain chemicals or blocking the depletion of certain brain chemicals, they are extremely powerful, so they need to be used in the proper way. They should never be started—nor stopped—without a doctor's knowledge. While you may be tempted to stop taking an antidepressant because you are feeling better, that is very likely to cause a relapse of depression.

As far as psychotherapy is concerned, it can come in numerous forms. Usually, a case of depression can be helped significantly by short-term varieties that last up to fifteen weeks.

Various Forms of Psychotherapy

Talking therapy. Also known as insight-oriented therapy, in talking therapy the therapist helps the patient explore his feelings about the depression and its root causes. Through a give and take between the therapist and patient, the patient gains a better, more in-depth understanding of his problems.

Behavior therapy. The patient is taught how to change his behaviors to create a more healthy lifestyle.

Cognitive/behavior therapy. This therapy works on the patient's negative thoughts and how they, along with his negative behaviors, can be changed to reshape his life in a more positive way.

Interpersonal therapy. As we all know, relationships can dictate how we feel about ourselves and the world. A person with depression can be helped to see how certain relationships in his life have caused or aggravated his depression.

Psychodynamic therapy. The therapist helps the patient focus on resolving emotional crises or conflicts, many of which may have started during childhood.

THERE'S NO WAY I CAN RELAX!
BASIC RELAXATION TECHNIQUES

After decades of job-related stress and tension, your muscles are probably as tight as bridge cables. It's time you learned how to relax—not only your body, but your mind as well.

Start with the right conditions: Wear loose-fitting clothes; find fifteen to thirty minutes of undisturbed time in a room with low, soft lighting (turn off that cell phone!); lie on a bed or the floor with a pillow under your head. Then try any or all of the following—they'll go a long way toward helping to relieve stress as well as keeping depression at bay:

- **Understand what relaxation feels like.** First tense a muscle, then release it (make a fist so your forearm muscles tighten, or curl your toes so your foot clenches up). When you suddenly release the muscle, the feeling you get is what relaxation is all about. Do this with all the muscles you're able to, from your head to your toes.

- **Breathe.** Take long, slow breaths while thinking that your tension and stress are leaving your body as you exhale. Exhale three times as long as you inhale, blowing gently with lips lightly parted (as if blowing on a lighted candle without putting it out).

- **Relax your mind.** Wipe away all thoughts except how peaceful and calm you feel. Or, think bland thoughts, about snow falling or waves breaking on a beach. Keep your breathing steady and deep.

When you reach a level of deep relaxation, your body should feel wonderfully heavy and numb. Don't worry if you fall asleep—you probably need it. And take your time coming back to life. Do a few slow stretches and wait a few minutes before getting back to work.

Drugs and Addictions

Flashback to the late sixties: a crowded basement room is rocking to the Rolling Stones playing on a stereo, the air is heavy with a sweet-smelling smoke, and a black light casts weird shadows on everything. A guy comes up with a Cheshire-cat grin and a little pill in his hand and says, "Hey, man, you gotta try this."

Most of us can probably remember some aspect of the drug culture that permeated the crazy, heady days of our youth. Whether or not you took the dude up on his generous (albeit dangerous) pharmaceutical offer—or even "inhaled" during those frenetic days—the vast majority of us can now agree that that part of the sixties and seventies is best long gone.

For those back then who actually did find the time and energy to do things other than party, there is another drug image, courtesy of Psych 101, that is hard to forget: the deranged, starving rat who couldn't stop pounding the pedal to get cocaine while ignoring the pedal for food.

What Is a Drug?

A drug is any chemical substance that affects the body's normal functioning. According to the Pharmaceutical Research and Manufacturers of America (as reported in the *AMA News*), there are 25,000 drugs in the world today. New ones are approved nearly every week. Particularly important in this section are psychoactive drugs—those chemical compounds that cause behavioral changes, such as extreme mood swings and hallucinations. Psychoactive drugs, all potentially addictive, come in four categories:

- **Depressants** that slow down the signals of the central nervous system. They include tranquilizers, barbiturates ("downers"), and alcohol.

- **Stimulants** that rev up the signals of the central nervous system. They include nicotine, caffeine, amphetamines ("uppers," or "speed"), cocaine, and even such dietary supplements as Metabolife (which contains ephedra).

- **Narcotics** that kill pain and generate a feeling of euphoria. They include opiates such as codeine, morphine, and their derivatives. Heroin is an opiate that has no legal medical use.

- **Hallucinogens** that distort the senses and can create hallucinations. They include cannabis (marijuana and hashish), mescaline, LSD, ecstasy, PCP, and psilocybin ("magic mushrooms").

What Is an Addiction?

Generally speaking, an addiction is the strong, if not irresistible, dependence on the use of a particular substance. It can be an actual physical dependence (like nicotine that the body comes to crave), and/or a psychological dependence (like needing a cigarette when you're nervous or anxious). Addiction, or dependence, can be characterized by an increased tolerance to the particular drug, so that more and more of the drug is needed to replicate the initial effects. If abrupt deprivation of the substance leads to withdrawal symptoms, it is a sure sign of addiction. Withdrawal symptoms can be physical and mental, can range from nearly insignificant to life-threatening, and can include anxiety, sweating, rapid heart rate, or convulsions.

Substances that can be addictive include:

• Many prescription-only drugs such as opiates (see above), amphetamines, sleeping pills, and benzodiazepines (Valium-like drugs), and illegal drugs such as marijuana, cocaine, and heroin.

• Alcohol, no matter what form it comes in.

• Other nonprescription substances, such as nicotine, caffeine, and even chocolate.

The critical words here are "can be addictive." Science has shown that there are addictive personalities—those who are much more prone to becoming hooked on addictive substances than others. While anyone—given the right conditions—can become addicted, approximately 5 to 10 percent of the American population can be classified as having addictive personalities.

The problem for doctors—and ourselves—is not knowing where you fall in this classification. That's one of the main reasons why many drugs require a doctor's prescription—objective control and monitoring of potentially addictive drugs helps ensure that most people don't become addicted. It should be noted, though, that two of the most widely abused drugs in the world are alcohol and tobacco— legal drugs that can cause as much damage as many illegal drugs.

As for men and addiction, the numbers aren't good. We seem to have the lion's share of problems in this field—more than eight million of the fourteen million alcoholics in America are men. Approximately twenty-six million men smoke.

It's a relatively safe bet, though, that if you've reached your fifties and you haven't had a problem with drugs, alcohol, gambling, or any other potentially addictive substances or situations, you're not likely to face such a problem. This doesn't mean, however, that it can't happen.

Environments Conducive to Addiction

• Loss of a close family member or friend (loss of a spouse may be a strong risk factor in men for developing an alcohol problem).

- Long-term pain situations, such as the onset of arthritis, may lead some to rely on painkillers for a sufficiently long time that they become dependent on them.

- Extended illness, even something as uncomplicated as a sinus infection, can bring on dependence upon the drugs (such as nasal spray) used to combat it.

- Starting—at any age—to experiment with illegal substances such as marijuana, cocaine, or heroin.

It should be noted that addiction to items such as caffeine and chocolate are relatively harmless, as long as they are not affecting your general health and fitness. (Do you act crazed after that tenth cup of coffee? How many pounds around your waist are attributable to that daily intake of chocolate?) If you think you—or someone close to you—have become addicted to a particular substance, ask the following questions:

1. **Can I stop using the substance without major side effects?** If your answer is yes, but you've never tried to stop, try immediately and see how well you do.

2. **Is the use of the substance negatively impacting my physical health, sleep patterns, or general mental well-being?**

3. **Is the use of the substance negatively impacting my relationships with others, or my ability to function normally in my life and job?**

If you—or the person you're concerned about—answered yes to any of these, there may be a problem that should be addressed immediately.

Treatment/Prevention. It is important to know that a serious addiction can be as devastating and life-threatening as a major illness. That's because addiction *is* a major illness and should be treated as such.

The first big step toward handling an addiction is acknowledging that it exists. This can be easier said than done. Friends, family members, medical practitioners, religious counselors, and various substance abuse support groups can help you face the reality of the situation. Groups such as Alcoholics Anonymous realize the importance of this personal acknowledgment when they insist that individuals start any remarks by stating: "I'm so-and-so, and I'm an alcoholic."

Your doctor can help to identify the problem and determine the best course of action to break the physical and mental dependence. Additionally, there is a broad base of substance abuse groups—many led by former addicts—ready to assist you. Inpatient detoxification is sometimes necessary.

Remember, help is out there.

Mental State and Changing Patterns

Psychosomatic Illness

"It's all in your head!"

How many times have you heard that? First it might have come from your mother when she thought you were trying to skip school with a fake stomachache (quickly revised when you threw up all over her new shoes). Then it was just as likely to be a coworker, friend, or partner when you whined about a headache or feeling run down.

Somehow, the simple act of identifying the mind as culprit—rather than a "real" cause—used to rob the entire ailment of its legitimacy. And if the problem was all in your head, then the symptoms must not be as intense as those brought on by "real" causes. Taking all this to its ultimate conclusion is the old joke about the hypochondriac whose tombstone simply reads: "I told you I was sick."

That guy would be happy to know that for years now science has been uncovering more and more evidence that there is a link between our emotional state and our immune system. When you're feeling down or depressed, your chances of contracting a cold are much greater than if you're feeling happy and upbeat. There is even a branch of medicine called psychneuroimmunology, or "psychosomatic medicine," that is concerned with how mental and emotional reactions affect the body's functioning and processes—in particular how emotional conflicts affect physical symptoms.

A growing number of people, prompted by the writings of such authors as Louise Hay (author of *You Can Heal Your Life*), Andrew Weil, and Deepak Chopra, take the mind-body connection to the extreme, believing that most, if not all ailments, no matter how severe, are initially triggered by mental attitudes. They feel that science hasn't yet proved what they already know to be true.

While most of us can now see the connection between feeling blue and the greater chance of getting simple ailments like colds, most of us would probably find it hard to believe that the mind can trigger—through negative thoughts and feelings—everything from dental problems to cancer.

While that debate will definitely be raging for generations (even we co-authors don't see eye-to-eye on the topic), most in the scientific community believe that the mind does play a tremendous role in our overall health and, generally speaking, symptoms are equally valid and intense no matter what causes them. An axiom in medicine—"even hypochondriacs can develop real disease"—indicates that doctors do approach each illness thoughtfully. Doctors have also seen how patients with strongly positive attitudes consistently show quicker recovery times, while statistics reveal that married people (both men and women) generally have better health and longer lives than single people—due, it is concluded, to the emotional stability and companionship of marriage.

Treatment/Prevention. Symptoms of any kind should not be ignored because you feel they might be in your head. Until a medical practitioner has said otherwise, take them seriously. And while a positive attitude does aid in recovery from any illness, don't forsake doctor-prescribed medicines. Science plus mental attitude is always a good combination; mental attitude minus science can possibly do real harm.

Alzheimer's Disease

Probably not one of us in our age group can honestly say he hasn't been pulled up short by the odd and seemingly random attacks of memory loss that first appeared in the late forties: "Where did I put my keys? What is that person's name? When did I present that report? What did I have for lunch yesterday? Why did I come into this room?"

At first these memory lapses simply generate jokes of "half-heimer's" or "sometime-er's," but soon the doubts creep in: "Are these the first signs of Alzheimer's?"

That's a tough one to answer, primarily because there are still so many unknowns about the disease.

What science does know is that Alzheimer's is a progressive degeneration of the brain's nerve cells, which leads to a loss of mental functioning that is usually accompanied by emotional instability and changes in personality.

Impairment of at Least Three of These Might Spell Alzheimer's Disease

- Language

- Memory

- Visual-spatial skills

- Emotions

- Personality

- Cognition (abstraction, calculation, judgment, or decision making)

Also called pre-senile dementia, Alzheimer's is a common disorder that affects men and women equally. The onset of Alzheimer's is slow and insidious, and, as such, it's difficult to put a finger on when it begins. Early symptoms include getting lost while traveling a familiar route and loss of ability to deal with family finances.

Memory lapses and changes in behavior can be followed by symptoms such as confusion, restlessness, and an inability to plan and carry out activities. Sometimes hallucinations and loss of bladder control are also present.

Known as a disease of the "elderly," it affects more than four million Americans. If you're over sixty-five, you have a one in ten chance of suffering from Alzheimer's, while if you're over eighty-five you have nearly a one in two chance; the mean age of onset being sixty-nine to seventy-one years old. While a full-blown case of Alzheimer's is rare in our age group, the early symptoms—memory lapses and changes in behavior—can be present in fifties men. The cause is unknown, but scientific research is closing in. Genetics seem to play a large role, because those with a family connection are more likely to suffer from it.

Medical evaluation of suspected Alzheimer's includes a review of the patient's general medical condition. Specific items that are checked include:

• Functions of the kidneys, liver, and thyroid.

• Possible deficiencies in vitamins (B12 and thiamine).

• The presence of HIV, syphilis, and tumors.

• Cerebral circulation.

• Abuse of drugs and alcohol.

Treatment/Prevention. There is no cure for Alzheimer's disease. Treatment with any of several drugs now available may slow progression of the disease and help maintain function, so early diagnosis is important. While positive identification of Alzheimer's used to be done only by examination of the brain after death, there is now a genetic test that can show a person's statistical likelihood of getting the disease in later life, but individual cases cannot be predicted.

Changing Patterns

Hair

Dreadlocks, ringlets, golden locks. Straight, wavy, curly. Red, blond, brown, black. Pubic hair, beard hair, nose hair. Samson's hair, Methuselah's hair, Don King's hair.

The diversity and range of hair within the human race—and on the human body—is simply staggering. Comprised mainly of a tough kind of protein called keratin, hair grows out of tubular hair follicles (pouchlike cavities) in the skin.

Little-Known Facts about Hair

• The number of hair follicles is set at birth, and no new ones are formed later on.

• The root of a hair is the only part that's actually alive, and as it grows it pushes the dead hair shaft out of the skin.

• Each hair follicle has a tiny strip of muscle attached. When these muscles contract, they produce the "goose flesh" effect.

• After the age of forty, hormonal changes in men increase hair production in all the wrong places—most notably the nose and ears.

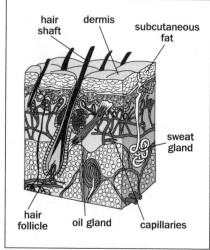

Hair serves important purposes, from insulation and heat retention for the top of your head, to corralling dirt, dust, and microbes so they don't get in your eyes, ears, and nose. For many people, hair (particularly scalp hair) also adds an important element to sexual attractiveness.

Three Basic Types of Hair

• **Scalp hair.** Similar to the body hair found on other mammals.

• **Human body hair.** Very fine, with little color.

• **Sexual hair.** Grows in the armpits, around the genitals, and, in men, on the face.

As most of us have figured out by now, hair can be found all over the human body, except on the palms, soles of the feet, lips, and a few other small areas. Hair goes through growth-rest cycles, which are different depending upon the type of hair and where it's located on the body.

Mental State and Changing Patterns

SCALP HAIR

Rightly or wrongly, after the penis, scalp hair is probably the likeliest body part to be tied to a man's feeling of masculinity. It also plays a huge role in how we perceive our attractiveness to others. Few men are really neutral on the subject—if they are, they're either comfortable with their baldness or still have a full head of hair.

While the number of hairs we have is very individual, most men start out with about 100,000 on their heads. For an average adult male scalp, the growth phase is about three years, with a rest period of approximately three months. On an average day, we lose about thirty to 100 scalp hairs, depending upon a tremendous number of factors. We only start noticing hair loss when it reaches about 200 per day.

Gray hair—something most of us have already begun to face—is caused when pigment production within each hair slows down. A gray hair contains little pigment, while a white hair contains no pigment at all. The term "premature graying" is somewhat misleading, because pigment production is based on genetics. The guy who starts turning gray in his twenties isn't doing it prematurely, it's part of his natural cycle (although he may not see it that way). Contrary to popular mythology, stress, tension, or fright cannot turn hair gray or white overnight, or even in the course of a few weeks.

Hair loss is another matter. It can happen quickly or over an extended period of time. Both men and women are constantly losing scalp hair, which is then usually replaced by more of the same. When the replacement hair is fine and downy, though, you know that balding is not far off. About 5 percent of men start losing their hair in their twenties. The rest of us usually have to wait a few more years or decades to see if we'll do the same. By seventy, approximately 80 percent of men are at least partially bald. Those who start losing their hair early are more prone to severe baldness than those who begin losing hair in later years. More than thirty-three million American men have experienced some form of hair loss.

The common myths that wearing a hat or washing your hair frequently will promote hair loss are simply not true.

Possible Reasons for Hair Loss

- **Skin problems.** Allergies, fungal infections, and skin diseases such as dermatitis and psoriasis can cause temporary hair loss, while burns or cuts to the scalp can destroy the hair follicles for good in the areas involved.

- **General ailments.** Diseases such as anemia and thyroid disorders can cause temporary hair loss.

- **Radiation and drug reactions.** Some forms of radiation and chemotherapy to treat various kinds of cancer can cause hair loss, usually temporarily.

- **Stress.** Because hair growth is linked to hormones, and hormone production can be affected by mental or emotional stress, your state of mind can cause hair loss. The good news: Once the stress is gone, the hair usually grows back. This type of hair loss, called telogen effluvium, is usually temporary.

- **Male-pattern baldness.** This accounts for 95 percent of hair loss in fifties males. Caused by male hormone levels in the skin that are influenced by hereditary aging factors, this condition cannot be reversed, stopped, or even retarded—other than by castration (a "stiff" price to pay for a head of hair).

A theory still being investigated is whether baldness in men is a sign of an increased risk of heart disease. This is because testosterone, the cause of much of what we perceive as "maleness," is also responsible for both male pattern baldness and a male's increased susceptibility to heart disease.

Treatment/Prevention. When it comes to the graying of your hair, once pigment production stops, there's no way to get it going again—hence the large number of hair-color options on the market today.

Baldness has its fair share of "remedies" as well. Your regular doctor can help you determine what the best option is and how to proceed.

Combating Baldness

A hairpiece. The good ones can hardly be detected; the bad ones look ridiculous. If you're contemplating a hairpiece, need we say more?

Drugs. Most men have heard or seen the ads for Rogaine, the brand name for the drug minoxidil, which comes in a lotion that you apply to the scalp daily. It has been shown to be effective in restoring thinning hair, especially in mild cases of baldness and in those who have just begun to lose hair. The downside is that if you stop using it, the hair will begin to thin again. An oral prescription drug, Propecia, does stop hair loss and can generate some regrowth, but only while it's being taken. Downsides of Propecia include diminished sex drive and difficulty achieving an erection—serious trade-offs. Neither drug works on completely bald spots, and not all users see good results.

A hair transplant. In this procedure, hair is taken from elsewhere on the scalp, usually the side of the head, and implanted into the bald areas. Besides the obvious downside that the procedure is rather painful, it is also expensive and baldness may recur.

Hair weaving. There are two different methods of hair weaving, which is also called hair linking, hair extension, and hair replacement. In both methods the living hair that surrounds the bald spot is woven into tight lines used as anchors. One method is to take a hairpiece and stitch it to the surrounding hair. The other is to string threads across the bald spot and then weave lumps of hair to the threads. Downsides to both options include difficulty in cleaning and combing the covered area, and having to be refitted every six to eight weeks.

Acceptance. For many, simply becoming comfortable with a "new" (albeit less hairy) visual image works. Take Sean Connery: His balding look certainly hasn't detracted from his sex appeal—that's because he doesn't allow it to. Other notables are Michael Jordan, Patrick Stewart, and even . . . Gordon Ehlers!

Remember, too, that trying to comb over a bald spot never fools anyone and looks a lot worse than what you can see in the mirror. Consider keeping your hair short, which gives a denser look to what you have. Some even take it a step further and shave off whatever's left in a "bald is beautiful" statement. A good hair stylist can help you find the best way to deal with your hair situation. Lastly, it should be noted that many women say that lack of scalp hair does not detract from a man's attractiveness—believe them.

Vision

Many of us, while traversing our forties, played the "trombone blues" with reading material as we struggled to find the best distance for our failing eyesight. Now, we have no doubt begrudgingly accepted some form of aid—whether it be simple reading glasses, bifocals, trifocals, contacts, or corrective surgery—while still not totally understanding what's happening.

When it comes to the eye, approximately 50 percent of the world's population has vision problems.

The Three Basic Types of Vision Problems

Nearsightedness, or myopia, means that you can see near but not far, due to an elongation of the eye ball or an error in refraction causing the image to focus in front of the retina, not on it. Age comes into play because the eye's lens become less flexible and the eye's muscles can no longer shape it into an efficient magnifier. Correction is by concave lenses.

Farsightedness, or hyperopia, is where you can see far but not near, due to an error in refraction where the image comes to focus behind the retina rather than on it. Correction is by convex lenses.

Astigmatism is a defect in vision in which the image is distorted because of an irregularity in the cornea. It is corrected by specially ground lenses or contact lenses.

For centuries the only correction for these three problems was glasses. Then contact lenses were developed, with improvements in convenience and appearance. For the past twenty years, a growing business has developed around corrective eye surgery.

Four Corrective Eye Surgeries

RK (radial keratotomy). This first of the corrective surgeries became available in America in 1978. A surgeon uses a scalpel to make six to eight radial slits in the cornea, like the spokes of a wheel. Too many complications made this a less than 100 percent successful procedure.

PRK (photorefractive keratectomy). Superseding RK, PRK is a scraping away of the outer surface of the cornea so that an ultraviolet beam can reshape the underlying corneal tissue. Reportedly, about 98 percent of people end up with 20/40 vision unaided—they can legally drive a car without glasses, and many obtain 20/20 perfect vision. A potential problem with PRK is that the scraping may cause scar formation and hazy vision later on.

LASIK (laser in situ keratomileusis). While PRK is still being performed, an advancement in the concept is LASIK. A hinged flap is cut into the cornea with a motorized blade, then the flap is lifted so a laser can reshape the cornea. The flap is then returned to its normal position. As with PRK, 98 percent of patients end up with at least 20/40 vision, while 80 percent or more have 20/20 vision. Complications are rare but do occur if the flap does not fall back into place properly.

Intacs. Two tiny, transparent polymer rings about the thickness of a contact lens are implanted around the edge of the cornea. They reshape the cornea without destroying any tissue and can be removed if necessary.

These corrective surgeries can be done on anyone from eighteen on up, as long as the patient is in good health. Anyone over forty might still need glasses for reading, and the cornea will still continue to age and change, so that more corrective surgery might be necessary years down the line.

Other than correcting for vision problems, we don't usually do much for our eyes, except use the occasional eye drops. While it's true that our eyes are normally low maintenance, eyestrain is one problem many of us face on a day-to-day basis. Eyestrain does not damage the eyesight, but because of our tendency to squint to clarify the image, fatigue and headaches are common.

While your eyes don't usually give you much trouble, that doesn't mean problems can't arise. There are three ailments in particular that you should be aware of: conjunctivitis, cataracts, and glaucoma.

CONJUNCTIVITIS (PINK EYE)

This is an inflammation of the membrane lining of the eyelids and front of the eye. Symptoms include pink-or red-looking eyes, eyelids stuck together in the morning, and a feeling of discomfort that is not pain. It can be caused by bacterial or viral infection, allergies or a simple irritant, and is common in children and their caregivers.

Treatment/Prevention. Treatment depends on the cause but usually involves antibiotic eye drops when the cause is bacterial. Prevention involves careful hand washing and attention to hygiene.

CATARACTS

The normally clear lens of the eye slowly becomes white and cloudy, so that light can't reach the retina, and vision progressively diminishes. It can happen in one eye or both, and the cause is usually degenerative changes that start taking place after fifty years old. Symptoms include cloudy vision, change in color vision, and increasing shortsightedness, but not blindness.

Treatment/Prevention. Treatment is surgical removal of the lens, with surgical placement of an intraocular lens chosen to restore sight to as close to normal as possible. Many people find that after cataract surgery, their vision is better than it's been in years.

GLAUCOMA

Fluid pressure builds up in the outer chamber of the eye, causes damage to the optic nerve, and can result in blindness. Most often it's due to a blockage in the channels that drain the eye of excess fluid. The condition is hereditary and usually attacks people fifty and older. Symptoms come on gradually and include loss of peripheral vision over a period of years that may be so insidious and free of other symptoms that considerable vision can be lost before it's noticed.

Treatment/Prevention. Treatment is with special eye drops. An acute or sudden form of glaucoma will cause symptoms such as a dull ache in or around the eye, reddening of the eye, foggy vision, and repeatedly seeing blue, green, orange, yellow, and red concentric circles around lights. These symptoms should be checked out by an ophthalmologist immediately. Starting at age forty, everyone should have their eye pressure checked yearly. An operation, called a trabeculectomy, is sometimes necessary to restore normal intraocular pressure (IOP).

Hearing and Balance

Back in those loud and heady rock-concert days of the sixties and seventies, we could not have cared less about our ears. When listening to music, the name of the game was: "Crank it up!"

Now, as we settle into mid-life, many of us have come to enjoy quieter pursuits—such as actual conversation and music played at decibel levels lower than those of a jet engine taking off; although the occasional oldies tune on the car radio does demand a nostalgic cranking up of the volume.

Unfortunately, some of us may have begun noticing that our hearing isn't as good as it used to be. We might not be able to hear as clearly or distinctly or be able to hear some of the tones at the high or low range of human hearing. Part of that has to do with age and/or maleness. Hearing does decline gradually with age, starting in the thirties and usually becoming noticeable or significant in the sixties or seventies. Men seem to experience hearing loss nearly twice as fast as women—although some of us might be suffering from the less serious "male pattern deafness" (domestic hearing loss associated with choosing what to hear and not hear from your partner).

But hearing loss can also be due to how much audio intensity we put our ears through in our younger years—or even today. Damage is cumulative and can end up causing significant hearing problems. Loud music, motorcycles, firearms, power tools, and snowmobiles are among the pastimes and toys that can be associated with nerve-damage hearing loss.

Biology is a good starting point for understanding.

The Ear's Three Basic Parts

The outer ear—consists of the cartilage on the outside of our head that we call our ears, and the ear canal, which gathers and funnels sound toward the eardrum.

Mental State and Changing Patterns

The middle ear—includes the eardrum, a thin membrane that vibrates to any sound; three delicate bones, commonly called the hammer, anvil, and stirrup that pass along the sound; and the eustachian tube that connects to the throat and keeps the air pressure in the middle ear equal to outside pressure. The middle ear is responsible for transferring sound from the outside air to the nerve receptors of the inner ear.

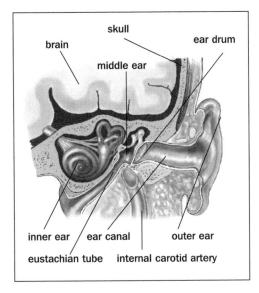

The inner ear—includes the cochlea, a snail-shaped structure filled with fluid and the organ that allows us to keep our balance. The inner ear transfers the sound from the middle ear to nerve cells that transmit the message to the brain, in addition to maintaining the mechanics of our balance.

Potential ear problems include earaches, muffled hearing, and a feeling of pressure building up in the ear. These symptoms are usually due to infection of the middle ear or the outer ear canal, or to an imbalance of air pressure on the inside of the eardrum due to swelling or congestion of the eustachian tube. An inner-ear infection, which is more serious, but less common, can cause dizziness and lack of balance. Normally, fifties males don't get many inner- or middle-ear infections, but they can get outer-ear infections.

Significant hearing loss and deafness may begin in our age group, but usually it's a problem faced more by people in their seventies and eighties. Hearing difficulties are growing less problematic, however, with scientific advances now being made in hearing aids. The days when hearing aids magnified all sounds, hindering rather than helping many users, are long gone. Today, sophisticated technology gives hearing aids the ability to enhance certain tones while leaving background static or noise unenhanced.

While the technology has improved, people's personal acceptance of hearing aids hasn't changed much—many people in their fifties or sixties who truly could benefit from hearing aids won't use them for a variety of reasons that can include vanity and the nuisance factor of not wanting to adjust to something new. One important point to consider: It's an established fact that the younger you are, the easier it is to adjust to something new. In this case, it's better to bite the bullet now and adjust to a hearing aid than to put it off for years and then really struggle with the adjustment when you're older.

All together, the ear is an incredibly delicate and sophisticated device. As such, it deserves a great deal of our respect and a little bit of our time. Until you're in your sixties, there is no need for an ear examination (audiogram) unless you're experiencing hearing problems. But in the meantime, your regular doctor will periodically examine your ear canals and eardrums.

What You Can Do for Your Ears

Carefully clean your ear and ear canal. Let ear wax (cerumen) do its job, which is to protect the ear canal and ear drum from microbes that might cause infections. If left alone, ear wax normally migrates to the outer portion of the canal, so you only need to clean the outer portion. Don't use cotton swabs or other pointed objects to reach into the canal, as there's a chance you could harm the ear drum. Once you know your ear is clear of major ear wax, you can periodically fill a dropper with rubbing alcohol and gently squeeze it into your ear to dissolve wax as it forms.

Practice pressurizing. Clamp your nose closed and *lightly* blow so that you pressurize your ears, then immediately swallow or move your jaw around to release the air pressure. This is what happens when changing altitudes, such as in an airplane. Doing this several times daily will help keep your eustachian tube open and clear. Do not do this if you have sinus problems, because you might make your condition worse.

Avoid headphones. Our ears weren't built for the intensity of focused loud noise conveyed by headphones. If you do use a Walkman or similar device, keep the level down and give your ears periodic breaks from the intensity.

Use ear protection around sustained, loud noises. Whether it be weekend warriors using loud equipment like chain saws, or full-time employees exposed to industrial-level noises, using good ear protection (ear plugs and/or headphones) is a must.

OUTER- AND MIDDLE-EAR INFECTIONS

Outer-ear infections are often called swimmer's ear. They can be painful and are usually caused by a build-up of moisture in the ear canal, which can foster bacterial or fungal growth.

Mental State and Changing Patterns

Middle-ear infections often accompany a cold and are due to fluid being trapped in the middle ear by swelling of the eustachian tube, the only conduit from the middle ear to the outside world. Bacterial infection may follow, but it's more common in children than adults.

Treatment/Prevention. Normally, swimmer's ear can be treated with antifungal ear drops or prescription antibiotics. Over-the-counter ear drops help prevent infection by cleaning the ear and evaporating trapped water from the ear canal.

Middle-ear infections can be cured with antibiotics.

TINNITUS

A more serious ear ailment is tinnitus, or ringing in the ears. Usually due to noise-related nerve damage, it doesn't cause hearing loss but can accompany it. Less commonly, tinnitus can be caused by certain drugs, including prolonged use of high doses of aspirin.

Treatment/Prevention. Depending upon the severity, tinnitus can be helped with a masking device (a so-called sound soother) when trying to sleep. But for many people treatment is learning to live with the background noise.

MÉNIÈRE'S DISEASE

This is a relatively rare ailment, but it does affect more men than women, and it does strike in middle age. A disease of the inner ear, its symptoms can include recurring attacks of dizziness, progressive hearing loss, tinnitus, nausea, and vomiting. The cause is unknown, but appears to be related to overproduction of fluid in the inner ear.

Treatment/Prevention. Using drugs, most notably OTC antihistamines and prescription diuretics, and control of the intake of liquids is the normal treatment. Surgery is occasionally necessary.

Headaches

We've all suffered through them; we all hate them. The pain can be dull and throbbing, pointed and sharp, in back or in front, one-sided or both-sided. Headaches can be like a discordant background note that you've come to ignore or like a full symphony that demands your complete attention. Headaches can also be lone warriors, or part of an army that includes numerous other symptoms besides pain.

The good news is that by the time we've reached our fifties, we've probably sorted out the kinds that we're prone to get and learned to avoid them, or at least learned to lessen their impact. Additionally, people actually outgrow one particularly nasty type of headache, the migraine.

MUSCULAR CONTRACTION (TENSION) HEADACHES

By far the commonest form, tension headaches come from the contracting of the muscles at the back of the neck and skull, the side of the skull, and/or the jaw. This tightening of your muscles is usually caused by stress and/or poor posture, such as hunching over a computer keyboard or sitting incorrectly while driving a car. As your muscles begin to rebel against what you're making them do, the pain begins to spread from the muscles until it covers part, or all, of the head. A classic tension headache starts at the back of the head and works its way forward.

With a tension headache there are no neurological changes (your brain activity doesn't change), no changes in vision, no feeling of nausea or vomiting—just a dull and throbbing pain. This kind of headache is not present when you wake up, but may show up as your day gets going and can reoccur on a nearly daily basis—as long as the stress and/or poor posture remain in place.

Treatment/Prevention. Treatments include taking OTC anti-inflammatories, using heat or ice on the affected areas (most notably the back of the neck and/or the forehead—see the heat and ice sidebar in chapter 2), stretching the neck and/or upper back/shoulder muscles, and taking a break from the behavior that has caused the muscle contractions. All these can also help prevent such headaches.

SINUS HEADACHES

As the name implies, these headaches are brought on by stuffed up or clogged sinuses or nasal passages, which create pressure in the delicate airways. The pressure inside your sinuses is what causes the pain, which turns into a sinus headache. Because the labyrinth of nasal sinuses is in your face, the pain is there as well—most notably right above your eyebrows and stretching out under your eyes and across your cheeks. If the pain is on both sides of your face, it's usually just a sinus headache, while if the pain is on one side only, it may be a sinus infection (see chapter 3 for sinus infection details). The causes of sinus headaches include allergies (seasonal and chronic) and/or air pollutants such as dust and smoke. Even a change in the weather can bring on sinus headaches. Besides pain, sinus headaches are usually accompanied by general nasal congestion and a running nose.

Treatment/Prevention. The standard course of treatment is to take antihistamines to stop or retard the allergic reaction that has caused the sinus headache. Over-the-counter antihistamines are usually able to treat mild allergic reactions,

Mental State and Changing Patterns

while prescription antihistamines are normally needed to handle severe or long-term allergies (see chapter 3's drug chart for details). These treatments also work for prevention. Topical prescription nasal sprays help, too.

MIGRAINE HEADACHES

Anyone who has experienced a migraine knows that these can be "monsters." Many times there are warning signs—a pre-headache "aura," consisting of a temporary irregular blind spot or other visual change, and sometimes numbness or tingling—that will last twenty to thirty minutes before the full migraine shows up. When a migraine hits, most people can't function due to the pain. If left untreated, a migraine can cause nausea and vomiting, and an aversion to light. Migraines can be triggered by stress and certain foods and beverages, such as cheese, chocolate, and alcohol. These headaches tend to run in families, are more prevalent in women than men, and can happen two or three times a week, month, or year, but never daily.

The good news is that most people actually grow out of migraines, so there's a good chance that if you had them in your younger years, you will be free of them in your fifties. And there's an even bigger chance that if you've never experienced a migraine by the time you've reached fifty, you'll never experience one.

Treatment/Prevention. Effective treatment does exist and includes the prescription "tryptan" drugs (such as Imitrex), that have revolutionized migraine treatment. For frequent migraines, preventive drugs are also available.

SEXUAL HEADACHES

Relatively rare, this is a kind of headache that comes on as you engage in sexual intercourse. While understandably an alarming event—especially because it's happening during an activity that's usually so pleasurable—a sexual headache is seldom serious, but it does warrant a trip to a doctor. The headache is normally a vascular phenomenon that is probably a variant of a migraine headache.

Treatment/Prevention. These are unusual and fleeting enough that treatment and prevention are seldom issues.

CLUSTER HEADACHES

The name refers to the frequency, rather than how the pain is. Usually cluster headaches will occur in bunches for two or three weeks and then be gone. Cluster headaches are almost exclusively the property of men; women rarely get them. A cluster headache will wake you up from a dead sleep and last one to two hours, but then is gone, and the sufferer feels fine. The pain is one-sided and extremely intense—so much so that cluster headaches are sometime referred to as "suicide headaches." The cause is, as yet, unknown, although another name for cluster headaches, "histamine headaches," indicates that many scientists think they may be related to allergic reactions. Others believe they are a variant of migraine headaches.

Treatment/Prevention. The "clusters" can often be "aborted" by breathing pure oxygen or taking prednisone (a corticosteroid drug).

STROKE HEADACHES

The name gives insight into what this headache is all about. A stroke occurs when bleeding happens in the brain. A stroke headache strikes when bleeding that is too small to cause a full-blown stroke occurs in the brain. Understandably, a stroke headache can actually be a warning sign that a severe, disabling stroke is not far away.

How does a stroke headache feel?

Medical students are taught that when a patient describes a headache as "the worst headache I've ever had" they should investigate the possibility that it's a stroke headache. The headache's pain is unbelievably intense and can last for several hours, then go away.

Treatment/Prevention. Prompt medical evaluation is essential, because a stroke headache may be a precursor to a hemorrhagic stroke.

BRAIN-TUMOR HEADACHES

This one tends to be unlike any headache you've ever had before, encompassing the entire head and often waking you up in the middle of the night. Another sign is vomiting without the sensation of nausea. A headache caused by a brain tumor may also include changes in your vision and possibly a weakness on one side of your body. No traditional headache remedies will work on this kind of headache.

A recurring worry for physicians is "missing" the early symptoms of a brain tumor, such as headaches that are increasing in severity and frequency, and headaches that are accompanied by neurologic symptoms, such as decreased coordination, mood changes, and confusion.

Treatment/Prevention. If possible, surgical removal of the tumor is the best course of action. If that's not possible (because of size, location, or fear of resulting brain damage), then traditional cancer therapies (chemotherapy and radiation) are used. There is no prevention known for a brain tumor or the headache caused by one.

Mental State and Changing Patterns

Sleep

We all need it, but we're not exactly sure why.

Scientists do know that when teenagers go to sleep, growth hormones spurt through their bodies—causing all the usual havoc when the little darlings wake up the next morning. It's also been proved that during sleep, energy is conserved: Most cells do major housecleaning, from getting rid of waste products to repairing any damage done during the day, and muscles, tendons, ligaments, and joints get some much needed R&R.

But all of those jobs could be accomplished simply by lying down, without sleep being involved, so why is sleep so important?

Simply put, it's because our brains are involved: the conscious and subconscious minds; the id and ego, super ego; dreams; and maintenance tasks such as repressing urges, reprogramming needs, and reducing memory overload. Scientists believe that all these diverse concepts are somehow served while we sleep. Suffice it to say that when you sleep, you not only recharge and rejuvenate your physical body, but somehow—in ways still being researched—you recharge and rejuvenate your psychological self.

While we might not know exactly why we sleep, we certainly know what happens when we don't get enough of it. Initially, we simply feel sleepy. The more sleep you lose, or don't get, the more your body craves, so you feel sleepy most of the day. If your sleep problems persist for any more than a week or so, you could move on to more serious symptoms.

Symptoms of Sleep Loss

- Reduction in overall thinking ability and performance

- General nervousness and irritability

- Fatigue and nearly constant grogginess

- Difficulty concentrating and making decisions

- Weakening of the immune system

- Loss of creativity

- Memory lapses

• Mood swings

• Even, in severe cases, hallucinations (sometimes seen in severely ill patients whose sleep has been impaired by a prolonged stay in an intensive care unit.)

What's an Adequate Amount of Sleep?

That differs with every person, but generally speaking, we should get between six and nine hours of sleep a night. That means we spend approximately one-third of our lives asleep—more than 172,000 hours sleeping by the time we reach the age of fifty-nine.

While it has been reported that a human body will die after about ten days without any sleep, it's doubtful that this has ever been self-imposed—at some point, no amount of personal willpower can keep a human awake.

This fail-safe mechanism means that if you are having difficulty sleeping, you should take heart, your body is ultimately going to force you to sleep. The psychological aspect of this point is important, because often those who are having trouble sleeping compound the problem by questioning their very ability to ever sleep normally again. If you tell yourself (and believe) that there is a point at which you will achieve sleep, then at least that particular psychological barrier will have been hurdled.

It's a barrier that many of us must face. The National Commission on Sleep Disorders and Research says that one in three Americans don't get enough sleep, while more than forty million people are plagued with chronic sleep disorders.

What are we all trying to achieve?

Sleep is a reduced state of consciousness in which the brain is still alert to certain aspects of its surroundings, such as noise and light, but the body's metabolism slows significantly. We all have a "biological clock," called the circadian rhythm, which controls the sleep-wake cycle in a person's twenty-four-hour day (that's what gets off kilter when we get jet lag).

The Two Phases of Sleep

1. **Nonrapid eye movement sleep (NREM).** Representing about 75 percent of our total sleep, NREM, or slow-wave sleep, occurs when our brain waves slow in frequency, there is little eye movement, and no dreams occur. This is the deepest, most restorative part of sleep, because the body and brain are at their most inactive.

2. **Rapid eye movement (REM) sleep.** In this phase of light sleep, our brain waves are similar to those when we're awake: We have rapid eye movements,

we dream, get erections (sometimes producing those nocturnal emissions called "wet dreams"), and our heartbeat, blood pressure, and breathing go through irregular changes.

Normally, we sleep in ninety-minute cycles. We start by taking thirty to forty-five minutes to get to the deep, NREM sleep, then the process reverses and it takes thirty to forty-five minutes to return to light, REM sleep. In the course of a regular seven or eight hours' sleep, we follow a cycle of thirty to ninety minutes of NREM sleep followed by ten to fifteen minutes of REM. Through the course of an eight-hour night, as we go through five or six ninety-minute sleep cycles, most of us wake up for a brief moment—usually just after the third hour of sleep and just before the sixth hour of sleep—but we normally aren't conscious of it. Those who sleep less than eight hours lose out on what some sleep researchers believe to be the most important sleep cycle: the one that happens between the seventh and eighth hours.

As we age, our sleep patterns change. One reason for this is melatonin, a sleep-inducing hormone secreted by the pineal gland (in the brain) that helps to control the circadian rhythm. The highest levels of melatonin are found in five- or six-year-olds who get the deep, rejuvenating kind of sleep many of us fifties males long for. Levels begin to decrease in the teenage years and are quite diminished by the time we're in our seventies or eighties.

Besides melatonin, there are other chemicals that are produced by the nervous system and help maintain our sleep-wake cycles.

Body Produced Sleep/Wake Chemicals

Cortisol, or hydrocortisone. As this decreases in your system, your body temperature falls and your mind becomes less alert, ready for sleep. The highest level usually occurs around 6 A.M., and by midnight it's fallen to much lower levels.

Serotonin. Also affecting body temperature, serotonin seems to control states of consciousness and mood.

Epinephrine, norepinephrine, and dopamine. All help keep you awake, especially during times of stress or emergency. This means that if you're lying in bed stressed out over some personal or business situation, you could be producing one of these "wake up" hormones at just the wrong time.

What should you expect, when it comes to sleep?

Remembering that our sleep requirements are individual, generally speaking, in our thirties, with melatonin already declining in our bodies, our sleep will have naturally become lighter, with much less NREM sleep than younger people experience. Because REM sleep picks up the slack, though, by the time we're in our fifties, we should still be getting seven to nine hours of sleep a night. Unfortunately, most adults actually report that they get less than seven hours. It's a situation we should all try to rectify.

INSOMNIA

There are a tremendous number of sleep disorders, including snoring and sleep apnea (see the following section for details). Most of them—especially those faced by men in their fifties—can be considered to be varying degrees of insomnia. The condition usually falls into three general categories: difficulty in falling asleep, dif-

YOU'RE NOT IN COLLEGE ANYMORE
DETERMINING YOUR SLEEP NEEDS

Two things can help you determine how much sleep you need and when you should be going to bed: (1) How you feel in the early afternoon; and (2) an alarm clock.

1. It is natural and normal to get a *slight* drop in energy and a slight feeling of tiredness sometime between one and three in the afternoon—especially after that heavy business lunch. But this should be easy to shake off without stimulants like coffee, and your normal amount of alertness and focus should return for the rest of the afternoon and into the evening.

2. In a perfect world your body should not need an alarm clock to wake up.

Combine these two concepts and you have a way of determining your sleep needs. If the alarm clock is waking you from a deep sleep, and you're overly tired in the early afternoon, and you can't shake that midday fatigue, then you need to adjust your schedule to create a better sleep pattern. Working in fifteen- or twenty-minute increments, start by giving yourself one more increment of sleep. Try it for a week or so. If this doesn't create the desired results, add another increment and then another until you find the optimum amount of sleep you need.

Once you determine that, you can easily figure out when you need to go to bed to obtain that amount of sleep—and still get to work on time.

Mental State and Changing Patterns

ficulty in staying asleep, or awaking too early (terminal sleep disorder) or experiencing seriously interrupted sleep, such as frequent short awakenings. Insomnia has numerous potential causes:

Possible Physiologically Based Causes of Insomnia

- Heart disease, kidney disease, arthritis, and/or urinary problems

- Circadian rhythm (internal time-clock) disorders

- Allergies

- Pain

- Abuse of alcohol, caffeine, or other substances

- Poor sleeping environment

- Jet lag

Possible Psychologically Based Causes of Insomnia

- Anxiety

- Stress

- Depression

While symptoms of sleep disorders can be obvious and pronounced (see the list in the previous section), sometimes the problem is chronic: It's been around so long that the sufferer doesn't even realize he has a form of insomnia. In fact, at one time or another, we have all faced a temporary lack of sleep or a problem sleeping. Beyond this, however, many people face a continual lack of sleep, or chronic sleep deprivation, that isn't deadly but certainly holds us back from functioning at peak levels.

A typical sleep routine that many of us follow is to get about one less hour of sleep per week night than we really need ("I have no choice, I need to get to work early"). Then we try to play catch up on the weekend by sleeping in as late as possible. This is definitely not a healthy approach to good sleep management. It simply perpetuates the problem, because prolonged sleep can actually lead to insomnia. And even if you do catch up on the weekend, you'll be losing sleep again during the weekdays if you don't change your schedule. Taking a realistic look at your sleep schedule and rearranging it to get better, longer amounts of sleep every night will ultimately pay handsome dividends in overall health and fitness—both mental and physical.

Treatment/Prevention. There are numerous steps toward returning to good sleep patterns, but the problem has to first be identified and classified. A physician is in the best position to identify what the cause of the insomnia is and how best to treat it. Treatments range from self-help options, herbal aids, and over-the-counter sleep aids, to—in severe cases—prescription sleeping pills and possibly some form of psychotherapy to alleviate the psychologically based causes. Many cases of insomnia can be cured with small measures developed over time.

Self-Help Options for Better Sleep

Exercise regularly. Periodic exercise during the day or in the early evening promotes good, deep sleep. Don't do any heavy exercise within three hours of bedtime, or it will keep you up. Some slight stretching or a short, nonstrenuous walk just before bed works well to help relax you in preparation for sleep.

Take a fifteen- to thirty-minute power nap during the day, if needed. The stress here is on the "if needed." A short nap will not disrupt your usual sleep at night, but more than thirty minutes probably will.

Make your bedroom a bedroom. Don't use it for work, eating, or even watching TV. Make the room sleep-inducing—cozy, peaceful, and restful—and conducive to your other passion: sex.

Determine your environmental needs. Window open or closed? Turn the furnace down or up at bedtime? Lots of blankets or no blankets? A sound-soother machine or complete silence? If necessary, experiment until you find the best conditions for you and your partner.

Establish a routine. Set a sleep schedule that works not only for the weekday but the weekend as well, then stick to it. Normal, regular routines are great for promoting good sleep patterns.

Wait about three hours between eating dinner and going to bed. Trying to sleep on a full stomach is tough for fifties males and is unhealthy to boot. It can cause acid reflux (see chapter 4 for digestive details) and can promote weight gain.

Mental State and Changing Patterns

Eat carbohydrates for dinner. They give you a quick energy high, followed by a sense of sleepiness. (See chapter 8 for carbohydrate details.)

Stay away from caffeine at least five hours before bedtime. Sure, some people can drink a gallon of coffee at 10 P.M. and sleep like a baby, but most of us are affected by this stimulant.

Stay away from alcohol and cigarettes at least two hours before bedtime. Initially, alcohol, a depressant, does bring on sleep, but within a few hours the alcohol level drops, resulting in wakefulness—not to mention that it stimulates your need to get up and urinate. Nicotine also promotes alertness, something you don't want when you're trying to sleep.

Take a warm bath. It's soothing, relaxing, and sleep-inducing.

Watch your intake of fluids a few hours before bedtime. Sleep isn't helped by having to get up a few times during the night to urinate.

Try herbs. Some of them are thought to have a calming, relaxing effect that acts as a mild sedative to promote sleep. They include anise, chamomile, cumin, garlic, honey, sage, and valerian, to name a few.

Try melatonin. Because our body's supply of this sleep-inducing hormone steadily declines as we get older, a popular belief is that sleep is induced by complementing our natural level with an artificial dose of melatonin. While it is a somewhat controversial idea, because it hasn't been fully studied, it has seemed to work for many people.

If you can't sleep, don't stay in bed. Get up, go into another room, and read, watch TV, or do relaxation exercises until you feel tired.

When it comes to pharmaceuticals, there are numerous over-the-counter sleep aids as well as prescription sleeping pills. Approach all of them with a little caution. Most over-the-counter products contain antihistamines, which have a sedative side effect, but remember they may cause urinary hesitancy. Antihistamines are intended for short-term use as a way of re-establishing good sleep and should not be taken for more than two weeks at a time. Prolonged use may lead to a psychological feeling of dependence. Prescription sleeping pills are much stronger, because they work to suppress nerve-cell activity within the brain. They, too, should be used for short periods of time and only under a doctor's supervision.

If you still have trouble with sleep, go talk to a physician.

SNORING AND SLEEP APNEA

We've probably all snored at one time or another. When we do it for any length of time, we probably get a swift elbow jab in the ribs or a not-so-gentle shove from our sleepless partner. Snoring, of course, has been the bane of many a good man ever since the caveman days. And, yes, in this case it's true what most women say—more men snore than women (probably due to our physical differences in the mouth, nasal passages, and throat)— although few women seem willing to admit they're capable of such a thing.

Snoring can be an old joke in many families—"Uncle Eddie's snoring is as loud as a John Philip Sousa march!"—but it can also be serious enough to cause major health problems, not to mention relationship difficulties. In most cases, snoring is the symptom and the ailment rolled into one. In fewer cases, snoring is a symptom of the serious ailment named sleep apnea, a disorder characterized by loud snoring and periodic breaks in breathing that causes the sufferer to wake up repeatedly through a night.

By the time we men have reached our age group, there's nothing much to laugh about when it comes to snoring. And, unfortunately, it's quite probably a condition many of us have had to deal with already—the fifties are a prime time for snoring to develop into a real problem.

How Snoring Occurs

It has to do with our mouth, nasal passages, and throat. The walls and airways within these three areas are relatively small, delicate, and/or precise. If anything partially blocks or narrows them, then the air that's going back and forth through them has a greater force than in unblocked passages. Many times that forced air is strong enough to vibrate surrounding tissues, which is what creates the snoring sound. The tissues that can be vibrated include the soft palate (the fleshy upper back part of the roof of the mouth), the uvula (the little dangling thing at the back of the throat), the tonsils, the adenoids (lymphatic tissue near the tonsils), and even the tongue.

Contributing Factors to Snoring

Obesity. If you are more than 20 percent above your ideal weight, you have a significantly higher chance of snoring than those who aren't. This is because all the tissues involved have gained weight along with the rest of your body and can end up partially blocking or narrowing the airways—especially when you're sleeping on your back (see below).

Mental State and Changing Patterns

Age. The tissues involved can lose their muscle tone and firmness as we age. When they get soft or floppy enough they can narrow or block the airways. In this condition, they are more susceptible to being vibrated.

Nasal obstructions. Even simple congestion within the nasal passages can shrink air passages, resulting in snoring.

A deviated septum or other deformities. If the center portion of the nose is not properly aligned, it's called a deviated septum, a condition that affects the airways and can lead to snoring.

Alcohol, along with sleeping pills and any other kinds of sedatives. They loosen or relax the muscular support of the soft tissues, which can get in the way of proper airflow.

Sleeping on your back. This gives gravity a better chance to pull down the soft tissues of the mouth, throat, and nose so that they restrict the airways.

Sleep Apnea

The difference between simple snoring and sleep apnea is, to a certain extent, a matter of degree. In simple snoring, it's more likely that the partner will be losing sleep, not the snorer. In sleep apnea, it's the snorer who will also be sleep-deprived. Additionally, though, sleep apnea includes the periodic cessation of breathing—the sufferer actually stops breathing for a few seconds. When breathing stops, the body quickly responds and the sleeper wakes up. But these wake ups can be so slight that the suffer may not be aware of the sleep disruption, only of the sense of never feeling adequately rested. All of this means that the person never gets a proper amount of sleep. In fact, he never reaches the deep, restorative sleep that is necessary for everyone to function properly, and he ends up experiencing true sleep deprivation. This chronic fatigue can sometimes be coupled with falling asleep at inappropriate times during the day. Such sleep problems can lead to other serious medical problems.

Treatment/Prevention. Treatment for snoring varies depending upon the exact cause. Some general treatments include:

• Losing weight, which will also reduce the size of the soft tissues and very well might solve the problem.

• Keeping the nasal passages moisturized via a saline spray or plain water. Properly moisturized tissues (especially in dry climates) are less likely to cause problems.

- Using nasal strips—the kind used by athletes—that are placed on the outside of the nose to help keep internal passageways open. They seem to help, especially in the case of a deviated septum or nasal congestion.

- Utilizing one of numerous prescription or over-the-counter drugs used for nasal congestion (though decongestants may cause insomnia).

- Inhaling nasal steroids (cortisone) through a prescription nasal spray. Sometimes this is helpful and necessary for unblocking the nasal passageways.

For those sufferers who find no relief with any of those, there is a relatively new surgical procedure that is a major breakthrough in the treatment of snoring. Usually done as a day surgery, it is performed by an ear, nose, and throat specialist who "debulks," or removes, part of the soft palate to create more room for the air to move freely. A laser is used so the amount and depth of tissue removed is precisely controlled—don't worry, even if the doctor has a shaky hand you won't end up with a hole through your neck. A sad reality, though, is that in some extreme cases in which snoring is coupled with obesity, a hole in the neck (a permanent tracheotomy) to aid breathing may be precisely what's needed.

Treating sleep apnea often requires a first step of going through a sleep study, where all body functions are monitored while you sleep. This will prove that breathing is actually stopping periodically and can determine the degree of severity.

For extreme cases of proven sleep apnea there is a treatment that may seem radical to nonsufferers but has actually solved the problem for those with the ailment. Called CPAP (continuous positive airway pressure), it's a face mask that provides, usually through the nose, a steady stream of air that's sometimes mixed with oxygen. The airflow from the mask opens up the soft tissues and allows air to get through. Most people would find it hard to believe than anyone could sleep with a mask buckled to their head and a steady stream of air constantly blowing on their face. But for the truly sleep-deprived sleep-apnea sufferer, who probably hasn't had a good night's sleep in years, it can bring full and restorative sleep on the first use.

Prevention of snoring and, to a lesser degree, sleep apnea involves basic issues, such as losing weight, sleeping on your side, watching your consumption of alcohol and sedatives, and maintaining healthy nasal passages. One home remedy that appears to have some success is singing—fifteen minutes a day for at least two or three months. The underlying principle seems sound: Singing can exercise and firm up the soft tissues in the throat so that they aren't so likely to vibrate into snoring. As long as you have a good voice—or an understanding partner with a good set of ear plugs—it might be worth a shot.

KNOWING WHAT YOU PUT IN YOUR MOUTH— A DRUG CHART

NAME	EXPLANATION AND USE	POSSIBLE SIDE EFFECTS

Antidepressants
  Selective Serotonin Reuptake Inhibitors (SSRIs)
  Fluoxetine (Prozac)
  Sertraline (Zoloft)
  Paroxetine (Paxil)
  Citalopram (Celexa)
	This class of drugs replenishes a depleted neurochemical transmitter called serotonin, in the synapses between brain cells—a condition with several possible causes (heredity, adverse events, hormonal influences) and with a strong correlation with depression and other emotional disorders (certain anxiety states, eating disorders, obsessive compulsive disorders, and others).	Nausea, headache (both usually mild and transient); drowsiness; dry mouth; increased sweating; sexual dysfunction (decreased libido, slowing of arousal, delayed or absent orgasm).

Miscellanous Drugs
  Venlafaxine (Effexor)
  Nefazodone (Serzone)
  Buproprion (Wellbutrin)
	These drugs function much like the SSRIs in effectiveness, indicated medical uses, and side effects. They differ primarily in affecting neurotransmitters in addition to serotonin, which gives a slightly different profile of side effects, which can be useful. For example, Wellbutrin and Serzone seldom cause the sexual side effects seen with the SSRIs. Wellbutrin, under the name Zyban, has been shown to help people quit smoking. Both Serzone and Effexor are sometimes used for chronic pain states to decrease the perceived severity of pain. Both these drugs seem to be more effective for this use than the SSRIs.	See the SSRI drugs on prior page.

NAME	EXPLANATION AND USE	POSSIBLE SIDE EFFECTS
Tricyclic Antidepressants *Amitriptyline (Elavil)* *Nortriptyline (Pamelor)* *Imipramine (Tofranil)* *Desipramine (Norpramin)*	This class of drugs, available as our first generation of effective antidepressants, has largely been supplanted by the SSRIs and a mixed category of antidepressants—mainly because of excessive side effects at the doses required to treat depression. They are now mainly used to treat chronic pain (as companions to the pain killers, they decrease the perceived severity of the pain), headache (particularly migraine headaches) and are useful in treating insomnia because they are not habit forming.	Sedation, dry mouth, visual blurring, constipation, urinary hesitancy, increased sweating, lowered blood pressure, and many others.
Tranquilizers *Benzodiazepines (Valium-like)* *Diazepam (Valium)* *Chlordiazepoxide (Librium)* *Clorazepate (Tranxene)* *Lorazepam (Ativan)* *Alprazolam (Xanax)* *Clonazepam (Klonopin)*	This class of drugs is the first of the so-called "safe" anti-anxiety drugs (relatively nonlethal in an overdose). Unfortunately, their usefulness is severely limited by their addiction potential. They are relatively safe and effective for occasional anxiety and periodic sleep disturbances, as well as for specialized medical uses (as adjuncts to anaesthesia, sedation in an intensive-care setting, muscle relaxation, tremors, certain kinds of epilepsy), but they're not especially useful for healthy fifties males.	Sedation, addictive potential.

THE GOOD NEWS

- Most of us reach our fifties without being struck by cancer, an on-coming train, or some life-threatening or life-changing disease.

- Your overall energy level and basic attitude toward life should not change drastically as you travel through your fifties—in fact, many report a kind of "second wind" that re-energizes them both physically and mentally.

- Stress, depression, and insomnia are very treatable ailments.

- Science and technology have teamed up like never before to help people with poor vision and/or poor hearing to restore both to near-perfect functioning.

7: CANCER

Standing Up to the Big "C" Fear

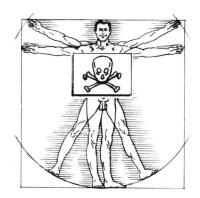

BACKGROUND BASICS

Like the long-ago playground bully we were afraid to face, cancer has an irrational hold on our minds. Just saying the word out loud brings a chill to many, as if stating the name will somehow conjure up the actual disease. Once cancer is confronted, though, its ability to frighten and intimidate disappears (like most playground bullies). In this case, the strength to confront cancer comes from knowledge—with the right information, we can:

• Put cancer in the proper perspective.

• Learn how to drastically cut our chances of contracting it.

• Free ourselves from needless worry.

The principles for all this are fairly straightforward: Certain environmental elements and lifestyle activities are known to increase the chances of contracting cancer, so staying away from them markedly decreases your chances of getting cancer.

The guy who eats right, exercises properly, stays out of the sun, does not smoke, and does not have a family history that includes cancer has a relatively small chance of contracting most kinds of cancers. Conversely, the man who eats poorly, never exercises, sits in the sun unprotected, smokes, and does have cancer in his family history has a far greater chance of contracting various kinds of cancer.

Overall, it's critical to remember that you do have *significant* control over your degree of cancer risk—approximately 80 percent of today's cancer cases come from environmental or lifestyle factors that can be moderated, controlled, and/or avoided. And even if you do have an unavoidable risk factor—such as heredity—the National Cancer Institute reports that most people at risk because of family history don't even get the disease.

Why Are We So Worried?

What ratchets up cancer's fear factor is the rather dubious "shit happens" category. Like lightening striking on a cloudless, blue-sky day, shit happens is the random, somewhat mysterious development of cancer in someone who is doing everything right. For a doctor, there are few things worse than telling a person who has chosen and maintained a good, healthy lifestyle that he suddenly has cancer.

Many doctors believe that the greatest negative impact of these "shit happens" cases (besides the actual cancer they bring to individuals) is the havoc they wreak on the personal motivation of the healthy general public toward even basic preventive measures. A lot of fifties males tell themselves: "Why should I go for a checkup or spend any time and energy quitting smoking, eating right, and exercising if cancer might show up anyway?"

This Doris Day "whatever will be will be" attitude comes mainly from feeling helpless against "shit happens." On a personal level, this helpless feeling is understandable; on a medical level, it's definitely bogus.

We *do* have ways of combating random acts of cancer—they're called testing and screening. Through numerous procedures—usually unobtrusive and inexpensive—many common cancers can be detected *before* symptoms appear. In the majority of cancers, early detection is the key to cancer survival—if a cancer can be discovered before symptoms show up, there's a very good chance the patient will live to see old age.

In 2000 the American Cancer Society reported that the five-year relative survival rate for many cancers was about 80 percent. That, in itself, is quite a positive statistic. More importantly, though, the society also pointed out that if all Americans participated in regular cancer screenings, this rate could increase to 95 percent—a drastic improvement, and one that would have great significance to you if you were part of that added 15 percent.

Cancer

In ancient times, Egyptians blamed cancer on the gods and believed it was untreatable. Science now knows better. Isn't it about time we put aside our irrational fears and start taking some sound medical advice?

(The specific cancers outlined in this chapter are those that are either unique to men or are the most common ones that men—especially those in their fifties—might face. This chapter is not meant to be a complete guide to all possible cancers.)

What Is Cancer and How Does It Happen— Knowing the Enemy

Cancer is about good cells going bad.

Normally, the body's cells grow, divide, and then die in a nice, neat, orderly fashion. When you're young, this process is quite rapid so your body can grow and mature into adulthood. Once you're a man, though, the process begins to slow and normal cells of most tissues divide only to repair injuries or replace worn out or dying cells.

In the case of cancer, normal cells become abnormal when they continue to grow and divide uncontrollably, forming masses of abnormal tissue called tumors, or neoplasms.

Three Classes of Tumors

Benign (noncancerous), which do *not* spread to other parts of the body. Normally, they are not life-threatening, can usually be removed, and do not grow back.

Precancerous lesions, which have the potential of becoming malignant but don't necessarily. At this stage, they are simply fast-growing normal cells and can be a result of an injury or disease. They are usually free of symptoms.

Malignant (cancerous), which, left untreated, do spread to other parts of the body where they then affect normal functioning. These potential killers spread, or metastasize, either by invading adjacent tissues or by spreading to distant sites via the blood and/or the lymphatic system, which is part of the body's immune system.

The primary way of determining which kind of cell is within a tumor is to have a biopsy. This is where a small piece of the tumor is removed—either via a needle or surgery—and studied in the laboratory to see if it's benign, precancerous, or malignant. From that determination, the best, most effective treatment can be chosen.

Why Good Cells Suddenly Become Abnormal

With newly acquired knowledge about DNA, medical science now understands that normal cells become abnormal when their DNA is damaged by mutations (changes or mistakes in genetic structure). A huge step in our understanding of cancer came with the discovery that, while normal cells with damaged DNA simply die, cancer cells with damaged DNA do not. They go on to grow, divide, and spread to become full-blown cancer.

What damages a cell's DNA are various substances, known as carcinogens, which are considered to be cancer-causing agents.

Known Carcinogens and Other Cancer Risk Factors

Tobacco. As most of us now acknowledge, smoking causes lung cancer, which is responsible for nearly three times as many American deaths as its nearest cancer competitor. Additionally, smokeless tobacco can cause numerous other cancers, such as mouth and tongue cancer. Taken all together, tobacco use is linked to approximately one-third of all cancer deaths in the United States.

Sunlight. The most common cancer in America is skin cancer, with more than one million new cases reported each year. The primary cause is the sun—more specifically, ultraviolet (UV) radiation. How important is it to avoid the sun? The American Cancer Society has estimated that 90 percent of cases could have been prevented by avoiding the sun (either staying out of it or being protected from it).

Diet. According to the American Cancer Society, researchers believe that about one-third of cancer deaths in America are due to the adult diet, including its effect on obesity. Being more than 20 percent over your ideal body weight can increase your chances of cancer of the prostate, pancreas, and colon. Consistently eating high-fat, low-fiber foods can increase your risk of colon cancer. Some studies show that people who eat few fruits and vegetables have twice the rate of lung cancer.

Alcohol. Drinking more than a moderate amount of alcohol (two or less drinks a day) can lead to a greater risk of cancer of the mouth, throat, esophagus, and larynx. Additionally, mixing alcohol with tobacco is dangerous business: According to the American Cancer Society, tobacco and alcohol have a synergistic effect—when used together, they're more dangerous than each individually would be.

Radiation. X rays you get in the dentist office or at the doctor's do have their effect, albeit minuscule (about the same as taking a coast-to-coast commercial flight). Properly chosen diagnostic X rays cause no cancer risk, but survivors of cancer that have been successfully treated with radiation can be vulnerable to other radiation-induced cancers.

Chemicals and Other Substances. Products such as asbestos, benzene, benzidine, cadmium, nickel, radon, and uranium have been shown to be carcinogens, or cancer-causing agents.

Viruses. Certain cancers are related to viral infections, such as hepatitis B and C, and human immunodeficiency virus (HIV). Many cases could be prevented through behavioral changes, such as having safe sex and using clean needles. Although *H. pylori* (the cause of many ulcers) is a bacterium, not a virus, prolonged infections of this kind are associated with an increased risk of stomach cancer.

Inherited Defective Genes. Cancers of the stomach, colon, prostate, and skin seem to appear in some families with greater frequency than in the general public, suggesting an inherited predisposition to these cancers. But according to the American Cancer Society, inheritance is responsible for only about 5 to 10 percent of all cancer cases.

With the exception of heredity, the list of cancer-causing agents above indicates how you can increase your chances of avoiding cancer. But even if you do adjust your life to decrease your risks, there is one more vital element that's critical to maximizing good health—periodic examinations and/or screenings.

Understanding the Principles of Prevention, Screening, and Early Detection— If I Feel Fine, Why Be Tested or Screened?

It can be a bit frightening to hear that half of all men will develop cancer sometime during their lifetimes, and that approximately 552,000 Americans will die each year from cancer (the second leading cause of death in the United States after heart disease).

Good News about Cancer

• Half of all cancer patients are cured.

• Literally millions of Americans are currently living successfully with cancer.

• Cancer can be prevented in many cases.

These positives are due in large part to tremendous advancements in the biological understanding of cancer; better treatment options, such as drugs, surgery, and gene therapy; earlier detection; and—most importantly—prevention.

With cancer, or any other life-threatening illness, doctors initially strive for "primary prevention," or preventing the disease in the first place. As a good backup, though, physicians also work on "secondary prevention," or detecting the ailment early enough to prevent death.

Both of these concepts are dependent upon periodic screening and testing of the patient. As we all know, every office visit includes many exams.

General Office Exams

• A nurse takes your "vital signs"—blood pressure, heartbeat, and temperature.

• The doctor does routine visual, physical, and verbal exams.

• Laboratory tests (when considered necessary) analyze blood, urine, and feces.

• X rays reveal underlying bone and tissue.

• Flexible miniature scopes have the ability to visually inspect, take samples, and do minor surgery of much of your digestive and urinary tracts.

Principles of Testing and Screening

Many of the weapons in a doctor's arsenal don't screen for just one particular ailment, but simultaneously test for numerous problems, situations, or diseases. When your blood or urine is analyzed, a tremendous amount of information is acquired that helps spot a multitude of potential problems, even if the doctor is not specifically looking for them. Examples of this include leukemia and adult diabetes—they are not usually tested for specifically, but normal blood and urine testing will indicate their presence.

How is it determined what to test and screen for, when symptoms are not yet present? There are three primary considerations:

1. How common the disease is.

Cancer

2. How effective the information will be in preserving the patient's quality and duration of life.

3. How expensive the test is.

Testing for lung cancer is a good example of how this works. For decades, chest X rays were often used to spot lung cancer, among other things. It fit two of the three criteria perfectly: Lung cancer was (and still is) one of the most common of cancers, and a chest X ray was inexpensive. It was also thought that chest X rays helped patients because they alerted doctors to lung cancer before symptoms appeared. Unfortunately, about ten or fifteen years ago, it was determined that by the time a chest X ray does detect lung cancer, it is already too late to save most patients. Because of that determination, chest X rays are rarely done in screenings today.

In the past few years, however, a spiral CT scan has been developed that appears to actually detect lung cancer at an early enough stage to make a difference in a patient's survival rate. As with the chest X ray, the CT scan fits two of the three criteria perfectly: Lung cancer is one of the most common of cancers, and a CT scan can definitely make a difference in a patient's life. Unfortunately, the cost of a CT scan test is too high for screening large populations. Once the cost issues are worked out, however, CT scanning may become usable as a screening test for symptom-less lung cancers in high risk populations.

Besides the CT scan, there are numerous exams that screen or test for cancer. For men in their fifties, the following is a list of periodic tests used to detect various kinds of cancer. Many of the tests are used not only for the cancers listed, but for other ailments as well.

Tests for Men 40 and Beyond

TEST	FREQUENCY	TESTING FOR WHAT
Visual skin exam	Once a year from 40 on	Skin cancer or precancerous conditions
Urinalysis	Once a year from 50 on	Blood in the urine, signaling possible bladder cancer, kidney cancer
Fecal occult blood test	Once a year from 50 on	Blood in the stool, signaling possible colon cancer

TEST	FREQUENCY	TESTING FOR WHAT
Spiral CT scan	Doctor or patient request; in high-risk individuals (30 pack years of cigarette use); (Not covered by insurance)	Lung cancer
Digital prostate exam	Once a year from 40 on	Prostate cancer
PSA blood test	Once a year from 50 to about 75; starts earlier in African-Americans and those with strong family risk profiles	Prostate cancer
Lower gastrointestinal (GI) X ray	When symptoms warrant	Colon cancer
Flexible Sigmoidoscopy	Every 3–5 years from 50 on	Colon cancer
Colonscopy	When symptoms warrant and in high-risk individuals based mainly on family history and previous polyp formation, and at detection of fecal blood	Colon cancer

While those tests and screenings are invaluable for early detection, another great agent of early detection is you, the patient. Be aware of your body and the changes it goes through.

Major Signs of Cancer

• Change in bladder or bowel functions.

• A sore that does not heal.

• A persistent cough or hoarseness.

• Unusual bleeding or discharge.

• Thickening or lump in the breast (yes, even in men) or some other part of the body, especially the neck, armpits, and groin.

• Persistent indigestion or difficulty swallowing.

• Unexpected weight loss (a doctor's old adage: Be suspicious when a diet works).

• Change in a wart or mole.

While most of these symptoms can also be related to other, less serious illnesses, they are nonetheless good starting points in cancer awareness and detection.

One symptom that's not mentioned is pain. That's because pain usually isn't a symptom in the early stages of any cancer. It's only in the later stages of the disease that pain begins to show itself, and by then treatment options may not be as effective as when the cancer just starts growing.

Cancer Prevention Tips

• Stay out of the sun and/or protect your skin when in it.

• Don't smoke, or stop if you're still a smoker.

• Choose most of your foods from plant sources, watch your fat intake, and cut down on red meat consumption.

• Exercise regularly, making sure to balance aerobics, stretching, and strengthening workouts.

• Limit alcoholic drinks to two or less per day.

• Be aware that certain lifestyle practices can increase your chances of cancer. Sharing dirty needles and participating in unsafe sex can lead to viral infections such as hepatitis B and C, which are linked to certain cancers.

If you combine lifestyle changes with periodic exams, you'll reduce your chances of cancer to the lowest possible level.

Treating Cancer—Each New Option Is More Effective

For many, the thought of a doctor announcing the presence of cancer is like receiving a death warrant, with the date of execution already penciled in.

In the not-so-distant past, that often was an accurate reflection of reality.

Within the past few generations, however, science has been able to change all that. Early in the twentieth century, the only curable cancers were those that were small and localized enough to be completely removed by surgery. Later, radiation was used after surgery to control small growths that could not be removed by the knife. Chemotherapy was added to destroy small tumors that had spread beyond the reach of the surgeon and radiotherapist. Now, the actual manipulation of genes has opened up a whole new world of treatment options.

Today, treatment can involve various options used in numerous combinations. A determination as to what to use, in what combination, is made only after considering the type of cancer, its stage, and the patient's age and overall health.

Major Cancer Treatment Options (and their possible side effects)

- **Surgery.** For many types of cancer, surgery is the primary weapon used. The standard method is to remove all, or as much as possible, of the tumor and any nearby lymph nodes (the "highway" by which many cancers spread) that have been invaded by the cancer. Many times other options, such as radiation or chemotherapy, are used in conjunction with surgery. Normally, the only side effects from surgery are possible bleeding, infection, and possible disfigurement or deformity, depending upon the extent of the surgery required.

- **Hormone Therapy.** The concept that one organ can control the workings of another is at the root of hormone therapy. The primary example for men involves the testicles. They, along with the male hormones they produce, have a tremendous effect on the prostate and the possible growth of prostate cancer. If cancer cells can be denied the hormones they need, the cancer can be stopped. Hormone therapy works either by surgically removing the hormone-producing organ, by using drugs to stop the hormone production, or by changing the way the hormone works. Temporary side effects can include nausea, vomiting, swelling, weight gain, infertility, lowered sex drive, tender breasts, and erection problems.

- **Radiation.** Only a few years after the discovery of X rays, radiation was used to combat cancer. While these early attempts proved that radiation itself can cause cancer, they did establish the therapeutic value of the new technology. Today, radiation is used with great precision to destroy malignant tumors throughout the body with minimal damage to adjacent, healthy tissue. It can be used by itself or in conjunction with other treatments, such as surgery and chemotherapy. Side effects can include nausea, vomiting, fatigue, and loss of appetite.

• **Chemotherapy.** Ironically, the first anticancer chemical (nitrogen mustard) was discovered by the U.S. Army when it was looking for a deadlier chemical than the mustard gas released by the Germans during World War I. Other chemicals have now been discovered that work in various ways to damage, retard, or kill off cancer cells—all of which fall under the heading of chemotherapy. Today, chemotherapy can be used by itself (with a single anti-cancer chemical or multiple chemicals) or with surgery and radiation. Temporary side effects include susceptibility to infection, fatigue, nausea, vomiting, mouth sores, loss of hair, infertility, and loss of appetite.

• **Immunotherapy.** Also called biological therapy or biological response modi-fier (BRM) therapy, it works by creating biological agents that boost or mimic the body's own immune system to fight particular types of cancer. Still in the developmental stages, immunotherapy shows great promise and will definite-ly be refined and improved within a few short years. Possible side effects are flu-like—fever, chills, muscle achiness, weakness, nausea, vomiting, diarrhea, and loss of appetite.

All of these procedures, separately or in concert, have been so successful at fighting cancer that nowadays approximately one-third of all patients with newly diagnosed cancers will ultimately be cured of their cancer. And this rate should only increase over the coming years, for, as the American Cancer Society stated on its Web site in 2001, "The growth in our knowledge of cancer biology and cancer treatment and prevention has been staggering in recent years. It is likely that sci-entists will learn more about cancer in the [1990s] than has been learned in all the centuries preceding. . . . "

WHERE AND HOW PROBLEMS OCCUR, TREATMENT OPTIONS, AND PREVENTIVE MEASURES

Skin Cancer

Lazy, hot summer afternoons in the 1950s. A cool dip in the community pool gave your skin goosebumps. Lying down on a towel that was warmed by the sun and the baking concrete made you feel good. With beads of water dripping from your face, and the sun warming your back, you dozed off to the sound of children's laughter, the dreams of summer romance, and the smell of chlorine, Coppertone, and just a hint of . . . frying flesh!

Ah, the good old days, when the sun was no enemy. It was the friend who turned your skin into a bronze tan—or red badge of courage—that your girlfriend would admire or help you soothe.

Wake up! Time to move ahead fifty-some years. Today the sun is not only the source of life-giving energy and warmth, but the cause of the most common form of cancer in America. Approximately 1.3 million new cases are forecast for America annually, according to the American Cancer Society. Not too surprising, really, when you think that the big culprit is sunlight—something we all need, and many of us crave. When Gordon was in medical school, skin cancer was regarded as being primarily an occupational risk—for farmers and sailors, especially.

What causes the most damage to our skin is the sun's ultraviolet (UV) radiation. As we all know from painful, personal experience, the damage initially comes in the form of a sunburn—the "cooking" of individual skin cells until they turn pink or red. Unfortunately, that's not all. While the sunburn ultimately fades and the skin sheds the dead cells and regrows new ones, the underlying damage from UV rays is permanent and cumulative over your lifetime.

In fact, researchers have now begun to connect some important dots—those who suffered numerous and severe sunburns as children have a far greater risk of developing skin cancer later in life. For those who did have such experiences, it's not time to panic; just be more aware and vigilant regarding your skin—both in avoiding or protecting yourself from the sun, and in watching for the early signs of skin cancer. And remember, even tanning causes skin cancer.

It should be noted—and stressed—that it does not matter where the UV rays come from; they still cause irreparable damage. This means, of course, that tanning booths and sun lamps can be just as dangerous as the sun. Maybe it's time to reconsider just how important having a tan is in your life?

Those with fair skin color and blond or red hair (generally, those whose ancestors originally came from colder climates) have a much greater risk of skin cancer than those with darker skin and darker hair color (generally, those whose ancestors originally came from warmer climates). Australians are an example of this—albeit an unfortunate one. Mainly English in origin, they currently lead the world in melanoma and other skin cancers. So, while the sun is the main culprit in causing skin cancer, genetics and family history also play a part in determining risk.

Three Main Forms of Skin Cancer

- **Basal Cell Carcinoma.** About three-quarters of all skin cancers are of this variety, which forms in the deepest layer of the skin. The most easily cured, it usually appears on the face and the ears (but can appear on any sun-exposed area) in the shape of a small, irregular mass that's white or gray. Sometimes it may become an open sore. If it spreads, it's usually to adjacent cells; it rarely spreads to distant sites.

- **Squamous Cell Carcinoma.** Originating in the top layer of skin, this faster-growing cancer comprises approximately 20 percent of all skin cancers. Usually, it starts as a small, round lump or flat, crusty, red spot, then develops into a wart-like mass. Squamous cell carcinoma is more likely than basal cell carcinoma to spread (metastasize) to distant sites.

- **Malignant Melanoma.** The deadliest form of skin cancer, malignant melanoma represents only about 5 percent of all cases (about 47,000 a year), but 75 percent of all skin cancer deaths (about 7,700 of a total 9,600). If caught early, it is very curable. If not, however, it can quickly spread throughout the body. Approximately ten times more prevalent in white men than in African-American males, it usually starts where there is a mole but can show up anywhere on the body. The most common locations are on the chest, back, and abdomen.

On the good news front, skin cancer is the most curable of cancers, given early detection. Even malignant melanoma has a 95 percent five-year relative survival rate if caught at the localized stage—which is done in more than 80 percent of cases, according to the American Cancer Society.

Treatment/Prevention. Depending upon the placement, size, and extent of the skin cancer found, treatment might include removal while under a local anesthetic or more involved surgery to make sure of complete removal. In advanced cases of melanoma, where the cancer has spread to other areas of the body, removal of nearby lymph nodes, radiation therapy, immunotherapy (gene manipulation), or chemotherapy might be necessary.

If you've reached your fifties without encountering skin cancer, it's no reason to be less vigilant. The American Cancer Society recommends that all adults over the age of forty should have a yearly skin exam by a doctor.

While this is a good idea, there is no reason why you—with the help of a friend or partner—can't do periodic self-exams. Even though looking for possible skin cancers is a serious thing, there's no reason why you can't mix that in with a little bit of fun. Why not play a little hide-and-seek with various body parts? Why not set up some exciting rewards for when you've completed a full body search? The possibilities can be as endless as your imagination.

What to Look for in Skin Cancer

Sexual fun aside, here's what you should be looking for: any changes or anything that appears unusual, including a change in the color or size of a mole or other dark-colored growth, nodule, or bump. Other signs to be aware of are spots of scaliness, bleeding, and/or oozing. The more often you check for such abnormalities, the better you'll get at spotting anything unusual. And keep in mind that pain is rarely associated with any skin cancer. Show all suspicious looking sites to your doctor.

The American Cancer Society has developed the "ABCD Rule" to aid in self-examination and to help you remember critical identifying marks of a melanoma. If a spot of your skin shows any of the following signs, see a doctor immediately:

A stands for asymmetry. One half of the suspicious mole doesn't match the other.

B stands for border irregularity. Edges ragged, notched, blurry, or rough.

C stands for color. Not uniform, has changed, or has varying degrees of tan, brown, or black.

D stands for diameter. Greater than six millimeters, progressively growing, or suddenly increasing in size.

Besides self-exams, you should try to stay out of the sun or wear adequate clothes and a hat for protection—remembering that being in a shady spot or out on a cloudy day does *not* completely protect you from the sun's dangerous UV radiation. There are plenty of reflected UV rays on a white, sandy beach. Sunscreen, with its varying degrees of solar protection factor (SPF), does partially shield you from UV radiation, but should be used with caution. Most people, if exposed to a noon-day sun, would burn within ten or twenty minutes. If you're using a 15-factor sunscreen, you get one-fifteenth of the UV exposure that you would get when unprotected, meaning you can stay out in the sun that much longer before getting burned. But remember, UV damage is cumulative, so ask yourself, is it worth it? Whenever possible, it's really best to use products that are SPF 30 or above, preferably even 45.

And avoid the sun from 10 A.M. to 4 P.M. The National Cancer Institute has an easy test for determining sun exposure safety. Called the "shadow method," it says that if your shadow is shorter than you are tall, then UV radiation is at its strongest, and you should stay out of the sun.

Lung Cancer

You couldn't get much cooler than the Marlboro Man. Back in the sixties, he rode onto our TV screens as one rugged dude. Not much older than us, he definitely was cool. But now he's dead, and we're not.

Let's see: cool and dead, or uncool and alive. What'll it be?

Few things in life are so cut and dried—so preventable—as lung cancer.

First the bad news: Lung cancer kills more Americans every year than any other form of cancer. The American Cancer Society predicts that more than 156,000 deaths (more than 93,000 of them men) will occur every year and that more than 160,000 cases will be reported annually.

Because this kind of cancer is common and very aggressive, diagnosis usually comes too late to do much good—only about one in twenty patients lives for more than two years after lung cancer has been detected.

The good news?

The incidence of lung cancer is declining significantly in men, from a high of 86.5 per 100,000 in 1984 to 70 per 100,000 in 1996, according to the American Cancer Society. And because smoking is linked to 90 percent of all lung cancer cases, the disease is also the most preventable cancer. It's simple: If people didn't smoke, lung cancer would barely rate a speck on any cancer death chart. This also means that if you've never smoked and aren't exposed to prolonged secondhand smoke, your chances of contracting lung cancer are quite low.

Scientifically speaking, lung cancer is the uncontrolled growth of abnormal cells of the lungs into tumors that can then spread to other parts of the body. Lung cancer usually starts in the walls of the bronchial passages, but it can also form in the body of the lungs.

One reason lung cancer has such a high mortality rate is that many times symptoms don't show themselves until the cancer is well-advanced.

Major Symptoms or Warning Signs of Lung Cancer

• Persistent cough

• Blood in the sputum (the stuff you hack up)

• Chest pain and/or breathlessness

• An unusually long case of pneumonia or frequent bouts of bronchitis or pneumonia

• Swollen lymph nodes in the neck

Another reason for lung cancer's high death rate is that, until recently, the primary diagnostic tool—the chest X ray—simply couldn't detect lung cancer at its earliest stage. The relatively new spiral CT scanner (mentioned earlier), however, can pick up lung cancer at its earliest stages.

While the expensive spiral CT scan is not covered by most insurance, male smokers in their fifties with more than thirty pack years of cigarette use should consider going to their doctor and requesting the test. While it's true they would personally have to pay for it, at the very least, it would put their minds at ease that lung cancer hasn't *yet* taken a foothold, or maybe motivate them to quit smoking before cancer does show up. At the very best, the test could catch lung cancer at its earliest stage, increasing the chance of survival. (A kind of catch-22 situation regarding insurance is that a test would likely be covered if cancer is found, while the same test would likely not be covered if everything is found to be normal.)

Treatment/Prevention. Because of the diagnostic problem mentioned above, treatment of lung cancer is many times a last-ditch effort to preserve even a small amount of time. Surgery (removal of up to an entire lung), radiation therapy, chemotherapy, and the new immunotherapy are normally tried in some form or combination. If the lung cancer has been found while it's still localized (meaning it hasn't spread beyond the lungs), there is a 49 percent chance the patient will live at least five more years. But only about 15 percent of all lung cancer is detected at this stage. The majority of cases are found after the cancer has spread, which translates into only a 14 percent chance of a patient living more than five years.

All of this puts greater emphasis on the word "prevention." As mentioned earlier, lung cancer is by far the most preventable of all cancers: Without tobacco use, lung cancer would be nearly nonexistent. (See chapter 8's smoking section for greater details about smoking and how to go about quitting.) Beyond not smoking, prevention also includes avoiding exposure to secondhand smoke, excessive air pollution, asbestos, arsenic, coal gas, high dosages of X rays, and radon gas (a radioactive gas considered by some to be second only to smoking in cancer-causing potential). Lastly, some studies have shown that daily intake of vitamins C and E may help to protect against lung cancer, although the results are not yet completely convincing, and other studies seem to indicate otherwise.

Prostate Cancer

As a male, you've probably heard all you want to hear about the prostate, prostate cancer, and those nasty side-effect words like impotence and incontinence. Hearing about them is like hearing about Lorena Bobbitt selling cutlery—you cringe and your "equipment" takes a couple steps back into the bat cave. You just don't want to listen, let alone deal with any of it.

But there's good reason for such media blitzing—prostate cancer is the second most common cancer in American males behind skin cancer, and the second most common cause of cancer deaths behind lung cancer. Annually, more than 170,000 are diagnosed with it (nearly twice the rate in African-American men as in white males), and more than 30,000 die each year, according to the American Cancer Society.

To give the media and medical community their due, they're only trying to do for prostate cancer what they did for breast cancer fifteen or twenty years ago—make the public more aware so that lives can be saved. Which means that you, for your own self interest, need to take a deep breath, gird up those loins, and read on.

To begin with, for those who have already spent years suffering through the pain and indignities of an enlarged prostate, prostatitis, or any other generalized infection of the prostate, it's important to stress that these ailments *do not* lead to prostate cancer. There is no convincing evidence to suggest that they predispose you to cancer. In fact, previous prostate problems might save your life, because your heightened prostate awareness might make you more vigilant and lead to early detection if prostate cancer does appear.

Currently, medical science doesn't know exactly what causes prostate cancer or how it gets a foothold. What scientists do know is that the cancer itself is the rampant, uncontrolled growth of abnormal cells within the walnut-sized prostate gland. Typically, symptoms do not appear until the disease is far advanced. If left untreated, the cancer can spread from the prostate to other sites in the body (most notably the groin, pelvis, and skeleton). When symptoms do show up, the disease is most likely incurable but not untreatable.

Risk Factors for Prostate Cancer

Age. The older you are the more likely you'll get it.

Race. Nearly twice as many African-American men contract the disease as white men.

Heredity. There seems to be a slightly higher risk if someone in your family has had it, especially if it was your father or brother.

Diet. It's not yet totally proven, but there seems to be evidence that a high-fat diet increases your chances of prostate cancer.

The good news is that with early detection a cure is quite possible. In fact, cure and survival rates are directly tied to detection times—the earlier the cancer is found, the better the chances of a complete cure and/or long survival. If the cancer is detected before it has spread to other parts of the body, you have nearly a 100 percent chance of survival. And, during the last twenty years, the overall five-year survival rate for all stages of prostate cancer has risen from 67 percent to 92 percent.

Two Kinds of Prostate Cancer

To fully understand the disease, it's important to know that, generally speaking, there are two varieties of prostate cancer. The more publicized of the two is a slow-growing one that strikes older men, while the lesser-known is a fast-growing, aggressive kind that often attacks younger men. The two varieties do not have different names, because they are similar in every way except for speed of advancement.

Because the vast majority of prostate cancer is of the slow-growing variety, it has gained the most media attention. The disease is usually diagnosed in someone seventy or older, with the average age of patients being seventy-two. Because this cancer's advancement is usually measured in decades rather than years, doctors take the patient's age and general health into consideration before determining the best course of treatment. In some cases, the most unobtrusive treatment is "watchful waiting," which means simply monitoring the disease's progress because the chances are that something else will take the patient before the cancer does. This has led to the somewhat catchy (and usually accurate) saying: "Most men die *with* prostate cancer, not *of* it."

Things are different with the fast-growing, aggressive kind of prostate cancer—the kind that took legendary rocker Frank Zappa in his fifties. This variety can strike at nearly any age—although it's usually in the fifties or sixties—and can kill within a few years. Time, in this case, is of the essence when it comes to detection and treatment.

Treatment/Prevention. Taking into account numerous factors, including age, general health of the patient, and progression of the disease, treatment of prostate cancer can include:

Cancer

Surgery. Because the prostate is small and honeycombed with little reservoirs, it is best to remove the entire organ if the cancer appears to be life-threatening. In the past, this nearly always resulted in impotence and in some cases incontinence, because certain vital nerves were cut when removing the organ. Now there is a nerve-saving technique that has proven successful in younger patients (men in their forties and fifties). Even if impotence or incontinence does occur, there are several ways of successfully treating both of them.

Radiation. Either separately or in conjunction with surgery.

Drugs. If the cancer has spread to other parts of the body, drug therapy will probably be necessary, including chemotherapy, which involves hormone manipulation (either a male hormone blocker or synthetic female hormones).

Watchful Waiting. Monitoring the disease and treating any symptoms as they arise.

Castration. This severe-sounding option is usually reserved for elderly men with recurrent (after treatment) prostate cancer. Removal of the testes eliminates the stimulating effects of testosterone on prostate cancer.

Detection of Prostate Cancer

Obviously, early detection is critical. This is done through periodic testing. While it would be wise for every male starting at forty to be checked, it's downright essential that every male should have his prostate checked annually once he turns fifty.

Currently, there are two major prostate tests: an old reliable one and a somewhat controversial one.

The first is the digital exam of the prostate. During a patient office visit, the doctor inserts his finger into your rectum and feels the organ through the rectal wall. If the prostate feels larger than normal, hard, or lumpy, other tests will be done. Remember, the digital exam does not diagnose cancer, it just finds abnormalities that might be cancerous.

The second, controversial test is the PSA (prostate-specific antigen), which measures a certain protein in your blood. Normal prostate cells produce this protein, while cancerous cells produce more of it. The scientific thought is that if your level is high, or suddenly becomes high, there's a likelihood of prostate cancer. Men usually should fall somewhere within a range of 0.3 to 4.0. If you're above that, it doesn't necessarily mean you have prostate cancer, it just means that you should have specific tests, such as an ultrasound, to see if you do. (See the prostate sidebar for details about its controversy.)

Because the cause of prostate cancer is still unknown, prevention primarily involves staying healthy, exercising, and watching what you eat. Some studies have shown that eating a low-fat, low-cholesterol diet may help, as may eating more tomatoes (the substance that makes them red is thought to help prevent prostate cancer). Daily intake of vitamins A, E, and D may help inhibit the growth of prostate tumors, and there has been some anecdotal evidence that the herb saw palmetto aids in healthy functioning of the prostate gland in general.

TO TEST OR NOT TO TEST, THAT IS THE QUESTION
THE PSA CONTROVERSY

Many doctors aren't sure of the value of the PSA (prostate-specific antigen) blood test. At first glance it seems straightforward: PSA registers the level of a certain protein that normal prostate cells produce and cancerous prostate cells produce more of. So a high PSA or a sudden spike from one reading to another should indicate the possibility of cancer.

Well, yes and no. The PSA is known for both false negatives (normal readings with cancer present) and false positives (elevated readings without cancer present). The problem is that PSA levels can be influenced by age, ethnic origins, presence of prostate enlargement, and even previously undetected prostate infection. Some resolution of this problem has come with the creation of age-adjusted PSA acceptable-level ranges and a separate chart for African-American males, who are twice as likely to contract prostate cancer as white males.

Age-Adjusted PSA Levels

WHITE MALES		AFRICAN-AMERICAN MALES	
40–49	2.5	40–49	2.0
50–59	3.5	50–59	4.0
60–69	4.5	60–69	4.5
70–79	6.5	70–79	5.5

Some doctors also question if a PSA truly helps the patient—if the cancer is so slow-growing that it probably won't kill him, the test results lead only to needless anxiety.

This point does not take into consideration the fast-growing, aggressive form of prostate cancer that can be detected via a PSA early enough to save lives. For this reason alone, Gordon believes every man should have a PSA test every year starting at age fifty.

Colon Cancer

While the incidence of colon cancer is slightly higher in women than in men, it still manages to be the third leading cause of cancer death in men behind lung cancer and prostate cancer. Around 6 percent of the male population is going to get colon cancer eventually, while 8 percent of women will get it. The American Cancer Society estimates that approximately 98,000 new cases (46,000 men) will be diagnosed annually, and more than 48,000 people (23,000 men) will die of it every year. For men, the fifties decade is where the disease really gains a foothold.

The good news is that, if caught early, colon cancer is very treatable.

The overwhelming majority—90-plus percent—of colon cancers start as a benign colon polyp. A polyp is usually a small outgrowth from the mucous membrane lining of the colon. Not all polyps turn into cancers—in fact, most don't—but almost all cancers start as polyps.

Unfortunately, polyps usually don't create symptoms. If they're large enough, they can create obstructive-type symptoms—recurring abdominal pain—but doctors want to catch the condition before that happens. In some cases, where the polyps have advanced to cancer, bleeding in the colon may take place and you may become anemic and feel generally weak. That's why it's important to have your stool checked every year so that any microscopic amounts of blood can be detected. And if your bowel habits change for more than a week, or you have unexplained weight loss, you should be checked out.

Besides Polyps, Other Possible Risk Factors for Colon Cancer

Family history. Some families seem to have an extraordinarily high incidence of polyps and colon cancer, giving the medical community a valuable clue as to who is most vulnerable. However, doctors can gain no particular reassurance from a lack of family, history since the overwhelming majority of cases come from people who have no past family incidences.

Inflammatory Bowel Disease. Ailments such as Crohn's disease and ulcerative colitis increase the chances of contracting colon cancer.

Lifestyle Choices. There is some evidence to show that obesity, being sedentary, high alcohol consumption (more than three drinks a day), and/or a high-fat, low-fiber diet might increase your chances of colon cancer.

Tests for Detecting Colon Cancer

Digital Exam. The doctor uses his finger to feel for abnormalities within the lowest portion of the colon and rectum.

Stool Sample. Officially called a fecal occult blood test (FOBT), this checks for blood in the stool, which may indicate colon cancer.

Lower Gastrointestinal (GI) Series. Also known as a barium enema, this test outlines the lower gastrointestinal tract with barium dye (introduced via the rectum), and is most often used nowadays as a supplement to a flexible sigmoidoscopy when a colonoscopy is not called for.

Flexible Sigmoidoscopy. Usually performed by your doctor during an office visit, an endoscope (a small tubelike device) is inserted into the rectum to inspect the lower portion of the colon for polyps or any other abnormalities. (See chapter 4 for greater detail.)

Colonoscopy. Normally done as out-patient day surgery, this is similar to a sigmoidoscopy, but includes the upper portion of the colon. (See chapter 4 for greater detail.)

Treatment/Prevention. If you have been diagnosed with colon cancer, treatment can include surgery, radiation therapy, and/or chemotherapy.

Because nearly all colon cancer starts with polyps, it's best to try and prevent polyps from forming on the colon's wall lining in the first place.

How is that done?

The medical community believes the time it takes food to travel through the large intestine may be a factor—the slower the movement, the more contact time possibly carcinogenic elements of the food have with the mucous membrane lining. To speed up the transit time, eat lots of roughage, drink plenty of water, exercise, and even take bulk additives such as Metamucil (see chapter 4's bulk additive sidebar for details).

Scientists also think—although they're not absolutely sure—that certain foods might prevent polyps. These include fiber, as well as vegetables such as broccoli, cauliflower, and Brussels sprouts. Perhaps daily intake of vitamin E helps, and some of the antioxidants, but it's best to get those from food rather than via supplements—in this case, it might not be the chemicals within the foods but the physical properties of the foods that are beneficial. Some say that a reduction of fats and red meat in the diet might be helpful. Regular use of aspirin or other NSAIDs (nonselective nonsteroidal anti-inflammatory drugs) may help prevent colon cancer.

Bladder Cancer

By far the most serious bladder ailment to be faced, bladder cancer is four times as likely to occur in men than women, especially if they're smokers. When smoke breaks down in the body, certain elements are excreted in the urine that can cause chronic bladder irritation that, in some cases, seems to lead to cancer. This may also apply to smokeless tobacco users.

The American Cancer Society estimates that approximately 53,000 new cases will be diagnosed each year, and approximately 12,000 deaths will occur annually from bladder cancer.

The good news is that the incidence of bladder cancer declined significantly in the 1990s, and since the 1970s mortality rates have decreased significantly as well. Today, the five-year survival rate for bladder cancer at the localized stage is 93 percent.

Bladder cancer is mostly symptomless early on. The only reliable warning sign is blood in the urine—a tremendously important sign, especially in men over fifty, that something, somewhere in your system is wrong. Blood in the urine should *never* be ignored. It can either pass as a clot or in microscopic amounts that can't be seen with the unaided eye. If it's a clot, it may be visible fleetingly, turning your urine momentarily red, maroon, or coffee-colored, and it normally will cause no pain. Most times, a man will not spot blood in his urine; it's more likely to be found during a routine urinalysis.

Treatment/Prevention. The best thing you can do to avoid bladder cancer is to not smoke. If you contract the disease, many times the cancerous bladder section is removed surgically. In severe cases the entire bladder is removed, meaning the patient will have to wear a bag to catch urine as it flows spontaneously through a surgical opening in the abdominal wall.

SORTING THE WHEAT FROM THE CHAFF
CANCER TREATMENT DEFINITIONS

For centuries, the fear of cancer has led many sufferers to seek out treatments that are beyond the normal, scientifically based methods used by physicians. While some have proved to be the hoped-for miracle cures, many others have only let the patient down. The American Cancer Society (ACS) offers some definitions as a way of helping people sort out what is what:

Proven Treatments. Evidence-based or mainstream medical treatments that have been evaluated via strict guidelines and found to be safe and effective.

Research or Investigational Treatments. Any therapies currently being studied in clinic trials. Tests start in test tubes, progress to animal trials, then human trials before being submitted to the Food and Drug Administration (FDA) for approval.

Complementary Treatments. Supportive methods that can be added to mainstream treatments. These are not to cure disease, but to help control symptoms and improve well-being. The ACS offers examples: meditation to reduce stress, peppermint tea for nausea, acupuncture for chronic back pain.

Integrative Therapy. The combining of proven and complementary treatments.

Unproven or Untested Treatments. Treatments with little basis in scientific fact, as well as treatments or tests under investigation.

Alternative Treatments. The ACS defines these as: "Treatments that are promoted as cancer cures. They are unproved because they have not been scientifically tested, or were tested and found to be ineffective. If used *instead* [emphasis by ACS] of evidence-based treatment, the patient may suffer, either from lack of helpful treatment or because the alternative treatment is actually harmful."

In this age of expanding consciousness beyond "norms," many cancer sufferers are trying one or more kinds of alternative and/or complementary therapies and finding varying degrees of success. It is critical that they not discontinue conventional treatments or begin alternative or complementary therapies without first talking things over with their doctors.

Testicular Cancer

Testicular cancer can occur in fifties males, but it's much more common in younger men, specifically those between fifteen and thirty-nine. Even so, the numbers indicate how unusual this cancer is: fewer than 8,000 new cases a year, and fewer than 500 deaths per year. If you've reached fifty with no sign of testicular cancer, you really shouldn't worry.

Nevertheless, this is a cancer where the help of the patient is best—periodically, every male should do a testicular self-examination, no matter what age he is. It takes no time at all and can be done in the shower. Just massage the scrotum and roll each testicle between your thumb and fingers. What you're feeling for is any change in the contour or heft (a feeling that your testicles are getting heavier). If you do feel anything different or unusual, have your doctor examine you immediately.

Treatment/Prevention. If cancer is strongly suggested, the usual treatment is surgery, followed by chemotherapy. If one testicle is suspected of having cancer, the surgeon will automatically remove it entirely, rather than taking a biopsy (tissue sample) first. This is done to reduce the risk of spreading the cancer to other tissues, and because the removal of one testicle does not interfere with the patient's fertility or ability to have an erection.

In the case of testicular cancer, chances of cure are excellent, as evidenced by American Lance Armstrong, who has not only survived testicular cancer but has gone on to win as overall champion in three Tour de France cycling contests.

Cancer of the Penis

Luckily, this type of cancer is rare and usually shows up only in uncircumcised men who don't keep their penis clean. It will first appear as a wart-like lump or ulcer on the foreskin or head of the penis. If left untreated, it will slowly develop into a growth that resembles a cauliflower.

Treatment/Prevention. Normally, early radiation makes surgery unnecessary.

Prevention means keeping the penis, especially under the foreskin, clean at all times.

REAL LIFE TALES

Number One: Shit *Does* Happen Even When Doing Everything Right

Alan is involved with state politics. At fifty-two years old, he's also in good physical shape—a real health nut who's into riding his bike and exercising a lot.

One night, while attending a baseball game, Alan is standing at a urinal and just happens to notice a little shred of blood disappear down the drain. There's no pain involved, just a quick view of a small blood clot, then it's gone. He thinks it odd, wonders if something's wrong, but quickly forgets about it.

Six months later, the same thing happens. Still no pain, and he feels perfectly fit and healthy. This time, though, he decides to find out what's going on. He goes in to see a doctor, who does a urinalysis. Nothing shows up. But the doctor doesn't take a chance. He sends Alan to a urologist, who puts a scope (a tubelike device) up through Alan's penis so he can see into the bladder. The urologist finds bladder cancer.

Because it's at a fairly early stage, the cancer is still curable. They surgically remove the cancer, taking out a portion of the bladder, but Alan is able to function fine without the use of a urine bag outside of his body.

Alan is an example of the "shit happens" category. He isn't a smoker, which is the biggest risk factor for bladder cancer. Risk factors do help doctors know who to watch, but a large number of serious diseases come out of nowhere.

Alan also had two other things going for him: luck and observation. He certainly was lucky to have spotted two times when he passed blood. Many times the passing goes unnoticed or is so minuscule that it can't be seen with the unaided eye—that's why periodic urinalyses are critical starting at fifty years old. Alan should also be congratulated for being observant—how many men ever look at their urine or their stools for that matter? Observation is a key component to maintaining good health and catching any ailments in the early stages, when cure rates are much higher.

Number Two: Some Real Tales are Short, Not So Sweet, and Follow a Logical Progression that Can't Be Ignored

Mike is a fifty-eight-year-old engineer who has had hypertension (high blood pressure) for years. He's never been good at taking the medicine that would control it. His cholesterol levels are good, he isn't overweight, but he doesn't exercise, and he's a heavy smoker, puffing away at almost two packs a day since he was fifteen. He doesn't want to listen when his doctor brings up smoking and how the odds will probably catch up with him someday.

To make matters worse, Mike's not too diligent about coming in to see a doctor on a regular basis. In fact, he probably never would see a doctor if it wasn't for his real love—flying. He's a private pilot who needs to get his FAA license renewed every two years. That means a physical exam.

At one of those biennial physicals, Mike complains about a cough that isn't going away. A chest X ray reveals an odd-looking pneumonia. More tests are warranted, especially with his history of smoking. Over the course of three weeks, it's found that Mike has a tumor—a malignant, inoperable tumor that's obstructing his breathing.

Within eight months, Mike is dead at fifty-eight years old.

Sometimes even modern medicine can't save a person from the consequences of personal choices.

Number Three: Without a Basis of PSA Comparison, the Result Might Have Been Very Different

Tim is fifty-four years old and a corporate executive of a large company. Generally in good health, he's a big fella—6'3" and 210 pounds—has never smoked, drinks only a minimal amount of alcohol, and is married with no children. Tim is also a believer in periodic exams, which, in this case, saved his life.

During one routine office visit, Tim had a PSA (prostate specific antigen) exam, which tests for prostate cancer. Tim's antigen level was significantly higher than a previous PSA test. While the new level was still within the "normal" bounds, it was, in fact, triple the last reading. Because PSA readings can sometimes be misleading, another test was done. The result was the same. A digital exam, where the doctor inserts a finger in the rectum and feels the prostate through the bowel wall, didn't reveal anything unusual.

Without previous PSA tests as a basis of comparison, Tim's elevated PSA score might have gone unnoticed, because it was within normal ranges. But because the doctor had a history with the patient, the PSA score warranted action. Tim was sent to a urologist, who repeated the test. Once again it was as high as before. A follow-up ultrasound showed abnormalities that warranted taking a tissue sample via a needle guided by an ultrasound. The lab results showed prostate cancer.

Tim was floored. His relatively young age meant that the cancer was probably the fast-growing aggressive kind that can kill quickly, as opposed to the slow-growing prostate cancer that many elderly men die *with* rather than *from*. His team of doctors recommended removal of the entire prostate as the safest, best course of action. Tim was warned that because of the hair-like network of prostatic nerves that are shot through the prostate, patients who undergo a prostatectomy may experience incontinence and/or erectile dysfunction (inability to get an erection) as a surgical side effect. Sometimes normal functioning returns with time; other times the incontinence and erectile dysfunction are permanent.

After long and involved talks with the doctors and his wife, Tim decided to go along with what was recommended. He made it through the operation with no problems and was cured of prostate cancer, but also found he couldn't get an erection. Happily, once Viagra was introduced in 1998, Tim found it to be as successful as the promotional literature suggested, and he resumed a satisfactory sex life with his wife.

Now, numerous years on, Tim's life has returned to being balanced, happy, and healthy—due mainly to good, periodic testing.

THE GOOD NEWS

- Most cancers can be prevented—about 80 percent of today's cancer cases come from environmental or lifestyle factors that can be moderated, controlled, and/or avoided.

- Half of all cancer patients are cured.

- Literally millions of Americans are currently living successfully with cancer.

- The National Cancer Institute reports that most people at risk for cancer never even get the disease.

- The American Cancer Society states that the five-year relative survival rate for many cancers is about 80 percent.

- If all Americans participated in regular cancer screenings, the five-year relative survival rate could increase to 95 percent.

- Approximately 90 percent of all skin cancers (the most common form of cancer) can be prevented by avoiding the sun or being protected from it.

- With early detection, skin cancer is the most curable of all cancers.

- Even though lung cancer is still the deadliest cancer, the incidence rate has been declining significantly in men since the 1980s.

Cancer

- If you've never smoked and aren't exposed to prolonged secondhand smoke, your chances of contracting lung cancer are virtually nil.

- If prostate cancer is found before it has spread to other parts of the body, there is nearly a 100 percent chance of survival.

- Most men die *with* prostate cancer, not *of* it.

- When bladder cancer is detected in the localized stage, it has a 93 percent five-year survival rate.

- Many tests, exams, and/or screenings for cancer can detect the disease before symptoms appear—ensuring the best possible survival rates.

- Recent DNA research has resulted in huge new knowledge of how and why cancer develops. Within a few years, this should translate into highly effective treatments.

8: WHAT YOU CAN DO

A Summary of Positive Choices That Make a Difference

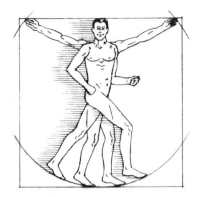

BACKGROUND BASICS

Think of your overall health as your retirement fund, and any effort you make toward good health as "saving" for retirement.

The big question is: Do you take the huge chance you're going to die early, which means you don't have to make the effort to "save" anything for your health retirement fund?

If you do die young, then you "win." Congratulations. But what happens if you live to be 100? Because you did nothing to "save" for the long haul, your chances are greatly increased that your last ten years of life will be spent in poor health.

The point, of course, is that if you put something into your health now (exercise, proper diet, periodic tests), there will be an important retirement "asset" (good health) waiting when you get older. Additionally, unlike a retirement program, the benefits can also be realized on a more immediate basis—more energy, better appearance, better sleep, better sex. Even a minimum amount of personal effort in diet, exercise, and health monitoring will bring some good results. But the more effort you choose to put in, the more rewards you'll get out. A concerted, sustained effort will bring good, visible, positive results; a tremendous amount of

305

work will bring a corresponding number of rewards. It's all up to you—you get back what you put in.

Where Do You Start?

Every New Year's Day, resolutions fly: "I'm going to stop smoking." "I'm going to exercise more." "I'm going to eat better; lose those extra pounds." By January 2 people are racing to smoking clinics, professional gyms, and diet programs like lemmings toward a cliff. At these various health centers the entire month of January is like shopping the day after Christmas, packed with people wanting— demanding—a change.

Unfortunately, by mid-February most people have returned to how they lived before. That's probably because most people put the cart before the horse. People who make a quick decision and jump into life-changing activities without fully understanding what truly motivates them are usually heading for a fall. Most people need to be completely motivated and inspired to maintain a good, healthy regimen of exercise and eating right.

How Do You Get Motivated?

Motivation is a real problem, mainly because it's so highly individualistic. What works for one person probably won't work for another. Go to a professional gym? Work out at home? Join a weight-loss clinic? Find friends to lose weight with? Exercise in the morning? In the afternoon? Find inspiration from within? Find it in a book? Do it for yourself? Do it for your kids? Do it for your spouse? To guarantee success we need to find out what gets us moving, what gets our heart pumping to the beat of full dedication and commitment. Finding that true motivation must come from inside you.

Once motivation is determined, the road to good health begins not with the first step but with deciding in your own mind what kind of first step it will be (what you want to achieve, both in short-term and long-term goals) and in what direction the step will go (how you will achieve those goals). Once those two critical components are decided, the rest of the health maintenance journey is just . . . a walk in the park.

Understanding What We Want to Achieve

But what is it that we are truly trying to achieve? Do we simply want to live as long as possible?

When we think about life and death, most of us would probably agree that it would be better to live only until eighty, if we had good health until seventy-nine-

and-a-half, than to live to be ninety with good health only up to eighty. Ten years of decrepitude is not most people's idea of quality living.

So, what we really want is to push back, or shrink, the amount of final poor health we must all endure so that it turns out to be the smallest portion of our lives—no matter how long we live.

That long-term goal is within our grasp, through preventive measures that often aren't too intrusive or difficult to implement once motivation is there. Keeping our final years of poor heath to a minimum is definitely within our grasp no matter how old we are, no matter how out of shape we are, no matter how bad our current medical condition is. Take heart, it's *never* too late to start taking control of your physical health—and the rewards begin almost immediately.

Keep in mind, though, that many times our minds do move faster than our bodies. We might have struggled for months with deciding it's finally time to start doing something about our health—struggling with inertia (getting up off that couch), struggling with exactly what tactics to use to get started, struggling to find the time to do it. If you've been grappling with these issues for a while on a mental level, you're probably mentally already several weeks or months into your health program even before you've completed the first actual week of physical work. Human nature dictates that we want to see results instantly, even though we've just started our program. We have to be patient, give our bodies time to catch up to our minds.

If we are patient with our bodies, the rewards will be huge.

Leaving Your Health Up to Fate— Is This Really the Best Option?

Why should you try to do all this "stuff"—denying yourself the foods you like, watching how much you drink, forcing yourself to exercise—when you had a grandfather who drank, smoked, ate what he wanted, never exercised, and still lived to be ninety?

Maybe you do come from sturdy stock. Maybe you actually are as impervious to long-term health problems as your grandfather seemed to be. Maybe—like a Winston Churchill—you can eat, drink, smoke all you want and live a great, high-quality life until you're in your nineties, then quietly drift off to sleep one night, after saying goodbyes to all your friends and loved ones, and never wake up.

And maybe not. That's the problem. We don't know what the future holds. And we don't know what our bodies can, or cannot, take.

What we do know is that only approximately 30 percent of overall health can be attributed to genetics. That means that a full 70 percent of general health is dictated by what you do or don't do. And even genetics aren't necessarily destiny. You can alter your destiny despite being subjected to immutable genetics, like a man with a genetic predisposition to heart disease who does everything right and, therefore, never suffers a heart attack.

On the other hand, ignoring the basic tenets of good health maintenance because you believe you have "good genes" is not a wise thing to do.

Working the Odds in Your Favor

To a large degree, health care can be distilled down to numbers—playing percentages, working the odds. Doctors are trying to stack the deck in the patient's favor when they recommend various courses of action to patients. People who do take an active role in maintaining their own health are also increasing their odds of a good, healthy life.

In a well-ordered world, no one would refute such logic. But because we don't live in such a world, there is a health category that we refer to as "shit happens." Many people find this category hard to accept. It's the out-of-the-blue lightening bolt that can't be explained, the seemingly random act of illness that fells someone who is doing everything right.

Such cases make many people stop and ask: "Why do all the work, if the effort will ultimately be for nothing?"

Our positive, proactive answer is:

- The "shit happens" category is already relatively small and getting smaller as medical technology continues to learn more about how our bodies function and malfunction.

- If you do the right things in terms of health maintenance, you decrease your likelihood of being in the "shit happens" category.

- You're not passive in other parts of life, so why be passive when it comes to your health?

- If you only have one life to live, do you want to make it a crap shoot?

Of course, the decision to take positive, preventive steps in your health care is up to you, but before you decide not to take action, consider these points.

Making a Case for Personal Effort

- In many cases, the "how you die" and even the "when you die" are, to a certain degree, within your general control—but only if you start taking control of your health care and maintenance.

- It's true that there's a lot more left to chance in life than any of us would like to believe, but it's also true that there's less left to chance than we are willing to sometimes acknowledge.

- Group statistics (especially those of death rates with diseases) apply to groups, not necessarily to individuals within the group—meaning that statistics aren't your personal health forecaster. A person who actively takes charge of his health care and maintenance can "beat the odds" nearly every time.

The critical point is that you can make a few relatively small corrections now and significantly affect the odds (not the certainty) of the long-term outcome.

Here They Are: The Twelve Most Important Steps You Can Take for Your Health

There are many activities you can do, and personal choices you can make, to increase your chances of having a good, healthy quality of life. Each of them can be broken into numerous subsections as well—meaning that there are literally hundreds of do's and don'ts. To bring a little focus to the situation, here is a list of the top twelve steps (in order of importance) that you, as a fifties male, can take to help yourself:

1. **Don't smoke.** It's the worst, most damaging thing you can do to your body.

2. **Have a health assessment.** If you don't already know, you need to find out where your general health stands before attempting to improve your health. It doesn't count that you think you're healthy—a doctor needs to check you out.

3. **Exercise.** Any kind of exercise is better than none, but try to incorporate all three critical elements: aerobics, stretching, and strengthening. Start slow and work up. (See the exercise section of this chapter for details.)

4. **Eat moderately from all food groups.** What goes in is critical to how healthy you are and how good you feel. (See the diet section of this chapter for details.)

5. **Drink alcohol in moderation.** Up to two glasses a day of beer, wine, or spirits. More and you lose the benefits and begin to adversely affect your health.

6. **Know your blood pressure.** High blood pressure is a major contributor to stroke and heart disease, the number one killer in America. If it's high, get on medication to lower it, then look into lifestyle changes, such as diet and exercise.

7. **Know your "good" and "bad" cholesterol levels.** Low levels of good and high levels of bad are major contributors to heart disease. Relatively unobtrusive drugs can lower your bad cholesterol, while eating right and exercising can increase your good cholesterol.

8. **Take an aspirin a day.** Only 81 mg a day can significantly reduce your risk of heart disease by thinning your blood. Check with your doctor first, and don't take aspirin if you're already taking the herb ginkgo, which also thins the blood. If regular aspirin upsets your stomach, try taking it with food, or try a coated aspirin.

9. **Have periodic medical examinations and tests done.** Doctors recommend that you start many critical ones at fifty. If you're past fifty and haven't had them done, get going! (See the following section for details.)

10. **Avoid the sun, and always use sunscreen when in the sun.** Skin cancer is the most common cancer in America.

11. **Wear a seat belt in a car, and a helmet when riding a motorcycle, bicycle, or horse.**

12. **Keep, or develop, a positive attitude toward life.** It goes a long way toward preventing minor illnesses, aiding in recuperation times, and generally improving the overall quality of your life. If you've never had a positive attitude before, but want to try and develop one now, remember: It takes practice.

Putting It On, Taking It Off—
Understanding Weight Gain and Loss

A few months ago you became fed up with how you looked and felt. You hated your "love handles" and flabby belly. You hated how you never seemed to have any get-up-and-go anymore. So you stepped up to the plate (home plate, that is, *not* the dinner plate) and decided to go on a diet.

Surprising even yourself, you found you had the motivation and the will power to follow one of those currently-popular diet plans, and you even started doing a little exercising—although the diet plan hardly mentioned exercise.

More surprising, you started losing weight during the first week. Within two or three weeks you had shed ten pounds and you were damn proud! Your image in the mirror hadn't changed that much—those love handles were still there, and you couldn't see a single stomach "ab" (abdominal muscle)—but you held on to that ten-pound stat as if your life depended on it.

Now, two months into your diet, you're still watching what you eat, you're still exercising a little, but you can't get rid of any more weight and you don't feel any different than you did before you started the diet. In fact, you're afraid to admit it, but you think you've put back a pound or two (it must be the scale). You're downright discouraged and thinking: "What the hell, why bother if nothing's working and I can't lose the weight I want?"

Welcome to the wonderful world of trendy diets and water weight loss.

Much of what people initially lose when they start a diet program is water weight. That's the easy stuff to get rid of. Once that's gone, though, real effort and dedication is needed to take off the fat pounds.

A Few Points Before Making an Effort to Lose Weight

- You're genetically programmed to put fat on in some places and not in others. Even if you have liposuction to get rid of fat in a fat-deposit area, that's where new fat will automatically go first to be stored. If you don't change your lifestyle, you'll probably have to have liposuction again.

- You cannot selectively remove inches of fat from a part of your body by selectively exercising that part of your body (such as trying to get rid of love handles). You need a complete program of diet and exercise to have a total impact.

- If you are doing everything right (exercising, eating correctly, and in the right amounts) and your weight won't drop below a certain range, then consider accepting that weight range as normal for you. We all can't have a "perfect" physique; few of us ever come close.

To Lose Weight, Know How Your Metabolism Works

To help you achieve your weight-loss goals, an understanding of your body's metabolism (a chemical and physical process necessary for storing and retrieving energy) is important. There are two distinct phases of metabolism:

1. **Anabolism**. (Loosely known also as anaerobic metabolism). During this "constructive" time the body takes the small molecules produced by the digestive

system's breakdown of food and forms them into more complex molecules that become tissues, organs, and fat. Additionally, anabolism is also known as the storage phase of metabolism because this is when the body packs away critical elements to be used later. Unfortunately, one of those elements is fat. On the good side, fat is a major source of energy for the body; we can't live without fat. On the downside (at least for those watching their weight), fat is stored until it's needed, and that storage is what translates into weight gain. For men, fat storage usually takes place on the belly and around the waist; for women, fat storage is normally on the thighs, buttocks, and belly.

2. **Catabolism.** (Loosely known also as aerobic metabolism.) During this "destructive" time the body retrieves fat from storage and breaks it down to get energy. The good news is that this retrieval and use of fat, if sustained for a long enough period of time, translates into weight loss.

Burning and Storing Fat

When we need energy, our bodies first burn the most readily available fuel source: sugar, which is normally floating around in our bloodstream. When we need energy over an extended period of time, such as when we're strenuously exercising, our bodies run out of easily available sugar. This usually happens after about twenty minutes of sustained, sweat-producing activity (such as aerobic exercise). Our bodies then turn to our fat reserves that have been stored. Slowly but surely, as we continue to exercise beyond the twenty-minute mark, fat is broken down and converted to usable fuel. If we do this long enough, over an extended period of time, we lose weight.

The key, in this case, is the shifting from anaerobic (fat-storing) metabolism to aerobic (fat-burning) metabolism. If the body's metabolism never makes this shift, no stored fat will be burned and, therefore, no weight will be lost. This is why a guy can walk all day, trudge up and down lots of stairs, but still not lose weight: His body has never been pushed into the aerobic, fat-burning stage.

Compounding the situation is that each of us has a general resting metabolic rate, which is like a thermostat that establishes how quickly or slowly our body's metabolism uses energy and stores fat. Those people who never get fat, no matter what they do, probably have a metabolic rate that runs "fast." Those people who seem to put on weight just thinking about food probably have a metabolic rate that runs "slow."

Resetting Your Metabolism

The obvious question is: Can an individual reset his metabolic rate so it runs faster and, therefore, burns more fat?

What You Can Do

The answer is a qualified yes. The bad news is that no pill or drug has yet been invented to safely reset a human metabolic rate—all the PR and hype suggesting otherwise is just that, PR and hype. The good news is that over time, and with lots of effort, we can raise our metabolic rate.

But resetting your metabolism takes work, pure and simple. You have to do aerobic exercise for twenty minutes or more at least three times a week (see the exercise section of this chapter for details). This kind of sustained exercise program will, ultimately, increase even your resting metabolic rate so that you burn more calories (energy). Additionally, a sustained exercise program has another weight-loss benefit—while you're doing all that exercise, muscles are being developed, and developed muscles burn more calories (energy), even when resting, than fat does.

Besides exercise, there is a dietary principle—simpler said than done—that can help with losing weight: You need to match your intake of calories to how much your body uses. If you exceed that amount, you gain weight; if you go below it, you lose weight. (See the diet section in this chapter for details.)

To sum up, there are two basic ways to lose weight: (1) watch your intake of calories (watch what you eat); and (2) exercise, so your body will shift from the storage mode into the fat-burning mode. The most effective method of weight loss is to do a combination of both.

Remember, though, the goal isn't to totally eliminate all the fat your body stores. We all need fat, and there is no way to get rid of all of it. You will always have some fat on your body, no matter how much you exercise and how much you watch what you eat. Ideally, men should carry approximately 20 percent or less of body fat, while women should have 30 to 35 percent or less.

Finding Your BMI

To find out how you stack up in the fat category, calculate your BMI (body mass index), which is a correlation between your height and weight. (BMI does *not* indicate your physical fitness.) Multiply your weight in pounds by 705; divide that number by your height in inches; then do that again—that's your BMI. For example, a six-foot man who weighs 195 pounds would have a BMI of 26.52 (195 × 705 = 137,475 divided by 72, then divided by 72 again). If your BMI is above twenty-five you're considered slightly overweight, while if you're above twenty-seven you definitely have too much body fat, and you're in trouble on various health fronts. The BMI is considered a good tool by many doctors, who don't think it should change as you get older, although for many it does as they put on weight.

BMI CHART

BODY MASS INDEX CHART

To find your BMI, find the column for your height and the row for your weight. The number at their intersection is your BMI.

If your weight or height is not on this chart, you can calculate your own BMI with this formula:

$$BMI = \frac{\text{Weight in pounds} \times 704}{(\text{Height in inches})^2}$$

HEIGHT																
FEET	5'	5'1"	5'2"	5'3"	5'4"	5'5"	5'6"	5'7"	5'8"	5'9"	5'10"	5'11"	6'	6'1"	6'2"	
INCHES	60	61	62	63	64	65	66	67	68	69	70	71	72	73	74	
WEIGHT CM	152	155	157	160	163	165	168	170	173	175	178	180	183	185	188	
LB KG																
100 45.5	19.6	18.9	18.3	17.8	17.2	16.7	16.2	15.7	15.2	14.8	14.4	14.0	13.6	13.2	12.9	
110 50.0	21.5	20.8	20.2	19.5	18.9	18.3	17.8	17.3	16.8	16.3	15.8	15.4	14.9	14.5	14.2	
120 54.5	23.5	22.7	22.0	21.3	20.6	20.0	19.4	18.8	18.3	17.8	17.3	16.8	16.3	15.9	15.4	
130 59.1	25.4	24.6	23.8	23.1	22.4	21.7	21.0	20.4	19.8	19.2	18.7	18.2	17.7	17.2	16.7	
140 63.6	27.4	26.5	25.7	24.9	24.1	23.3	22.6	22.0	21.3	20.7	20.1	19.6	19.0	18.5	18.0	
150 68.2	29.4	28.4	27.5	26.6	25.8	25.0	24.3	23.5	22.9	22.2	21.6	21.0	20.4	19.8	19.3	
160 72.7	31.3	30.3	29.3	28.4	27.5	26.7	25.9	25.1	24.4	23.7	23.0	22.4	21.7	21.2	20.6	
170 77.3	33.5	32.2	31.2	30.2	29.2	28.3	27.5	26.7	25.9	25.2	24.4	23.8	23.1	22.5	21.9	
180 81.8	35.2	34.1	33.0	32.0	31.0	30.0	29.1	28.3	27.4	26.6	25.9	25.2	24.5	23.8	23.2	
190 86.4	37.2	36.0	34.8	33.7	32.7	31.7	30.7	29.8	28.9	28.1	27.3	26.6	25.8	25.1	24.4	
200 90.9	39.1	37.9	36.7	35.5	34.4	33.4	32.3	31.4	30.5	29.6	28.8	28.0	27.2	26.4	25.7	
210 95.5	41.1	39.8	38.5	37.3	36.1	35.0	34.0	33.0	32.0	31.1	30.2	29.4	28.5	27.8	27.0	
220 100.0	43.1	41.7	40.3	39.1	37.8	36.7	35.6	34.5	33.5	32.6	31.6	30.7	29.9	2.91	28.3	
230 104.5	45.0	43.5	42.2	40.8	39.6	38.4	37.2	36.1	35.0	34.0	33.1	32.1	31.3	30.4	29.6	
240 109.1	47.0	45.4	44.0	42.6	41.3	40.0	38.8	37.7	36.6	35.5	34.5	33.5	32.6	31.7	30.9	
250 113.6	48.9	47.3	45.8	44.4	43.0	41.7	40.4	39.2	38.1	37.0	35.9	34.9	34.0	33.1	32.2	
260 118.2	50.9	49.2	47.7	46.2	44.7	43.4	42.1	40.8	39.6	38.5	37.4	36.3	35.3	34.4	33.5	
270 122.7	52.8	51.1	49.5	47.9	46.4	45.0	43.7	42.4	41.1	40.0	38.8	37.7	36.7	35.7	34.7	
280 127.3	54.8	53.0	51.3	49.7	48.2	46.7	45.3	43.9	42.7	41.4	40.3	39.1	38.1	37.0	36.0	
290 131.8	56.8	54.9	53.2	51.5	49.9	48.4	46.9	45.5	44.2	42.9	41.7	40.5	39.4	38.3	37.3	
300 136.4	58.7	56.8	55.0	53.3	51.6	50.0	48.5	47.1	45.7	44.4	43.1	41.9	40.8	39.7	38.6	

TESTS AND SCREENINGS: WHAT, WHEN, AND WHY

"Why do I need a test? I feel fine."

That manly refrain is heard countless times around America every day. But we need to face facts: We're not avoiding medical screenings and tests because we feel fine, we're avoiding them because they strike fear in the hearts of even the stoutest lumberjacks. Most of us have this irrational fear of the tests themselves and a fear of what the tests might uncover. So we hide behind, "I'm feeling fine; why should I have tests done?"

The obvious answer is to increase your odds of living a complete and healthy life. Numerous illnesses and diseases can be handled, if not downright cured, if they are discovered early enough. Often that means even before visible symptoms have developed. Without certain tests, this would not be possible.

The flip side of the male fear of tests is that when something does go wrong with our health, we immediately want to have every test possible to find out exactly what's wrong and what the best course of treatment should be.

Somewhere, somehow, a balance needs to be struck.

Getting the Right Perspective on Tests

Just as lawyers know that we've become a society that sues at the mere thought of an alleged wrong, doctors realize we're becoming a society that wants a test at the first sign of any ailment, no matter how minor. That sinus infection might be the early warning symptom of a brain tumor, or maybe not. Either way, the patient wants it tested.

In the last fifty to seventy-five years, medical technology has surpassed everyone's wildest dreams. We now have machines that can see into our bodies better than most of us can see across a room; we have probes that can travel into the deepest reaches of our vital organs, stopping to take pictures and tissue samples before treating the ailment at its source; and we have lab tests that analyze body fluids so well that many illnesses can be detected before they cause real problems.

This technology has improved our quality of life immeasurably, helping to take what once were life-threatening or life-changing diseases and injuries and turning many of them into minor inconveniences.

Unfortunately, these technologically marvelous machines, and the tests they perform, are not cheap. While doctors don't dictate how much tests cost, they are on the front line of determining which test is done to whom. Because of this situation, the doctor has a responsibility to put tests in their proper perspective for the patient being treated. It's critical that patients understand there is a time and a place for testing and a time and a place for not testing—and that insurance companies demand every test be justified by a specific ailment.

MRI Testing as Example

The expensive MRI (magnetic resonance imaging) test is interesting to highlight. Many men experience a disc or lower back problem for the first time in their fifties. When such an ailment strikes, many sufferers think they should immediately have an MRI to define exactly what's going on. They think that because some professional football player gets an MRI every time he's hurt, they need one too.

The truth is, for most back problems, the majority of patients don't need an MRI initially. An expensive MRI test doesn't give any information that the patient or the doctor needs at the time. In fact, an MRI is not going to change what most doctors initially prescribe or why they prescribe it. While an MRI is an essential test when surgery is required, an MRI is usually not needed until the possibility of surgery enters the picture.

With most back problems before the doctor considers surgery as a viable option, he or she needs to take the patient through two or three steps that are relatively easy, nonintrusive, and usually work (see "Real Life Tale Number One" in chapter 2 as an example). These steps include seeing if the patient responds to taking anti-inflammatories, getting on a proper exercise program, and maybe even making some lifestyle changes—all before an expensive MRI test is ordered. Even the passage of time, all by itself, is often beneficial.

Doing an MRI too early may even confuse the issue. A doctor's decision on whether a person is going to require surgery is usually based on how that person responds to the initial treatment, rather than on what the MRI looks like. A doctor can sometimes see a horrendous-looking MRI in a patient that is getting better with anti-inflammatories and a good exercise program, or is even getting better spontaneously. Should that doctor decide on surgery based on what the MRI looks like, or on what the patient looks like? If the back problem is improving (usually within several weeks), the information that the MRI gives is basically useless, and the money spent on the test was wasted.

The What, When, and Why of Tests and Screenings

Although you may not need an MRI test for your back problem (see the previous section for details), there are numerous exams, screenings, tests, and self-exams all fifties men should do—or have done—on a periodic basis. They've been mentioned throughout this book and are now brought together to help you keep track of what needs to be done, when, and why. Before they're listed, however, a few explanatory notes are in order:

What You Can Do

When it comes to the blood chemistry screen, or "panel," mentioned below, keep in mind that numerous tests can be done with one vial of blood. This means that blood sugar can be checked at the same time cholesterol levels can be determined.

Before computer technology, a doctor would order individual tests that were done by hand. If a doctor wanted to check your potassium level, he'd order a potassium test; if he wanted to check your sugar level, he'd order a sugar test. That changed when computer analysis was developed in the 1960s. Doctors were able to get a whole series of tests (called "channels" when they're part of an automated "panel" of tests) done at the same time from a single vial of blood. And the beauty of it was that a big, twenty-four channel workup didn't cost any more than a panel with six channels (tests) on it.

Unfortunately—for both doctors and patients—the federal government, in a battle with larger commercial laboratories over "unnecessary testing" in Medicare patients, has, in effect, made twenty-four-channel "autoanalyses" less available, even to non-Medicare patients. Patients should be aware of this, because checking for such important items as cholesterol levels, which used to be standard with practically any blood test, are no longer part of a routine blood chemistry panel. Unusual diseases, such as parathyroid disease and hemochromatosis (an iron-storage disease affecting mostly men) are now much less likely to be diagnosed in their early, easily treatable, stages because they aren't automatically tested for in a blood analysis.

Some of the tests/screenings listed below are usually done in combination with other tests, but they have been broken out as individual items to signify their importance in monitoring your health. The tests have also been put in a general hierarchy of importance.

Doctor-Related Tests/Screenings:

WHAT	WHEN	WHY—SCREENING FOR
1. General physical (exam and Q & A time with doctor)	Once a year	General signs of problems (stress, tension, drug or alcohol abuse, etc.)
2. Blood pressure (via an inflatable band around the arm)	Once a year	High blood pressure, which can lead to heart disease and strokes
3. Cholesterol levels (via blood chemistry analysis), including HDL (good) and LDL (bad)	Once a year	High levels, which can lead to heart disease and strokes

317

WHAT	WHEN	WHY—SCREENING FOR
4. Blood sugar or glucose (via blood chemistry analysis)	Once a year	Diabetes
5. Other blood chemistry analysis	Periodically (yearly for those taking medication regularly)	Kidney disease, liver disease
6. Urine analysis test, or urinalysis	Once a year	Blood (possible cancer), microorganisms (urinary tract infections), crystals (possible kidney stones), excess sugar (diabetes), protein (kidney disease)
7. Thyroid screen, or TSH	At least once beyond age fifty	Disorders of the thyroid
8. Prostate specific antigen or PSA test (via blood chemistry analysis)	Once a year until age seventy or seventy-five, then less often	Prostate cancer
9. Digital exam of prostate (doctor inserts finger past anus to feel prostate through rectal wall)	Once a year	Prostate cancer, or other abnormalities
10. Electrocardiogram, or EKG (electrodes on chest, wrists, legs)	Periodically after at least one baseline test at fifty	Heart disease, heart abnormalities
11. Flexible sigmoidoscopy (doctor's office exam of lower bowel via a flexible scope)	Every 3 to 5 years	Colon polyps, which can be precursors to colon cancer
12. Stool test for blood.	Yearly	For blood (colon cancer)
13. Chest X Ray	Every year, only if you smoke—controversial	Lung cancer, lung abnormalities
14. Eye exam	Every year	Vision correction, glaucoma, eye abnormalities

What You Can Do

WHAT	WHEN	WHY—SCREENING FOR
15. HIV test (via blood chemistry analysis)	At least once for anyone who has engaged in risky sexual behavior or injected recreational drugs	HIV, which can lead to AIDS
16. Hep B and C screen (via blood chemistry analysis)	At least once for anyone who has engaged in risky sexual behavior, injected recreational drugs, or received a blood transfusion before 1993 (hep C)	For hepatitis B and C
17. Audiogram (hearing exam)	Only if problems exist	Hearing loss or abnormalities
18. Dental cleaning and exam	Every six months	Cavities, mouth cancer, gum disease

Self-Exams and Preventive Measures

WHAT	WHEN	WHY—SCREENING FOR
1. Skin exam (look for anything new or changes in size, shape, color of existing skin abnormalities)	Every month	Skin cancer, precancerous abnormalities
2. Testicular self-exam (roll testes between thumb/fingers for change in size, heft, or feel)	Every month	Testicular cancer, abnormalities
3. Flu shot	Every October	To prevent influenza
4. Pneumonia shot (discuss with your doctor first)	One shot at 50; one booster 5–7 years	To prevent potentially lethal infection by the pneumococcal bacterium

WHAT	WHEN	WHY—SCREENING FOR
5. Immunization shots for hepatitis A and B.	Immediately	Even when not traveling or into high risk activities (shared needles, unsafe sex), it's definitely recommended because accidental exposure is relatively easy and can cause numerous medical problems that are totally avoidable with immunization
6. Tetanus/diptheria booster	Every 10 years	To prevent life-threatening tetanus and diptheria

These screening recommendations are based on the recommendations of the Preventive Health Task Force and the Advisory Committee on Immunization Practices, and are modified considerably by Gordon's own medical practice and experience, as well as his own biases.

EXERCISE

It's 5:45 A.M. You're lying in bed, comfortable and warm, and sound asleep. Pamela Lee Anderson is asking you to rub some tanning lotion on her back.

Suddenly the alarm goes off.

What the hell . . . the alarm usually goes off at 6:30. Then it hits you, you set the alarm to ring earlier because today you're going to start exercising. But, man, the bed feels so good, and Pamela is beckoning.

Are you going to break through inertia and get going, or are you going to roll over and go back to sleep?

That's the critical moment of any exercise program. Once you've gotten up and started working out, there's little chance you'll break off your routine in the middle because you're lazy, tired, or uninterested. The moment of truth is right there at the very beginning. That's where you have to distill your intentions down to the purest possible form and concentrate on your goal: "I need to get myself in shape; I want to look and feel better."

You also need to choose wisely the kind of exercises you're going to do. If you've

What You Can Do

always hated running, don't pick running as your fitness activity. Be realistic. If you think maybe you like swimming, but you haven't been in the water in fifteen years, you're probably not going to stick with it for long. Most men in their fifties find that walking is very realistic, either outside or on a treadmill. Keep in mind, though, that the best kind of exercise is the one that you'll keep doing.

Once you've decided to start an exercise program, the options are nearly endless: professional gym, personal trainer, in-home fitness equipment, jogging, walking. Because a personal trainer or a gym's trainer will guide patrons through the exercise process, this section is written for those of you who have not exercised before or are returning to exercise after years away, and are planning to exercise on your own. All the exercises suggested in this section are ones that can be done at home, at the office, or in a hotel room, and without the use of specialized equipment or devices.

Before you start actually exercising, though, the first step is to visit a doctor. No man in his fifties—if he hasn't exercised before or only did it years before—should start an exercise program without first checking with his doctor for potential problems (specifically heart-related), as well as for suggestions on how to proceed. Once you've been given a clean bill of health, you can start exercising.

General Points on Exercise

- Motivation is the key factor to starting and maintaining an exercise routine. Find some reason(s) that will get you exercising every day (or at least three times a week).

- Make your exercise program part of your regular daily routine, so that you actually miss it if you don't do it. You want to reach the point where you don't feel like your day is complete without your exercise session. This is called a "positive addiction."

- Actively resist boredom by using a Walkman, the radio, recorded books, or the TV—all of which can make time pass more quickly during your exercise routines.

- Set reachable short-term goals for positive reinforcement early in the effort, as well as long-term goals to keep you stimulated even after you've obtained your short-term goals.

- Be realistic about results. Know that you won't see or feel results for many weeks, if not months, depending on your exercise regimen and what you hope to accomplish.

- Start with some kind of aerobic exercise (walking, jogging, bike riding), making sure that stretching is also in your routine. Strengthening can come later, once you're well on your way.

- Start slow and small and work your way up. Remember, even a small amount of exercise helps.

- Just getting up off the couch is critical, because then inertia is broken, and you can start riding a little of your own momentum.

- Don't expect to feel the "endorphin rush" that exercisers talk about for quite some time. You have to be in pretty good shape to get the good feelings that come from your body's production of those brain chemicals involved in reducing pain and enhancing pleasure.

- Don't exercise within three hours of bedtime, or you might end up struggling to sleep.

When exercising, the most important parts of a fifties male body to protect are the joints, specifically the shoulders, ankles, knees, and hips. Properly conditioned feet and spine are also critical to being able to maintain and increase incrementally your exercise program. If you prepare these body parts properly, they will take you to whatever exercise goals you have set. It's not the lungs that ultimately dictate how much exercise you can do, it's your joints, ligaments, and tendons (see chapter 2 for details).

The three basic kinds of exercise are aerobics, stretching, and strengthening.

Aerobic Exercises

Aerobics is, by far, the most critical type of exercise. It is defined as any rhythmic form of exercise, involving groups of large muscles, that can be sustained for a long enough period to raise the heart rate and shift your anaerobic (storing) metabolism into aerobic (burning) metabolism. Basically, aerobic exercise is anything that can get your heart pumping more than normal. Walking, jogging, stationary bicycling, treadmill walking, cross-country skiing, swimming, and rowing can all be aerobic exercises.

The real "magic" about aerobic exercise takes place when it shifts your metabolism from a storage mode into a fat-burning mode. This only happens, however, after at least 20 minutes of sustained aerobic exercise. To get the full beneficial impact of aerobic exercise, it's best to exercise at least thirty minutes a day, at least three times a week. That's when you'll start to see some weight loss (as long as you're not overcompensating by eating lots more food).

When exercising aerobically, a long-range goal should be to sustain exercise at approximately 65 to 85 percent of your maximum heart rate, while *never* taking your heart rate to its maximum.

How do you find your maximum heart rate?

It's roughly calculated at 220 minus your age. For a fifty-five-year-old man, the maximum heart rate is 165—a figure that should never be reached. When aerobically exercising, this man should consistently get his heart rate up between 107 and 140 beats per minute (best at 120–140), which is approximately 65 to 85 percent of his maximum heart rate.

Many pieces of fitness equipment have heart monitoring devices attached, or you can buy a strap-on monitor. Or you can count your pulse. To count your own pulse, first find your pulse either in your neck (under your jaw, in the notch between your side neck muscle and your wind pipe), or on the thumb side of the inside of your arm, just below your wrist. Count the beats for ten seconds and multiply by six, or count them for fifteen seconds and multiply by four.

After you've been exercising for a few months, and checking your heart rate regularly, you should be able to sense the feeling when you're working out at 65 to 85 percent of your maximum heart rate. A good general rule: While you're exercising you should have enough "wind" to talk, but not enough wind to sing. Additionally, if you're relatively fit and stop exercising for a minute, your heart rate should slow down significantly from the start of that minute to the end of the minute.

Some Good Aerobic Exercises

Cross-country skiing (stationary or outdoors). Probably the best aerobic exercise because of the vigorous movement of the large leg muscle groups and the large arm and upper chest muscle groups.

Downhill skiing. A good aerobic workout if pursued vigorously, but depending on your intensity (and propensity to fall), skiing can be hard on your joints, especially your knees. The "cruising" down easy slopes that's done by many skiers in their fifties will never get you into the fat-burning aerobic metabolism. Keep in mind your age, and be honest about your current abilities—can you really handle that double black diamond run, or is that your evil, twenty-year-old self whispering in your ear?

Jogging and speed walking. Excellent aerobic exercises. (See the sidebar in this chapter for details.)

Stationary bicycle. Good for aerobic exercise with low impact on joints, tendons, and ligaments, because your legs don't go through the entire range of motion that can cause damage. Especially good for people with bad knees or those recuperating from knee surgery. You can get as good a workout as you want on a stationary bike, because you can set the tension of the bicycle to your level of fitness.

Outdoor bicycling. While bicycling is good exercise (see above), outdoor bicycling is not recommended because of the potential for accidents—slipping, sliding, hitting immovable objects, collisions with cars—and even death. Additionally, street bike rides are not as aerobically beneficial as a stationary bike workout—there's too much "coasting" involved. If you do ride, make sure to wear a good, protective helmet, and obey all traffic laws.

Swimming and pool exercises. Because of the body's natural buoyancy, pool activities aren't as good aerobically as other exercises, but they are excellent for anyone with joint problems, such as arthritis, because there's less impact on the joints than with out-of-the-water activities.

Rowing machine. If used correctly (maintaining the right posture and form), rowing is an excellent aerobic exercise with a minimal chance of joint damage.

Team sports. By the time most men reach our age group, they've hung up their cleats, put away their mitts, stored their Air Jordans. Most of us know that many team sports have a high injury potential for guys in their fifties. For those of you who haven't learned—the guys who have joined the weekend softball team—remember to do a substantial amount of warming up and stretching before playing, try not to sprint or make sudden twisting moves (major causes of injuries), and generally cut your body some slack. Don't ask your body to perform as it did when it was eighteen; your body's likely to let you down if you do. Age-group team sports (the over-fifty league) may be the safest way to continue to compete in a beloved sport.

Tennis and other racket sports. Racket sports are good, because you can completely control how much exercise you get, although it can be hard on joints (especially knees). Remember to do lots of stretching and warming up before playing, and be careful of sudden moves, twists, or turns (where injuries most often occur).

What You Can Do

Golf. Not exactly exercise, but at least golf gets you away from the office, makes you walk around outside, and, if you can control your temper, helps you unwind from the daily stresses of life. If your pulse starts imitating your score (100 or higher), you might want to consider some other "leisure" activity.

Stretching Exercises

You're in the middle of a long stressful day at the office. You're exhausted from a sleepless night. You're two-thirds of the way home on a long flight. You're zoned out from lounging on a couch watching a full day of TV football.

SO WHAT'S YOUR POISON?
TO WALK OR TO RUN?

Walkers and joggers are a little like cross-country skiers and downhill skiers, Democrats and Republicans—neither side is ever going to fully appreciate the other's viewpoint.

Walking—as defined by always having at least one foot on the ground—is a less jarring exercise for the joints, tendons, ligaments, feet, and spine than running. It is easier for those who have never exercised before to start walking. There's less chance of injury or accident. The downside is that even with speed walking, it's difficult to get the heart rate up to levels needed for a complete aerobic workout. Swinging your arms, especially if you're carrying weights, will raise your heart rate, or if you're walking on a treadmill, increase the incline for a heavier workout.

Running—as defined by periodically having both feet off the ground at the same time—definitely gives a better aerobic workout than walking. And, if properly conditioned and prepared, the joints, tendons, ligaments, feet, and spine can handle the rigors of jogging, even if you start in your fifties. The downsides are that more injuries and accidents do occur with running, and it is normally more difficult for those who have never exercised to start jogging than walking.

Proper foot gear is extremely important for both walking and running, as is finding a physician who is interested in treating any injury while keeping you active in your chosen sport.

A runner's question for walkers: Do you ever break a sweat?

A walker's question for joggers: Why don't you ever look like you're having fun? (Gordon is a jogger; Jeff is a walker.)

No matter the scenario, physically and mentally, you feel beat. Suddenly your body, of its own accord, begins a long and luxurious cat-like stretch. It feels as if every muscle and bone is getting into the act, moving separately and yet as one. When it's done, you feel surprisingly refreshed—maybe it is time to get off the couch and do something.

Welcome to the benefits of stretching—an underrated but highly important part of any serious exerciser's routine. In fact, every man in his fifties should be doing some kind of stretching. While you can reach a reasonable level of fitness without doing any strengthening exercises, you can't reach that same level without doing some kind of stretching.

Stretching is important because the natural tendency of muscle at rest is to shorten, or stiffen. When you stretch you help to keep your muscles—and your joints, tendons, and ligaments—loose and supple, which protects them from being damaged or injured at times of sudden moves, twists, turns, or impacts.

It's best to stretch after you've done a few warmup activities, such as walking, to get the circulation going and to soften up the muscles a bit. It's not a good idea to stretch the moment you get out of bed. You get more benefit from stretching if you do it either during, or after, aerobic exercise. Try breaking up your exercise routine with a little stretching.

All stretching should be done with a slow and steady pressure to a point just this side of discomfort. Stretching is not supposed to hurt. When you reach that point just short of discomfort, hold the position for ten to fifteen seconds, then slowly release. Never do "ballistic stretches," where you bounce the body part you're stretching—that bouncing can cause damage.

A good stretching program only takes about five to ten minutes a day, and yet it can be tremendously beneficial. The sport or activity you're doing will determine what muscle groups need to be stretched, although, generally speaking, the most critical muscle groups are the lower back, the hamstrings, the upper back, shoulders, and neck.

Stretching of the Lower Back

This is critical because the lower back is so important in sitting, standing, lying down, and overall structural health. Here are some specific exercises that stretch the lower back, but in different ways (all are equally good for you):

- Lie on your back, draw both knees to your chest, bringing them closer and holding them to your chest with your arms.

- Lie on your back and push that reverse curve you have in your lower back flat against the floor. This not only stretches the lower back, but also strengthens

What You Can Do

the stomach—it's the stomach muscles that you're working to flatten that back curve.

- Lie on your left side. The left leg should be straight out in line with your body. Bend the right leg so the knee is touching the floor at a point parallel to your waist. Stretch the left arm out in front of you as if you're pointing to something. The right arm should be bent at the elbow. Move that right elbow so it is reaching back behind you—meaning you're twisting your upper body in the opposite direction from your hips. Move to where the position is a little uncomfortable, then hold it for ten seconds. Change sides and repeat.

Stretching the Hamstrings

Many people think the hamstrings run along the inside of the upper thigh and into the groin. In fact, hamstrings run from the back of the buttocks down the back of the legs and connect to the back of the knee. Here are some exercises to stretch the hamstrings, but in different ways (all are equally good for you):

- Stand on your left leg with your right leg outstretched and propped on a table, fence, or something that's about waist high. Then lean forward slowly from the waist, which stretches the hamstring of the right leg. Change legs and repeat.

- Stand about three feet from a wall. Put both hands on the wall at a point about chest high. Move your left leg forward so the knee is bent and the foot is flat on the floor. Keeping your right foot flat on the floor, lean your upper body forward into the wall, which stretches your right leg's hamstring. Change legs and repeat.

- Sit on the floor with both legs outstretched in line with your body, but with the right leg slightly bent at the knee so that it's raised off the floor. Slowly bring your head down toward the bent right knee, which stretches the left leg's hamstring. Change legs and repeat.

- Sit upright in a chair, take your left leg and do a man's leg cross where your left ankle is resting on your right knee. Keeping the left ankle on your right knee (to use as a pivot point), take your left hand and push your left knee up and over toward the right leg. You should feel your left outer butt stretching, which means your "glutes" and upper hamstring are being stretched. To intensify the effort, at the same time move your upper body in the opposite direction. Change legs and repeat.

- Lie on your back, bend the left leg at the knee and bring the knee up to your chest. Wrap your arms around it and gently pull to your chest, which stretches the right leg's hamstring. Change legs and repeat.

Stretching for the Upper Back, Shoulders, and Neck

This is where much of daily tension is registered. Here are some stretches to relieve these areas, but in different ways (all equally good for you):

- Take your left hand and reach back behind your head as if you're trying to scratch your right shoulder blade. Your elbow should be behind your head and the highest point in the air. Try to reach further and further back in slow, steady efforts. Change arms and repeat.

- With your left hand behind your head, grasp your left wrist with your right hand, or grip the left elbow with your right hand; then pull slowly and steadily. Change arms and repeat.

- Take a towel and stretch it tight between your hands. Raise your hands over your head and pull from side to side so that the towel and your hands sway from side to side.

- Take the left hand and reach across your chest to grasp the opposite shoulder. The right hand should then grasp the left elbow and slowly pull the elbow further to the right. Change arms and repeat.

- Sit or stand upright and let your head fall forward so your chin is nearly touching your chest. Using no hands, slowly pull your head as far down as possible, then gently move your head in a clockwise, then counterclockwise, rotation, stretching as far as possible with each rotation, rolling your head over your shoulders.

Stretching for Other Areas of the Body

Every body part does need some kind of stretching, although certain areas are harder to stretch than others. These are some recommended stretches for various parts of the body (all are equally good for you):

- **For the Achilles tendon.** Sit on the floor with your legs outstretched in line with your body, take a towel, and wrap it around the left foot's toes, then pull the towel toward you. Repeat with the right leg.

What You Can Do

- **To strengthen and stretch the sole of your foot, which helps plantar fasciitis** (see chapter 2 for details). Sit in a chair with your shoes off and place a towel on the floor in front of you. Keeping your left heel in one place, pull the towel toward you with your left toes.

DON'T LET THE CATTLE CAR STOP YOU
STRETCHING ON LONG AIRPLANE FLIGHTS

During any flight of more than two hours, passengers should stretch their feet, legs, and thighs. This will not only relieve the boredom and give you a feeling of refreshment, it will also help guard against a potentially deadly ailment—a deep-vein thrombosis—in which a blood clot forms in the lower extremities during periods of prolonged inactivity. (Taking an aspirin before a flight can also help prevent a deep-vein thrombosis, but check with your doctor first.) While in your seat, every twenty minutes or so:

- Stretch out a leg as far as you can, then rotate your foot in wide circles. Using only your foot and leg muscles, pull back your toes toward your shin as far as possible, then thrust them forward like a ballerina. Repeat with the other foot.

- Flex your feet muscles by pulling your toes in toward the soles of your feet.

- Contract your calf muscles repeatedly, without moving your legs.

- Contract your thigh muscles repeatedly, without moving your legs.

- Clench and unclench your buttock muscles.

Walk up and down the aisle every hour or so, if possible. When you're standing in the aisle or waiting in line for the lavatory:

- Rise up and down on your toes to stretch your leg muscles.

- Bring one knee up to your waist, then pull it up toward your chest with your arms.

- Stretch your arms and twist your upper body around to loosen tight muscles.

- Pump or clench all the muscle groups that you did while you were sitting.

• **For carpal tunnel (repetitive motion) problems,** such as with typing or using a computer mouse. Stop every hour or so to stretch your shoulders and forearms. Hold your left arm out straight and cock your hand up or down so your fingers are perpendicular to your arm. Then, with the right hand, push the cocked left hand toward your body to the point where there's discomfort, but not pain. Hold it there for ten to fifteen seconds, then release. Repeat, cocking with right hand and pushing with left.

Strengthening Exercises

Is rising from your chair unaided an important issue to you?

If you're a healthy fifties male, probably not.

And yet, when you get to be ninety, it just might be. We can learn a lot from a group of ninety-year-olds in New England who were put on a muscle-strengthening program (see chapter 2 for details). With no other changes to their lifestyle, these men and women experienced significant health benefits from strengthening exercises—not the least of which was that a substantial number were once again able to rise out of their chairs unaided and walk without the use of a cane—important issues when you get to be that age.

What's the lesson for us healthy fifties males?

Strengthening should play a part in any exercise program, along with aerobic exercise and stretching. Strengthening actually helps build stamina, something that most people want more of. The more muscle strength, the greater the stamina. And, as a real incentive, strengthening can allow you to eat more—bigger muscles burn more calories, even at rest, than fat does.

Three Methods of Strengthening Exercises

Isometric exercises. You create the resistance for the muscle to push or pull against, which will strengthen it. Good for beginners and those working at home, but benefits aren't as big or as quick as with other strengthening methods.

Weight-lifting or weight-resistance machines. Found in professional gyms or health clubs, they are highly effective for targeting specific muscles for strengthening. They're safe to use, because professionals at the club will set you up and monitor your progress.

What You Can Do

Free weights. Also called barbells or dumbbells. They are a little more versatile than exercise machines, but there is a greater chance of injury. It is also difficult for beginners and/or people working out at home to handle free weights correctly and safely.

It takes a high level of understanding and knowledge to do strengthening exercises correctly so that you avoid injury and get the most out of the workout. This is why strengthening routines can be best developed, nurtured, and monitored in a professional gym. (Many community colleges and neighborhood recreation centers also offer weight-lifting classes.) The next best option is to use professional weight-lifting/weight-resistance home equipment (following all instructions to the letter). The third option is to create your own home strengthening program of free weights, correctly and safely.

What muscles should you concentrate on?

For general fitness, the strengthening of the back side of your lower extremities is important, as is the strengthening of the quadriceps on the front of your thighs and the stomach muscles. For more aesthetic reasons, many people also work to strengthen their biceps (upper arms), pectorals (upper chest muscles), and latissimus dorsi (the side chest muscles that run vertically from your underarm down to your waist).

Strengthening Exercises for Lower Extremity Backside Muscles

These include those of your butt, your hamstrings, and calves.

• Bicycling, walking, or running—all good to strengthen backside muscles.

Strengthening Exercises for the Quadriceps (Thigh) Muscles

A tremendously important set of muscles for fifties men is the "quads"—the four-part muscle group on the front of your thighs. Used in walking to pick up your legs, the quads also help to keep your knees properly stabilized and supported, especially in the back and forth motion of the knee. If you feel your knees hurting after downhill skiing or even walking downhill, it may be, in part, due to weak quads. Most people don't realize that walking and running don't do anything to improve or strengthen the quads. The best way to exercise quads is through a Nautilus or Cybex machine, but that takes going to a gym. For those working at home, try these exercises:

• Stand with your feet a little away from the wall and with your back against the wall, then slide down the wall until your knees are bent, as if in a sitting position. Hold this position for as long as your quads can take it.

• Sit in a chair, and bring your left knee up toward your chest. Take a towel in both hands and throw it around your left shin. Then try to push your left leg out straight as you hold the towel tight with both hands. You should see your quads bulge as they fight to push through the towel. Repeat with the right leg.

• Sit in a chair, with both feet flat on the floor, and put on ankle weights. Lift the left foot a few inches off the floor. Swing the lower left leg out so it lines up with the thigh, straightening your entire leg. That's moving your lower leg from 90 degrees (the lower leg at a right angle to the thigh) to 180 degrees (the lower leg straight out in line with the thigh). When you start doing repetitions of this exercise, do *not* put your leg through this entire motion (90 degrees to 180 degrees), because it puts unnecessary stress on your knee joint. Work your lower left leg from about 120 degrees to 180 degrees. The amount of weight on your ankles should vary with your level of fitness (greater weights for higher level of fitness). Repeat with the right leg.

Strengthening Exercises for Stomach Muscles

Your stomach muscles are critical to giving proper support to your lower back.

• **Crunches, or sit-ups.** Lie on your back and keep your knees bent, then bring your head and shoulders up toward your waist. Your arms can be at your side, lying across your chest, or clasped behind your head, but don't cheat and pull your head up with your arms.

• **Push-ups.** Old fashioned, maybe, but they are effective in strengthening the stomach muscles, the arm muscles, and the chest muscles. Remember, no stomach touching the floor—the stomach should be held tight in place so that your chest gets closest to the ground.

A Specific Exercise Plan for an Average Guy

Okay, you've found motivating factors or reasons that will keep you focused on an exercise program. Now what?

What You Can Do

It's time to build a program.

Remember to be realistic about what you can do and tie your program into what interests you. So, if you've never been a runner, don't suddenly decide to become one. Also, realize that everyone will start out differently, depending upon overall health factors. The 300-pound man who has a hard time walking from the parking lot to his workplace is going to start out at a much lower level than the man who is relatively fit and only ten to fifteen pounds overweight. A doctor can help you determine where you stand in this regard.

Following is an exercise program example that you can work from to create your own unique and individual routine. It has been created for Sam, a fifty-five-year-old man, generally in good health, carrying fifteen pounds of extra weight, who did play some sports in high school, has not worked out or exercised since college, but does weekend yard work. He's now motivated to get back into some kind of shape, but is worried about what he should do and how he can keep from accidently hurting himself.

The Ultimate Goal

To reach thirty to forty-five minutes of aerobic exercise four to five days a week. During each workout, Sam's heart rate should hit 107 to 140 beats per minute (65 to 85 percent of his maximum heart rate) and stay there for most of the workout.

The Specific Walking Exercise Program

After a full health assessment from his doctor, Sam should:

1. Go to a good fitness shoe store and talk with a knowledgeable salesperson about what he hopes to do, so he can find the best exercise shoe for his regimen. Remember that much of a shoe's beneficial support structure breaks down before the tread wears out.

2. Start walking. It's the easiest, least obtrusive exercise around. Maybe it's outside, in a shopping mall, or on a home treadmill or NordicTrack. No matter what the method, walking is the best way for a beginner like Sam to start. Sam should determine the best time to do his walking (before work, lunch time, after work), then stick to that time—make the walking part of his everyday routines.

3. Start walking at a reasonable pace and walk for ten minutes, at least three days a week. Initially, he should be a little out of breath by the end of each walk, and maybe a little sore in the joints, feet, muscles, and back. The soreness should not be so much that he has trouble getting around; if it is, he's pushing too hard and should back off a little.

4. Swing his arms while walking, which helps increase aerobic exercise.

5. Keep walking at the same speed and the same length of time until he's had a few days of not being out of breath at the end of the walk and is not feeling sore. This might take a week or two, which is good because it not only conditions his lungs, but also helps condition the most important parts of the body when it comes to exercise—the feet, legs, knees, hips, and back.

6. Be able to walk for ten minutes comfortably. Sam should then slowly increase his walking speed and the duration of his walk, so he's back to being a little out of breath by the end of the walk. He might even feel slight soreness returning to his joints, feet, or back.

7. Remember that before any new increase in his routine's speed or length, he should go at least three to four days without breathlessness or soreness.

8. Take a couple of months or longer to go from ten minutes to thirty minutes of walking. But that's okay—the most important thing is to continue to exercise as frequently as possible.

9. Try to increase the frequency of his walks to at least four or five times a week. While three days a week of walking is the minimum, there is no maximum, as long as Sam likes the walking and it feels good.

10. Incorporate stretching into his routine as he increases his walking. The best time to stretch is after he's walked a few minutes or at the end of the walk. All he needs is ten minutes or so of stretching. (See the previous section on stretching.)

11. Begin to incorporate a little strengthening into his walking and stretching program. This can be done at a separate time and place (see the previous section on strengthening), or it can be incorporated into his walking routine by the use of wrist or ankle weights (check with the doctor before using them).

12. Also do other healthy activities throughout his day, such as taking stairs wherever and whenever he can, and parking as far from building entrances as possible.

13. Be very conscious of what he eats (see the following diet section), so he can maximize his exercise efforts and lose the extra fifteen pounds he's carrying around.

How will Sam be able to tell if his walking program is working?

If he has been able to increase his walking increments faster and faster with little soreness, this is a sign he's getting into better and better shape. If Sam is watching what he eats as well, he should have dropped at least half of his excess fifteen pounds within a month or so. By that same time, Sam also should begin to feel significantly better in an overall healthy sort of way. The good feelings generated by the exercise should last well into the rest of the day, should help him sleep better at night, and maybe even put a new spring in his step.

Even if Sam has reached part of his goal—the thirty to forty-five minutes of walking four to five days a week—he might not be able to reach the other part of his goal: keeping his heart rate at 107-140 beats per minutes for a short time. To do this, Sam either needs to do some serious speed walking during his routine, or consider upping the ante—shifting to jogging, moving to a NordicTrack machine, or otherwise engaging in a more strenuous aerobic workout of some kind. While the effort is definitely more intense, the rewards are far greater than from just walking.

DIET

Nearly every minute of every day it seems as if another fad diet is being born, hyped, then forgotten. Eat certain foods only at certain times. Eat a grapefruit before and after every meal. Eat mostly proteins. Eat mostly carbohydrates. Return to a caveman diet of twigs and berries.

No doubt there are numerous good diet books out there, but often they are buried in the avalanche of misguided, inaccurate, and sometimes downright dangerous self-help diet books. Rather than wade into the morass of diet-book critiquing, we're going to offer some general, sound principles of eating right. You can take it from there.

To begin with, you should drop the concept of "going on a diet." If somebody "goes on" a diet, that implies that someday he will probably "go off" the diet as well. Additionally, both experience and logic show that the more extreme a diet seems to be—the more it deviates from what we all tend to know is a fairly conventional, middle-of-the-road, well-balanced diet—the harder it will be to sustain over a long period of time. Which means the more resounding your failure is going to be when you fall off such a dietary band wagon. So why even climb aboard?

What you need to do—if you are truly committed to losing weight and eating right as a way of maintaining good health over a lifetime—is to develop eating habits that are sustainable for an entire lifetime, not just until you've lost those extra fifteen pounds. This takes an understanding of how nutrition and your body work together.

Nutrition Basics

Our bodies need a variety of nutrients to function properly, all of which we get from the various foods we eat and drink. Nutrients include:

Water. Without this we could not exist for more than a few days. About 60 percent of a man's body weight is water, and practically every one of the millions of chemical reactions that goes on in the body needs water as a base. It is also critical for absorption, digestion, circulation, and waste removal. Drink six to eight ten-ounce glasses a day (see the hydration sidebar in chapter 4 for details).

Protein. The body's primary building material. Digestion breaks down protein into smaller components that become the main building blocks for bones, muscle, blood, antibodies, skin, hair, and the like.

Fat. The primary storage form of energy, fat also combines with protein to form the membrane around every cell in the body. Fat comes from either animals or plants. While we all need fat in our diet, too much fat can be dangerous to our health, because it increases our chances of heart disease. Fat comes in four types:

1. **Saturated fats.** Found in meats and dairy products, such as butter, ice cream, cheese, and whole milk, these are the worst kinds of fat because they raise the level of bad cholesterol (LDL) in our blood. Saturated fats are usually solid at room temperature, although they are liquid in coconut and palm oils. Many food manufacturers use saturated fats in their processing, so if you don't read labels, you can be consuming saturated fats without realizing it.

2. **Trans-fatty acids.** Found in vegetable shortening and some types of margarine that have been processed with hydrogen (hydrogenated) to make them solid and to help preserve them, these are almost as bad for you as

saturated fats, because they raise bad cholesterol levels and lower good cholesterol (HDL). Manufactured foods like cookies, crackers, pastries, and other "convenience" foods are usually made with trans-fatty acids.

3. **Polyunsaturated fats.** Found in vegetable oils like corn, safflower, sunflower, cottonseed, and soybean, they aren't too bad, although they do lower HDL while not affecting LDL. They are liquid at room temperature.

4. **Monounsaturated fats.** Found in canola and olive oils, these are the fats that are good for you, helping your body to lower bad cholesterol without affecting your good cholesterol levels. These are also liquid at room temperature.

Carbohydrates. The main source of energy for our body, "carbs" or "carbos" are also a major source of vitamins and minerals. There are two kinds of carbohydrates:

1. **Simple.** These are sugars such as sucrose, fructose, and galactose, which are the primary fuel sources of the body.

2. **Complex.** These are starches and fibers. Fiber can be soluble (dissolves in water) or insoluble (doesn't dissolve). Fiber helps relieve constipation by keeping everything moving during digestion. Fiber-rich diets may delay the absorption of carbohydrates, thus preventing post-meal "spikes" of elevated blood sugar (very important to avoid spikes if you're a diabetic).

Vitamins. A group of organic compounds necessary for normal growth, development, and metabolism. The "circular" definition of a vitamin is a substance required in trace amounts to prevent a well-defined vitamin deficiency. Vitamins need to be consumed because, with a few exceptions, the body cannot make them.

Minerals. Inorganic substances, such as iron and zinc, are necessary for proper growth and functioning. They need to be consumed. (See the following section for details.)

Calories: Where They Fit In

Strictly speaking, they're a unit of measurement for the energy our bodies generate or "burn." For the sake of simplicity, think of calories as energy.

Our bodies constantly require energy for the complex systems and functions they run, from brain activity to jumping jacks. While it's obvious that our bodies need and use energy when we're exercising, it's not so obvious that, even when we're sleeping, our bodies need energy to maintain various life-support systems, like heartbeat, respiration, and cell repair.

Our bodies get their energy (calories) from three types of nutrients: carbohydrates, proteins, and fats. One gram of carbohydrates provides about four calories. One gram of protein also supplies about four calories. On the other hand, one gram of fat provides a whopping nine calories. Alcohol—which if you indulge, needs to be remembered, when creating an eating plan—is not a nutrient, but it provides energy, too—about seven calories per gram.

Critical to the entire process is that most calories not used relatively soon after consumption are stored as fat for the body's future energy needs.

This means that any health-conscious person needs to keep track of calories—where you get them, how many you eat, and how many your body uses (burns). For those trying to control their weight, it's a straightforward equation: If you take in more calories than you use, you are going to gain weight. If you use more calories than you take in, you're going to lose weight.

Complicating matters is the fact that this calorie intake/use relationship is not static. Our bodies have been designed to adjust and react to feast or famine. If there is a drastic limiting of calories (as when food is scarce or you go on a crash diet), the body's survival mechanism (our metabolism) senses that we're heading for a famine, so it makes the body run a little leaner and starts storing reserves of fat for the upcoming famine. On the other hand, if calories are abundant (we have lots to eat), the body is a little bit more reckless in its use of calories, and we don't store as much fat.

Additionally, the tendency to put on weight is partly genetic, through the so-called "thrifty gene" trait. If you have this gene, it means your body handles calories very efficiently (burning calories judiciously; storing the rest as fat). While this means your body will be less likely to perish in a famine, it also means your body is much more likely to become obese during times of plenty. Looking around at the general size of our American population today, guess what era (famine or plenty) we're living in now?

It would seem obvious from studying calories that the most efficient gathering of calories would be from eating mostly fats and drinking mostly alcohol—the two substances that provide the greatest number of calories per gram. Sounds like a great diet—deep-fried cheese balls, ice cream, and booze—right?

The problem is that it isn't just a matter of calories. For one thing, our bodies can't live without the nutrition provided by carbos, proteins, vitamins, and minerals. And fat may provide calories, but saturated fat also provides the building blocks for the body to produce cholesterol, which is a major contributor to heart disease. When it comes to cholesterol, keep in mind that it isn't so much the amount of cholesterol you eat that's important or that registers as your cholesterol level, it's how much your body produces and whether or not it can flush any excess from the system. Cholesterol in our diet is a nearly negligible source of cholesterol in our blood stream—which means that when a product is advertised as being cholesterol-free, the information isn't as important as most people think.

How Many Calories Should You Consume Daily?

Many health organizations, including the American Heart Association, agree that no more than 30 percent of calories should come from fat (with less than 10 percent of that 30 percent being from saturated fats). To put that in perspective, today's average eater gets about 40 to 50 percent of calories from fat, while some extreme diets advocate a meager 10 to 20 percent. To some people, a diet restricted to 10 to 20 percent percent fat is like eating sticks and bark. The sad truth is that fat is tasty—greasy burgers, chips, ice cream—and it's what ends up on our waistlines.

What about the remaining 70 percent of calories—where should we get them?

Dietary experts say that at least half of your daily calories should come from carbohydrates, with the remaining 20 percent coming from various other sources. If you don't have carbs in your system, your body will draw its energy from fat or protein. This is okay in the short run (you lose weight by burning stored fat), but in the long run it can lead to muscle tissue breakdown and a dangerous condition called "starvation ketosis."

How do you make sense of any of this? What does it mean to you?

Let's put it in a perspective most can understand. In a world where a Big Mac is 550 calories (mostly from fat), the average fifties guy who's not watching what he eats is probably consuming anywhere from 2,000 to 3,000 calories in a day.

That would be fine, if the average fifties male burned 2,500 to 3,000 calories a day. Unfortunately, that's not the case. Take the corporate executive who doesn't really exercise, spends most of his weekday at the office, or sitting at home watching TV, and does only the occasional weekend warrior thing with yard work. He probably burns from 1,500 to 2,000 calories in an average day. If he takes a fifteen- to twenty-minute brisk walk, he'll probably burn a few hundred more calories.

If you do the math (eat 2,000 to 3,000 calories a day; burn 1,500 to 2,000), that still leaves anywhere from 500 to 1,500 extra calories that the corporate executive has eaten in a day that very well might end up as part of his ever-expanding waistline. A general guideline is that a fairly active, middle-aged man will probably gain weight if he takes in more than about 2,400 calories per day, while he'll lose weight at about 2,000 or fewer calories a day.

Don't forget that you will burn more calories when you exercise (see the exercise section for details), not only during the initial effort, but through the long-term building of muscles, which burn more calories, even at rest, than fat does. Additionally, if you exercise regularly over a period of time, your metabolic set point changes, meaning you will burn more calories even when asleep.

So what should you eat?

Read on to find out.

The Food Guide Pyramid and Federal Nutrition Guidelines

Most Americans have heard about the food guide pyramid. Put out by the U.S. Departments of Agriculture and Health and Human Services and based on *Nutrition and Your Health: Dietary Guidelines for Americans,* the pyramid is an outline of what to eat each day. All foods are placed within six categories, and recommendations are made for a daily amount of servings within each category. The category with the most servings is at the bottom of the pyramid, while the one with the fewest number of servings is at the top.

According to this pyramid, most of your daily servings of food should fall into the two bottom tiers (grains, fruits, and vegetables), while the next tier (meats, diary products) should make up a moderate portion of your daily servings, and the top (fats, oils, and sugars) should be such a small portion of your daily intake that there are no recommended daily servings.

Fats, Oils, & Sweets
(USE SPARINGLY)

Milk, Yogurt, & Cheese Group
(2-3 SERVINGS)

Meat, Poultry, Fish, Dry Beans, Eggs, & Nuts Groups
(2-3 SERVINGS)

Vegetable Group
(3-5 SERVINGS)

Fruit Group
(2-4 SERVINGS)

Bread, Cereal, Rice, & Pasta Group
(6-11 SERVINGS)

Source: U.S. Department of Agriculture/U.S. Department of Health and Human Services

What Constitutes One Serving

Bread, Cereal, Rice, and Pasta: a slice of bread; an ounce of ready-to-eat cereal; one-half cup of cooked cereal, rice, or pasta.

Fruit: a medium apple, banana, orange; one-half cup of chopped, cooked, or canned fruit; three-quarter cup of fruit juice.

Vegetables: a cup of raw leafy vegetables; one-half cup of other vegetables, cooked or chopped raw.

What You Can Do

Meat, Poultry, Fish, Dry Beans, Eggs, and Nuts: two to three ounces of cooked lean meat, poultry, or fish (one-half cup of cooked dry beans, one egg, or two tablespoons of peanut butter count as one ounce of lean meat).

Milk, Yogurt, and Cheese: a cup of milk or yogurt; 1½ ounces of natural cheese; two ounces of processed cheese.

If you try to adapt your eating to the pyramid, you'll find that you will increase your intake of complex carbohydrates and cut down on sugar and fat, especially the saturated fats.

If you're a vegetarian, you can still get all the required amounts of nutrients, but it takes a little bit more work and a greater understanding of the principles of nutrition. You especially have to make sure you're getting enough protein, iron, calcium, and vitamin B12.

Remember that processing often changes what a food has to offer. A perfect example is the lowly potato. When it's raw, baked, steamed, or boiled, it contains approximately 32 calories. When it's turned into French fries, that same potato now has sixty-eight calories—mostly from the fat in which it was fried. When the potato is made into potato chips, it has a whopping 159 calories, mostly from fat used in processing.

Dietary Recommendations

When you're setting up your eating plan, acknowledge that you're only human, that you have food weaknesses, and that your resolve occasionally buckles. Build this into your eating plan by giving yourself a 10- or 15-percent exemption time. Then make sure that the time counts.

For example, if you just love ice cream and believe you can't live without it, use that weakness to keep yourself focused. Tell yourself that you'll reward yourself for staying on the plan all week by indulging in an ice cream fix once during the weekend. Make a ceremony of it. Build up the excitement over having earned this reward through hard work and discipline.

Remember, too, that planning ahead for your entire day will help you avoid moments where you're starving, and when the only food available is fast food (chips, fries, burgers). As we all know, fast food is probably the worst in terms of fat content.

Other General Eating Guidelines

• It's better to have frequent smaller meals during the day than three big meals. We function and feel better if we eat smaller amounts of nutrients on a regular basis.

WHAT IS NATURAL?
PUTTING MODERN HEALTH CARE INTO PERSPECTIVE

A vocal part of today's society supports "natural" things such as herbs, vitamin supplements, and natural methods of healing, such as aromatherapy and reflexology. Much of this movement has developed into a big business that plays off the "natural" theme to sell more product.

While it's true that some items and practices have been shown to have value (see the following vitamin and mineral sections for details), most of what is hyped as "natural" has not yet been proven useful or, in some cases, is actually harmful (e.g., megadoses of vitamin C and certain B vitamins). We only have to look back 100 or so years to see that "natural" was:

- Fifty percent of the childhood population dying before they reached the age of five.

- Epidemics of water-borne diseases such as cholera and typhoid.

- Epidemics of contagious diseases, such as polio, tuberculosis, and rheumatic fever.

- Average life expectancies in the forties.

Doctors, when they save lives, usually use "unnatural" procedures or products (surgery, blood transfusions, antibiotics). In fact, a doctor's working life is dedicated to cheating mother nature as often as possible by preventing "natural" death and disease.

So when it comes to your health, if you feel so inclined, go ahead and take natural substances and try natural healing techniques (making sure to inform your doctor about all of them), but don't do so at the expense of modern medications and scientific practices, or you just might find real nature catching up with you.

- Consume most of your calories at the beginning of the day (about one-third of the day's total calorie intake), for breakfast or lunch. Make dinner the smallest meal of the day, since evening is when your body's in a storage mode and packs away more fat than it burns. This will also help alleviate indigestion and heartburn problems. And don't "graze" between dinner and bedtime.

- Eat slowly. If you eat faster than your "satisfied" mechanism can kick in, you will stuff yourself beyond what you really need. So try to eat a small meal, followed by a ten-minute break. By then, your satisfied mechanism should have kicked in and you probably won't feel the need for more food.

• Eat sitting down. It's easier to eat beyond your needs if you're standing up.

• Fill your plate only two-thirds full, and don't go back for seconds.

• If you eat less, you'll want less. While your stomach doesn't actually "shrink" as you eat smaller portions at every meal, your appetite will "shrink." Within the first week you might feel momentary pangs of hunger, but if you stick to your plan, your appetite will adjust and adapt to the smaller amounts of food. It will then begin signaling that it's satisfied at an earlier point in time than before.

Specific Food Preparation Recommendations

• Trim off all visible fat before you fry up that bacon, or put that steak on the grill.

• Avoid "utility" meats—cold cuts, hot dogs, sausages—which are high in fat.

• Drink a glass of water a few minutes before a meal. It not only helps to keep your body hydrated, but will help give you a satisfied feeling before you eat too much.

• Don't spread butter, jam, margarine, peanut butter, or cheese half an inch thick. Think of the spread as only a flavor- and moisture-enhancer, nothing else. Keep the spreading thin and light.

• Order salads with the dressing on the side, and skip the extras, such as egg, meat, and cheese. Eat only salads made with vegetables and the greens, and use only a slight sprinkling of dressing.

• Skip that sixteen-ounce sirloin—three or four ounces of meat is enough for one meal.

• Eat only nonfat or low-fat dairy products (including low-fat cheese and low-fat cottage cheese).

• Switch to diet soft drinks, or go without. You don't need the 150 calories in regularly sweetened soft drinks.

• Use artificial sweeteners instead of sugar.

• Remember that the less fat you consume the better.

• Avoid nondairy coffee creamer, because it is laden with trans-fatty acids (some of the worst fats).

• Control your alcohol intake. Remember that alcohol is a source of calories that many forget to add into their eating plan. Four ounces of wine, one-and-a-half ounces of hard liquor, and one twelve-ounce beer each have around 150 calories, while a light beer can have around 110. Don't ignore the fact that drinks can make you less likely to follow your eating plan because you lose your inhibitions—you get a case of the "screw its" and end up pigging out.

Some Specific Recommendations on Dieting to Lose Weight

• Make sure your scale works accurately, then check your weight at the same time every day, preferably in the morning.

• Be realistic in setting your weight goal. You're in your fifties, you aren't as athletic as you were in your twenties, and your time is limited.

• Don't set a specific target weight. Set a five-pound range because your weight does fluctuate daily with numerous factors, such as fluid balances.

• Remember that muscle is denser and weighs more than fat, so you might end up staying the same weight or even gaining weight while getting into better and better physical shape.

• Don't berate yourself if you fall off your eating plan. Think of your plan as a sixty-minute game. That means you've only blown a play or two; you still have the rest of the game to play. The situation is definitely salvageable—successful people are those who overcome their setbacks.

Vitamins and Minerals

With only a few exceptions, all vitamins and minerals need to be consumed because the body cannot manufacture them.

What You Can Do

Vitamins are organic compounds that are either water-soluble (any excess is flushed from the body—the B vitamins and vitamin C) or fat-soluble (any excess is stored—vitamins A, D, and E).

Minerals are inorganic substances.

Both vitamins and minerals are necessary for the body's normal growth and functions. In some cases, too much of a vitamin or mineral can be toxic, so a balance must be maintained within the body for proper functioning.

To help people find the correct balance of vitamins and minerals, "recommended dietary allowances" (RDA) have been established. We've all seen product labels telling us what percentage of the RDA of such-and-such vitamin or mineral is satisfied if you eat what's inside.

RDAs come from standards set in 1968 and approved by the Food and Drug Administration. Today, more than thirty years later, those standards have finally been updated. In January 2001 the Institute of Medicine, a private science organization that establishes the nation's RDAs for nutrients, released new figures, which came from four years of reviewing scientific research into vitamins and minerals. Additionally, the Institute has listed, for the first time ever, which popular megadose vitamins can be harmful.

In 2002 the Institute plans to issue another report on how much protein, fat, and fiber we should eat. After that report comes out, the FDA will begin steps to add the new vitamin RDAs to all food labels. Until then, food labels will continue to use the 1968 standards.

To find out what the new RDAs are, go to the Institute of Medicine's Web site (www.iom.edu). Once you've learned what the recommended daily doses are, you can then go to an Agriculture Department site (www.nal.usda.gov/fnic/food-comp) and find out the vitamin and mineral content of certain amounts of certain foods.

Many of the RDAs have not changed drastically, and you can still get most of your daily requirements from a healthy diet that includes at least five servings of fruits or vegetables (see previous section for details). Remember, though, that vitamin supplements are aptly named—they should be used as a supplement to, not a replacement for, your dietary intake. Keep in mind: *A bad diet plus vitamins is still a bad diet.*

Following are some of the most popular nutrients, why they are needed, their new RDAs, any possible harmful effects from mega-doses, and where they can be found in nature.

Vitamin A. Essential for normal vision and immune system function. RDA: 900 micrograms for men, 700 for women. More than 3,000 micrograms a day creates risks of birth defects in pregnant women and liver damage in others. Found in carrots and other dark-colored vegetables and fruits.

Vitamin B12. Aids in red blood cell production. RDA: 2.4 micrograms. People over fifty may have trouble absorbing B12 from natural food sources, so they should eat foods fortified with it (such as breakfast cereals) or take a daily supplement. Found in red meat, eggs, and fish.

Vitamin C. Prevents scurvy (weakness, joint swelling, and bleeding gums). RDA: 75 mg for women, 90 for men, 35 more for smokers. More than 2,000 mg a day can cause diarrhea. Recent studies have suggested that greater than 500 mg of vitamin C per day may have long-term adverse health effects. Found in fresh fruits and vegetables, most notably citrus fruits.

Vitamin D. Essential for normal bone formation and use of calcium and phosphorus in the body. RDA: 200 international units (IU) for people under fifty; 400 IUs for people fifty to seventy. Found in fortified milk, egg yolks, butter, and exposure to sunlight.

Vitamin E. Essential for reproduction, muscle development, and other functions. RDA: 15 mg. Beyond 1,000 mg there is a chance of uncontrolled bleeding. Found in egg yolks, beef liver, and cereals.

Folic Acid. One of the B-complex vitamins, folic acid is essential for cell growth. A deficiency of folic acid may predispose a person to cardiac problems and to certain birth defects in pregnant women. A folic acid deficiency can easily be tested for. RDA: 400 micrograms. Found in green, leafy vegetables, liver, kidney, and whole grain cereals.

Calcium. Needed for bone and tooth formation. RDA for most adults up to fifty: 1,000 mg; for anyone over fifty, 1,200 mg a day. Found in dairy products and calcium-fortified orange juice.

Iron. Necessary for carrying oxygen to cells and for the formation of hemoglobin in the blood. RDA: 8 mg for men and postmenopausal women. Stomach upset can occur with dosages beyond 45 mg. Found in eggs, meat, pigmented vegetables. Except in very unusual circumstances (consult your doctor), men should *never* take iron supplements.

Zinc. An essential component of certain enzymes; needed for proper functioning of taste, smell, and male sexual organs. RDA: 11 mg for men; 8 for women. More than 40 mg a day can block absorption of copper. Found in meat, eggs, nuts, milk, peanut butter, and whole grains.

What You Can Do

A Warning about Vitamins and Minerals

In the last few decades, many people have begun to use vitamins, minerals, and certain herbs (see the following section) more as drugs than as dietary supplements—taking them in much higher doses (megadoses) than the medical community recommends. This trend can be traced back to Nobel prizewinner Linus Pauling, who advocated gigantic doses (ten to twenty grams per day) of vitamin C as a way of preventing everything from colds to cancer. One part of his argument was that any vitamin C the body didn't use was harmlessly flushed from the system. Today, some studies have suggested that such massive doses can create problems, even with this flushing mechanism. The moral, in this case, is that untested megadoses of any vitamin, mineral, or herb are not a good idea.

This is especially true because the FDA views these substances as dietary supplements, not drugs, so they are less rigorously scrutinized. Manufacturing and inspection standards are at a food level rather than the much higher pharmaceutical level. Basically, when it comes to vitamins, minerals, and herbs, the FDA cares only if they are reasonably wholesome—which they are at recommended doses.

L-tryptophan, the melatonin of a few decades ago, is a sad example of what can happen when a dietary supplement starts being taken like a drug. An amino acid, it was used as a sedative and was produced in fairly large amounts by a fairly small number of producers—none of whom had strict quality controls to follow, because L-tryptophan was a dietary supplement, not a drug. Unfortunately a batch became tainted in production, and the end result was a couple of dozen deaths and several hundred extreme disabilities.

An axiom in medicine is that anything doctors give people that produces a good effect can also produce a bad effect in someone. It's naive to think otherwise. That's why it's important that patients tell their doctors what vitamins and food supplements they are taking, and in what doses, so that the doctor can help observe and monitor the situation.

Herbal Supplements

In the last thirty years, people have been rediscovering some of the herbal "medicines" that our distant ancestors used to treat those who were sick. The famous 5,300-year-old iceman, who was found frozen and preserved in the European Alps a few years ago, carried a pouch containing various herbs that have now been shown to have true medicinal effects. Some of our ancestors really did know just how to use roots, twigs, bark, and berries to ease suffering and in some cases, actually cure illnesses.

347

Today, a generation looking for natural remedies has embraced some of that ancient knowledge, causing a multibillion dollar business of herbal, vitamin, and mineral supplements to flourish.

On the bad side of the business, many supposed herbal remedies are still not scientifically proven to be curative, or even beneficial. Many times, demand for such untested products is driven merely by anecdotal evidence (personal experiences).

On the good side of the business, a growing number of herbal supplements have been tested and found to be beneficial for a wide array of ailments, from mild depression to male sexual organ problems.

No matter what the herb, however, everyone should be cautious when initially deciding to taking any herbal supplement. Ask these questions: Have true clinical trials been done on the product? Are there any warnings about who should or should not take the herb? Are there any side effects listed or known? What are the minimum and maximum doses recommended? Is there standardization of the potency or quantity of the active ingredient found in each batch? And, most importantly, what does your doctor say about taking the herb?

Before taking an herbal supplement, remember these principles:

• Herbal supplements, like vitamins, are not closely regulated by the FDA. Not only are medical claims regarding herbals unscrutinized, but there is no way for a consumer to know how much of, or even what, substance is actually present in each batch.

• If you're taking an herb to achieve an effect that can also be achieved by a regulated drug, the drug is nearly always preferable because: (1) FDA regulation ensures that the purity and potency of each drug are uniform, (2) dosing ranges, benefits, and side effects are usually well defined, and (3) you have an ally in managing your condition and its treatment: your doctor.

Herbal/Dietary Supplements That Seem to Have Benefits

Cranberry or blueberry (juice or supplement)—Helps to prevent urinary tract infections because chemicals within them prevent bacteria from "clumping," which is necessary for scattered bacteria in the bladder to invade the bladder wall and cause an actual infection. Large amounts (more than three or four pints a day) often result in diarrhea and other gastrointestinal symptoms.

Echinacea (herb extract)—Taken to prevent colds and/or to reduce the duration and severity of a cold, although no scientific proof exists as yet. Not suggested for those with auto-immune diseases.

Ginkgo biloba (leaf extract)—Has been shown to thin blood, which can have a beneficial effect on arterial disease, blood flow, and even vertigo and tinnitus (ringing in the ears) problems. Reported by some to be beneficial for memory. Side effects can be stomach upset, headaches, or allergic skin reaction. Should not be taken in combination with blood-thinning drugs, including aspirin. May cause unexpected bleeding problems in those undergoing surgery.

Glucosamine and chondroitin sulfate (not herbs)—Marketed for the treatment of arthritis and taken either separately or together, both are compounds found in healthy joints. A Belgian study reported in the medical journal *The Lancet* in January 2001 suggested glucosamine sulfate could be the first treatment to actually slow the progression of osteoarthritis (degenerative arthritis).

Saw palmetto (berry extract)—It may have some benefit for symptoms of benign prostatic hypertrophy (enlargement of the prostate), and it does seem to aid in the healthy functioning of the prostate gland in general, but the scientific evidence is still somewhat sketchy.

St. John's wort (herb extract)—Actually recommended by many doctors in Europe for cases of mild depression, it appears to be fairly effective. Should not be used with prescription antidepressants. Possible side effects at high dosages include photosensitivity, especially in fair-skinned individuals, and allergic reactions in some.

Valerian (root extract)—An aid for restlessness or for sleeping disorders that are based on nervous conditions. No known side effects other than mild stomach upset.

SMOKING AND YOUR DELIVERY SYSTEM

Well, here it is—the lecture on smoking. We're sure you've heard it all before, but we promise it won't be too long or too severe, and we hope you'll find a few new spins on the subject that give you a fresh perspective. For those of you who do still smoke, we hope you'll take a moment to read the following; for those of you who have stopped recently, we'd also suggest you read on.

It should be stated that all sides of the smoking issue have been personally covered by the authors: Gordon has never smoked, but has treated and helped numerous smokers quit; Jeff smoked two packs a day for fifteen years before he quit in

1982 on his own after two unsuccessful attempts. Gordon was instrumental in Jeff's quitting.

The first step for any fifties male smoker is to assess where you and your smoking stand now. In the medical community, the standardized system of measurement is "pack years." It's simple: If you have smoked one pack a day for ten years, then you have accumulated ten pack years. Unfortunately, this also means that if you have consistently smoked two packs a day for ten years, then you have chalked up twenty pack years in the same time. Conversely, though, if you have only smoked a half a pack a day for ten years, then you have accumulated only five pack years.

Before you strike up a cigarette in celebration of how little you have accumulated in pack years, one point should be made. Many doctors agree that there are three things that most male patients lie about to their doctors (and probably to themselves): their sex lives, how much they drink, and how much they smoke. Please remember that doctors cannot do their job fully and completely without accurate information.

This goes double for you—you're not going to get anywhere lying to yourself about your smoking consumption. Don't kid yourself that you don't have to count all your cigarettes because you leave so many burning in the ashtray. We strongly recommend that all smokers use the amount of cigarettes they actually *buy* as an accurate indication of how much they truly smoke.

What Your Total "Pack Years" Means

- One to ten pack years: If you stop now, you should return to normal within the range of a few months to a year or two.

- Ten to twenty pack years: Usually is associated with reversible changes in the lungs and upper respiratory tract, but arterial changes may be more permanent.

- Over twenty pack years: This is the point at which all bets are off. You're treading on ice that's wafer thin. The medical community generally believes the twenty-pack-year mark is where your chances of developing everything from emphysema to lung cancer start skyrocketing.

Smoking Related Stats (this will be as bad as our scare tactics get)

- The National Cancer Institute reports that one-third of all cancer deaths in America are attributable to tobacco use.

What You Can Do

• Cigarette smokers are seventy times more likely to develop lung cancer than nonsmokers.

• Men who smoke increase their risk of death from lung cancer by more than twenty-two times and their risk from bronchitis and emphysema by nearly ten times over nonsmoking men.

• Two out of every five smokers die before sixty-five, compared to only one out of five nonsmokers.

• Smoking is the greatest single risk factor for death that occurs suddenly and unexpectedly.

• Smokers have twice the chance of a heart attack than nonsmokers, and those smokers who do have a heart attack are more likely to die within the hour than nonsmokers.

• Smokers with other risk factors (high cholesterol, high blood pressure) are at higher heart attack risk.

• A nonsmoker who has a partner who smokes has a 30 percent greater chance of developing lung cancer than a nonsmoker with a nonsmoking partner.

• Men in their fifties are much more susceptible to smoking-related problems, because their lungs have already begun the natural aging process, which decreases some of their elasticity and vigor.

Why does tobacco smoke have such wide-ranging and devastating effects on us? There are three major reasons. Cigarette and cigar smoke contain:

1. **Tar**—which is comprised of more than 4,000 chemicals. So far, scientists have been able to identify at least forty-two of those as being carcinogens (cancer-causing agents).

2. **Carbon monoxide**—a toxic gas that reduces the amount of oxygen the lungs carry to the blood. Smokers have been found to have up to ten times the amount of carbon monoxide in their blood than nonsmokers.

3. **Nicotine**—one of the strongest known addictive substances in the world is also a powerful blood vessel constrictor.

351

Smoking's Impact Beyond the Respiratory System

Your blood vessels. Smoke restricts, or tightens, blood vessels. Translation: your blood pressure goes up and increases the chance of heart disease, heart attack, and stroke.

Your healing powers. Because smokers have less oxygen in their blood, it can take longer for them to heal from wounds or surgery.

Your back. No one really knows why, but smoking seems to cause back pain. Maybe it's the restriction of blood vessels or the fact that smokers cough more. Reportedly, smokers have three times greater chance of developing disc problems in the lower back than non-smokers. Smoking also contributes to osteoporosis.

Your skin. Smoking causes wrinkles, especially around the mouth.

Your digestive tract. Smoking can promote indigestion and heartburn. Smokers also have five times greater risk of suffering from gastric ulcers, and twice as great a chance of suffering from duodenal ulcers than nonsmokers. Reasons are not clear, but it might be because of swallowed smoke residue, reduced blood supply to the stomach surface, or the slower healing time of smokers.

Your head. Excessive smoking has been shown to contribute to migraine headaches.

Your sperm count. Male smokers have less sperm, and many of the ones that are still swimming won't win any medals, because they're more likely to be damaged. Not a huge concern or priority for men in their fifties, but something to think about.

Your accident rate. Smokers are four times as likely as nonsmokers to get into accidents. The reasons aren't really clear—although images of fumbling a lit cigarette into your lap as you're driving seventy-five miles an hour come to mind.

Your death or injury by fire. Smokers run a higher risk because of smoking in bed.

Your incidence of respiratory infection. This includes ailments such as sinusitis, bronchitis, and ear infections.

Your children's or grandchildren's health. Young people who live in a household with smokers have a much higher risk of asthma, ear infections, and other respiratory infections.

How Smoking Affects Your Lungs

It took generations for tobacco companies, the medical community, and the public to officially agree that smoking is harmful to your lungs. That's something that any thinking smoker could have told you after one coughing fit or after hacking up the first wad of "something." Even if you don't think too much about smoking, the statistics can make you sit up and take notice. Lung cancer is the most common cause of cancer death in the world, and nearly 85 percent of all lung cancers in men worldwide are related to—guess what!—smoking.

The mechanics of the situation are pretty straightforward. As smoke is inhaled into the lungs, the chemicals in smoke begin to wreak their havoc.

Inhaled Smoke Can:

• Irritate the bronchial tubes (which carry air to the lungs) so much that they cause "smoker's cough," which ultimately can lead to bronchitis and chronic bronchitis. The constant cough of smoker's cough is the lungs' attempt to rid themselves of tobacco tar and the overproduction of phlegm that comes from smoking. Healthy lungs don't get such phlegm build up, and their healthy cilia (see below) can handle normal phlegm production.

• Inhibit the immune system of your lungs, allowing infection and disease, such as pneumonia, easy access.

• Destroy the tiny cilia of your lungs—the little wavy sweepers that are responsible for getting rid of harmful material from your lungs. Without them as a major line of defense, your lungs are much more susceptible to disease.

• Gradually destroy the elasticity of the alveoli (the tiny air sacs where the transfer of oxygen and carbon dioxide takes place between the lungs and the blood). This will, eventually, lead to rupture of the alveoli, which begins the progressive, irreversible, and ultimately deadly disease called emphysema.

How Smoking Affects Your Cardiovascular System

While even the most adamant pro-smokers will admit that smoking probably hurts their lungs, few smokers consider what kind of damage smoking is doing to their blood vessels.

Most of the scare tactics against smokers usually revolve around the respiratory system: Do you want to get lung cancer? Do you want to be on oxygen the rest of your life?

We think these arguments pale in comparison to a vascular one: If you had a choice between smoking or having an erection, which would you take?

Yep! Smoking can, in fact, cause the loss of your pride and joy. It happens when the lower extremity blood vessels start hardening (arteriosclerosis) and/or clogging (atherosclerosis). These two conditions are directly linked to smoking (or diabetes), and if the blood flow is too restricted, the ability to get an erection is lost because not enough blood can get to the penis.

In fact, there's a saying in the medical community: vascular (blood vessel) and thoracic (chest) surgeons, who deal with respiratory/circulatory problems, wouldn't have anything to do if there weren't smokers and diabetics in the world.

So, how does smoking work on the cardiovascular system?

Mainly through carbon monoxide, which is the most concentrated gas in tobacco smoke. Because it combines more readily with your blood than oxygen, it pushes oxygen out of the way, so when your body needs oxygen it gets less than desired or useless carbon monoxide in its place. Some scientists report that the amount of oxygen in a smoker's bloodstream can be reduced by up to 8 percent— a significant amount that the smoker will feel in less endurance and stamina, not to mention reduced immune function. Even more important, this reduction of oxygen also means that the heart has to work harder to get the same amount of oxygen to the rest of the body.

Then there's nicotine. Its most negative contribution is that it constricts blood vessels, which can cause a host of blood vessel damage.

In addition to the effects of nicotine and carbon monoxide, smoking raises the level of fatty acids and cholesterol in the blood and encourages platelets, which aid in clotting, to stick to each other and to blood vessel walls, creating the potential for dangerous blood clots.

The combination of a heart that has to work harder with the increase in cholesterol and clotting can be a deadly one. They are all contributors to arteriosclerosis (hardening of the arteries) and atherosclerosis (clogging of the arteries), which can lead to coronary heart disease—all of which can ultimately lead to heart attack and stroke. In fact, coronary heart disease occurs, on average, seven years earlier in smokers than in nonsmokers.

Steps to Stopping

To quit smoking is to tap into the fastest and easiest way to improve your overall health, primarily because smoking is the largest single avoidable cause of ill-health and death in the world. It's as simple as this: The sooner you quit, the longer you'll live.

But, as we all know, you'll never quit until you really want to quit. There has to be an inner desire, an inner commitment that is the foundation for all the external quitting activities you'll be doing.

Suggestions to Help Stop Smoking

• Seek support before you try it. Talk with a doctor about your desire to quit and your plan of attack in doing so. Having a long-term relationship with one physician can be especially helpful when trying to quit smoking. You can also sign up for a smoking-cessation program, if you think that might help—there are excellent and varied programs out there. Talk to nonsmoking friends about getting their continued help, or quit at the same time as another friend.

• Orally (out loud to yourself in a mirror) and in writing, commit to stopping in strong, declarative sentences: "I am quitting for my health and happiness." "I no longer need cigarettes." "Smoking no longer controls me." Remember that quitting is *not* self-denial, it is an act of self-determination.

• Get rid of all things associated with smoking, including ashtrays, lighters, and, of course, any cigars, cigarettes, or chewing tobacco lying around the house.

• Take stock of your smoking. How many cigars or cigarettes do you smoke? How many are just habit and how many are really desired? When is the toughest time of the day for you? Know your weaknesses and your strengths, and work with them to help yourself set up a good, personalized plan of quitting that avoids behaviors or habits that might promote smoking.

- Make a motivation list. Motivation is a key ingredient in stopping successfully. Make a list of the positive reasons why you want to stop smoking and post them in a prominent place where you will see them every morning.

- Consider, in discussions with your doctor, whether or not a nicotine patch, nicotine chewing gum, prescription drugs such as Zyban, or other nonsmoking aids might be helpful. Keep in mind that Zyban is also an antidepressant, which could be just the added muscle necessary to help you get over the initial hurdle of quitting.

- Go cold turkey. Many doctors—and recovering smokers—feel this is the best way to break the tremendously strong nicotine addiction. And use those first few days of difficulty as a reason to continue not to smoke—you don't want to go through the agony of those first few days again, do you?

- Use an illness to springboard to success. Even the hardiest of smokers usually stop (or nearly so) when they get a respiratory illness such as a chest cold or bronchitis. Why not use those days as your first days of quitting? By the time you're healthy enough to want a smoke, you will have already been off them for a few days, if not a week or more. This means that you will have already "survived" what is considered the hardest part of quitting—the first week or so.

- If you fail, acknowledge and admit that you did so, but don't berate yourself. You're human; you're allowed to make mistakes. Cut yourself some slack and just analyze why you failed, then work the answer into a new plan for stopping. While you're in the transition between the failed plan and the new one, try to keep your smoking to the barest minimum, which should help when you begin your next assault.

- In this day and age of support groups and medical aids for quitting smoking, we believe that anyone who's not mentally ill can quit. It might take numerous tries and tremendous physical and psychological effort, but it can be done.

- Remind yourself, it is *never* too late to quit smoking.

If You Stop, What Can You Expect?

Depending on how long and how much you've been smoking, there are certain things you will notice over the course of the first few weeks and months of non-smoking. As with everything in life, there's good news and bad news in this regard:

What You Can Do

- **Initially Not Feeling Better.** We're not going to lie to you. A discouraging element to quitting is that within the first two weeks of stopping you may not necessarily feel better. In fact, you may feel worse as your lungs start to kick-start themselves back to life. This could involve some serious coughing and the bringing up of some seriously ugly phlegm.

- **Physical Manifestations.** Possible physical side effects of quitting can include sweating, drop in blood pressure and heart rate, gastrointestinal changes, sleeplessness, and cravings—although rarely are any of these more than mild. Additionally, once your lungs have cleared, you might find that you now suffer from various allergies. The quitting has not stimulated allergies; the smoking was actually masking your allergies.

- **Mental Manifestations.** Possible initial side effects can include irritability, anxiety, even depression—although rarely are any of these more than mild.

- **Healing Does Begin at Once.** Despite how you might be feeling, rest assured that as soon as you do stop, your lungs will begin almost immediately to repair and heal themselves. And the long-term results are impressive: After ten years of nonsmoking, your risk of lung cancer drops to 30 to 50 percent of that of smokers who haven't quit. After fifteen to twenty years, your lung cancer risk becomes similar to someone who never smoked.

The concept of positive changes taking place within hours of quitting is a tremendous motivator for some people.

American Lung Association Outline of What Happens When You Stop

Twenty minutes after quitting:
- Blood pressure decreases.
- Pulse rate drops.
- Body temperature of hands and feet increases.

Eight hours:
- Carbon monoxide level in blood drops to normal.
- Oxygen level in blood increases to normal.

Twenty-four hours:
- Chance of heart attack decreases.

Forty-eight hours:
• Nerve endings start regrowing.
• Ability to smell and taste is enhanced.

Two weeks to three months:
• Circulation improves.
• Walking becomes easier.
• Lung function increases.

One to nine months:
• Coughing, sinus congestion, fatigue, shortness of breath decrease.

One year:
• Excess risk of coronary heart disease is decreased to half that of a smoker.

Five years:
• From five to fifteen years after quitting, stroke risk is reduced to that of people who have never smoked.

Ten years:
• Risk of lung cancer drops to as little as one-half that of continuing smokers.
• Risk of cancer of the mouth, throat, esophagus, bladder, kidney, and pancreas decreases.
• Risk of ulcer decreases.

Fifteen years:
• Risk of coronary heart disease is now similar to that of people who have never smoked.
• Risk of death returns to nearly the level of people who have never smoked.

EPILOGUE
Now What?

In the end, we all want the same thing: to live healthy lives for as long as we can.

We hope that we've helped you move toward that worthy goal of long-term good health by outlining what lies ahead, detailing how to handle specific problems, and describing what preventive measures can be taken.

Now, it's up to you.

Remember, though, that you should approach the goal of life-long good health like you should approach the goal of losing weight. In the diet section of chapter 8 we explain that anyone who wants to permanently lose weight should throw out the idea of going on a diet (which automatically brings up the concept of falling off a diet). Instead, those who want to lose weight need to establish life-long good eating habits and exercise routines.

Similarly, life-long good health is rarely achieved if approached via temporary measures, half-hearted commitments that are quickly forgotten, or a defeatist attitude of "what's the use." Yes, it's true that life-long good health does take some work, does take some resolve, and no small amount of sweat, but most importantly, it takes a shift in perspective that says: "This is how I want to live the rest of my life." The rewards from this kind of personal commitment are immeasurable.

Such a commitment, we believe, should also include a relative acceptance of the aging process and the need to periodically redefine your physical limitations. You aren't twenty anymore. You can't play sports like you used to. You can't stay up all night and be completely alert the next morning.

Those facts of life can come as quite a shock to many of us as we enter our fifties. But if you think about it, they're not that lamentable, especially when we realize that age has given us a greater appreciation of the world around us and the ability to smooth out some of life's roller coasters. We've even matured a little. And even the limitations of age can be stretched and manipulated to a large degree by individual effort and personal commitment.

As we're all coming to realize, the fifties—like every phase of life— has its unique rewards and challenges. In the end, our own aging is not an opponent to fight, but rather an ally to work with to maximize our overall health and enjoyment of life.

Another ally who is critical to the equation of good health is your physician. It's no exaggeration that a long-term relationship with a physician you can trust and be honest with will add tremendous quality to your life and could quite literally add years as well.

Finally, one last piece of advice—maybe the best piece of advice in this entire book. Once you've had a physical assessment, once you've taken the preventive exams and tests, once you've implemented a sound, life-long program of good eating, exercise, and periodic physician visits, then remember:

Don't Obsess about Your Health.
Simply Live Your Life to the Fullest.

ABOUT THE AUTHORS

Gordon Ehlers, M.D.

Dr. Gordon Ehlers has been practicing medicine for more than twenty-five years. A former Air Force flight surgeon, he is certified in sports medicine and family practice, emphasizing adult and geriatric medicine. From his practice he's gained an unusually broad experience base, which has included treating more than 100,000 outpatients and 5,000 hospital patients. Having provided medical care for thousands of men as they've aged, Dr. Ehlers has recognized the pivotal importance of the decade of the fifties in the transition from youth to maturity.

Currently, Dr. Ehlers is a faculty member at the Swedish Hospital Family Medicine Residency, a University of Colorado-affiliated family practice teaching program, where he teaches medical residents.

Dr. Ehlers has also held leadership positions in the medical profession—most notably, he is past president of a sixty-physician group practice and vice chairman of a 1,400-physician affiliation. In his spare time, he jogs, climbs Colorado's 14,000-foot mountain peaks, and recently was surprised (as many fifties males are) to find he has heart disease. Dr. Ehlers lives in a Denver suburb with his wife, Michele, and children Megan, Greta, and Erik.

Jeff Miller

Jeff Miller has been a professional writer, magazine editor, and author for more than twenty years. He spent ten years as a magazine editor specializing in national publication start-ups in the real-estate, cable, satellite TV, and entertainment fields.

Able to write on topics ranging from business to entertainment, history to health, Miller was also editor-in-chief of five in-flight airline magazines.

For the past ten years Miller has been a freelance writer. His articles have appeared in more than 130 magazines and newspapers, including *Better Homes & Gardens, Country Living, New York Daily News, Chicago Tribune, Los Angeles Times, The Dallas Morning News*, and the in-flight magazines for U.S. Air, Delta, British Airways, Singapore Airlines, and Qantas.

Additionally, Miller researched and wrote the hardbound history book *Stapleton International Airport: The First Fifty Years* and a World War I historical novel, *Behind the Lines*. Miller came up with the idea for *Facing Your Fifties* because he knew—just like the average Boomer male—that he should be doing more for his health, but didn't know where to start. He's still not doing everything he should, but he's working on it. He lives in Denver with his wife, Susan Burdick.

INDEX

363

Index

Index

Index